ADVANCES IN RADIATION RESEARCH

BIOLOGY AND MEDICINE

VOLUME 2

ADVANCES IN RADIATION RESEARCH

J.F. DUPLAN and A. CHAPIRO, Editors

BIOLOGY AND MEDICINE

Volume I
Volume II
Volume III

PHYSICS AND CHEMISTRY

Volume I
Volume II

Advances in Radiation Research

BIOLOGY AND MEDICINE

Editors

J.F. DUPLAN and A. CHAPIRO

Laboratoire Pasteur de l'Institut du Radium

VOLUME 2

GORDON AND BREACH SCIENCE PUBLISHERS

New York   London   Paris

Editorial office for the United Kingdom

   Gordon and Breach, Science Publishers Ltd.
   42 William IV Street
   London W. C. 2

Editorial office for France

   Gordon & Breach
   7-9 rue Emile Dubois
   Paris 14e

Library of Congress Catalog card number: 72-92724
ISBN 0 677 30560 5 set of five volumes
0 677 30880 9 vol. 1; 0 677 30890 6 vol.2
0 677 30900 7 vol. 3

Printed in the German Democratic Republic by Druckwerke Zwickau

VOLUME II

CHAPTER 1

CHAPTER 2

ix

THE INFLUENCE OF RADIATION QUALITY ON BASIC MECHANISMS OF RADIOBIOLOGICAL PROCESSES

G.J. NEARY

M.R.C. Radiobiology Unit, Harwell, Berkshire, England

1. INTRODUCTION

In the development of radiobiology, the comparative study of different kinds of ionizing radiation has played an important part. It was recognized that this approach was a necessary and fruitful one since any understanding of the mechanisms of action of any one radiation type was likely to be incomplete if the quantitative and qualitative differences between the effects of different radiations were ignored, particularly as the commonly used radiations such as hard X or gamma rays do in fact represent rather broad distributions of quality. An important concept [1] was the sequential character of radiation damage, starting with the initial absorption of energy in a molecule (an activation event [22]), followed by possible physico-chemical reactions between activated centres within or between nearby molecules (metionic reactions) producing the final state of chemical change. The concept included recognition of the possibility that the final molecular damage produced by a high LET track giving a high local concentration of activation events might be more extensive and more disturbing to cell function than that produced by a low LET track giving more dispersed activation events. Therefore, radiation quality might well be an important factor at all three stages of production of radiation damage, namely the production of initial lesions, the production of fixed post-metionic lesions, and the residual lesions,which the cell was unable to repair or by-pass in the post-irradi-

ation period [16]. It was expected that as the LET and
therefore the local concentration of activation events
increased, some or all of these three stages of lesion
production could occur with greater effectiveness, though
when the local concentration of activation events became
needlessly larger than required, the effectiveness per
unit dose would progressively decrease, the phenomenon of
so-called 'overkill', just as observed experimentally for
cellular effects.

Thus, although some other aspects of relative biological effectiveness have been considered [18], attempts
to explain the influence of radiation quality on cellular
effects have been mainly by consideration of the influence
on processes at the molecular level. The determination of
cellular effects by the character of the molecular events
must be expected to be important and has been discussed
frequently and extensively but the precise relationship
is still quite uncertain. In the first place, knowledge
of the nature of the molecular lesions which are important is limited though there are strong indications that
the site of at least some of these lesions is the DNA [8,
9,10]. Secondly, there is only limited knowledge of the
influence of radiation quality on effects on molecules in
general [17], and, in particular on the various physico-
chemical lesions in DNA which could conceivably be important. Nevertheless, within this limited framework of
knowledge, there appears to be a discrepancy between the
influence of radiation quality on cellular effects and
molecular effects. The effectiveness per unit dose for
cellular effects may rise with increasing LET but always
reaches a maximum, usually around 100 keV/μm, whereas for
some simple molecules, effectiveness appears to go on increasing even up to the highest attainable LET's [4, 12].
In DNA itself, the limited data on double-strand breaks
[21] show that effectiveness at 255 keV/μm is about twice
as great as at 100 keV/μm (Fig. 1); there are no adequate
data on the LET dependence of other lesions in DNA, either
simple or compound, for example, a strand break and base
damage produced in close proximity by the same track.

A possible partial explanation of this discrepancy
between the radiation quality dependence of cellular and

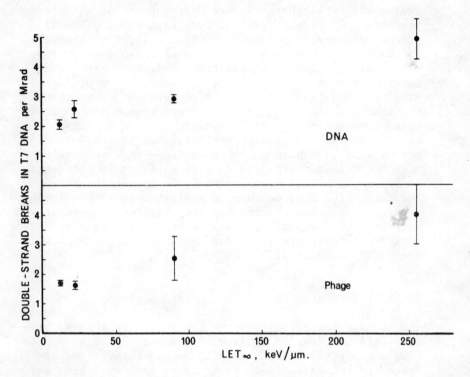

Fig. 1.   Double-strand breaks per molecule of dry T7 DNA (2.5×10^7 Daltons)
per Mrad at various track-segment LET values; above, irradiation of
isolated DNA; below, irradiation of phage particles.
(Data of ref. [21]).

molecular effects is that even if there were no 'overkill' at high LET for the cellularly - important individual molecular lesions themselves, there could still
be an 'overkill' for the cell as a whole through production of several lesions in a cell by a track which
crosses it.   Such a track will, for example intersect
the DNA of the cell several times on average [14, 15]
and the higher the LET the greater the chance of occurrence of a primary lesion (and therefore of a metionically-fixed lesion) at an intersection.   If only one
residual lesion, that is, an unrepaired or un-by-passed

lesion will kill the cell, the consequences of multiple
production of primary lesions by a high LET track will
depend on the repair capacity of the cell, for this will
determine the mean number of residual lesions which result from the passage of the track. If the mean number
is greater than one, then there is some degree of 'overkill' and consequent reduced effectiveness per unit dose
for that quality of radiation. Obviously, the mean numbers of residual lesions in a cell crossed by a track
will also depend on the probability that the relevant
molecular lesion will occur at any one track intersection
with the DNA, but provided this probability is not small,
it may in some cell types cease to be the dominant factor
for the cellular dependence on radiation quality. Thus
some general considerations of the cellular response to
radiation quality may be possible without knowing the detailed nature of the individual molecular lesions or
their LET dependence.

2.   EXPERIMENTAL EVIDENCE ON MULTIPLE LESIONS

Some evidence on the effect of multiple lesions within a cell is afforded by data of the author and R.J. Preston, not yet reported in detail, on the comparative effects of protons and soft X-ray in killing sensitive and
resistant variants of *E.coli* B bacteria. The total range
of the protons was much greater than the linear dimensions
of a bacterium; the LET in the track segment of the proton
as it crossed a bacterium was 22 keV/μm. The soft X-rays
had a quantum energy of 1.5 keV and the mean free path for
absorption was also large compared to the bacterial dimensions; absorption of any one quantum would occur at random
in a bacterium and would give rise to an electron track
with a track-average LET of 21 keV/μm and a total range of
only 0.07 μm, that is, much smaller than the linear dimensions of the nuclear body of the bacterium, of the order
of 1 μm [14]. The DNA of a bacterial chromatid is dispersed throughout the nuclear body and it would be inter-
sected about 5 times on average by a proton track crossing
the nuclear body of the cells used [14], but normally at
not more than one place by one of the short electron
tracks generated by absorption of a soft X-ray quantum.

In view of the comparable LET's of the two kinds of
track, lesion production at a single intersection of the
DNA should be quantitatively and qualitatively equal [21].
If a population of bacteria is irradiated with equal doses
of the two radiations, the same total number of primary
lesions should be produced in the two cases, but whereas
those due to the soft X-rays will be randomly distributed
between cells, those due to the protons will not, being
concentrated into clusters of several lesions in those
cells though which a proton track happens to pass. Therefore, there will be more cells free from primary lesions
after the proton irradiation than after the soft X-rays.
If the cells have little repair capacity, virtually any
cell which starts with a primary lesion will fail to survive and the protons will be less effective than the soft
X-rays; this is 'overkill' on the cellular scale, not the
molecular scale. If the repair capacity of the cells is
high and if the chance of repair of a lesion is independent of the total number of lesions in a cell, then in
the proton case most of the primary lesions in those cells
through which a proton has passed will be repaired and the
distribution of the residual lesions in the cells of the
population will be random just as for the soft X-rays; the
two radiations will then be equally effective. For brev-
ity, the argument has been presented without making a distinction between cells, nuclear bodies, or chromatids, but
the principle is unchanged.

These predictions are born out by the experimental
results shown in Fig. 2, where survival from the two kinds
of radiation is compared for $E.coli$ B_{s-1} and $E.coli$ B/r,
a sensitive and a resistant pair of genetic variants,
which differ only at three loci, hcr, exr and fil which
influence radiosensitivity. For B_{s-1}, the slope of the
log-survival curve for protons is only half that for soft
X-rays; for B/r, the slopes of the straight parts of the
log-survival curves are equal. Exactly the same picture
was found for the pair of genetic variants $E.coli$ K12 AB
2463 rec⁻ and K12 AB 1157 rec⁺ which differ only at the
rec locus which also influences radiosensitivity.

The preceding qualitative argument explaining these
experimental findings can be expressed more concisely in

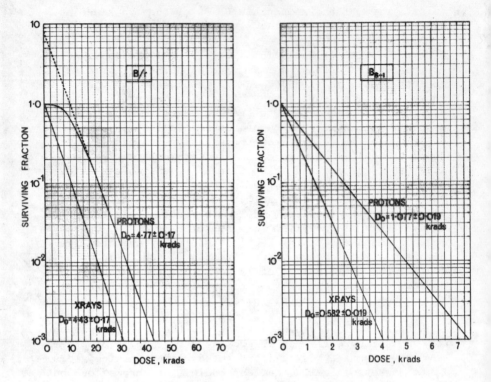

Fig. 2.   Survival of *E.coli* B/r and B$_{s-1}$, cultured in rich medium and ir-
          radiated in log phase by soft X rays of quantum energy 1.5 KeV,
          track average LET 21 keV/µm, or protons of track sebment LET 22
          keV/µm.
          (Data of Neary and Preston).

quantitative mathematical terms.   It is assumed as an approximation that the number of intersections with a bacterial chromatid by a proton track passing through the
region containing the chromatid has a Poisson distribution.   It then follows that the distribution of residual lesion in chromatids after a dose D is a double
Poisson and the probability that there will be no residual lesions in a chromatid, i.e. that there will be a
surviving cell is

$$\exp\{-(DA/16L)\,[1 - \exp(-usK)]\} \tag{1}$$

where D is the dose in rads, A the mean projected area in
$(\mu m)^2$ of the region containing the chromatid, L the LET
in keV/μm of the track segment, u the probability that a
metionically-fixed lesion will not be repaired, s the
mean number of intersections of the track with the chromatid, and K the probability that a metionically-fixed
lesion of the relevant type will be formed at any one intersection; K will not be specified further except to note
that for any one type of lesion its value will tend to increase as the LET increases. The radiosensitivity, the
reciprocal of D_0 is from equation (1)

$$(A/16L) \ [1 - \exp(-usK)] \tag{2}$$

With soft X-rays, multiple intersections of a chromatid
by any one short electron track are very unlikely and the
distribution of residual lesions in chromatids approximates to a simple Poisson; the probability of survival is

$$\exp[-(DA/16\bar{L})usK] \tag{3}$$

where $\bar{L}$ is the track average LET in keV/μm of the
electron track; the radiosensitivity is

$$(A/16\bar{L})usK \tag{4}$$

Thus the ratio of the radiosensitivities to soft X-rays
and protons where L and $\bar{L}$ were chosen to be equal is from
equations (2) and (4)

$$(usK)/[1 - \exp(-usK)] \tag{5}$$

This ratio approaches a minimum value of unity when usK
approaches zero, e.g. in a cell with high repair capacity
where u is very small; it could be appreciably greater
than unity if usK were not very small, e.g. in a cell
with no repair capacity so that $u = 1$ provided K were not
very small. The observed value of the ratio for $E.coli$
B_{s-1} in Fig. 2 is 1.85 and this implies a value of $\sim$1.5
for usK; if u were unity (no repair) and s were $\sim$5, K
would be $\sim$0.3. The observed equality of radiosensitivity
of $E.coli$ B/r to the two radiations would follow from
equation (5) with this same value of K provided u were
not much greater than 0.1.

3. GENERAL DISCUSSION

The data on the soft X-ray and proton comparisons appear to be explicable with the simple assumption that K represents the same molecular lesion in sensitive and resistant bacteria though the possibility is not ruled out that K is much smaller in resistant than in sensitive bacteria. This possibility has been suggested [14] as an explanation of the different LET dependence of radiosensitivity in track segment experiments with sensitive and resistant bacteria where it was assumed that there are two different kinds of lesions with different K and u values, which are of different importance in the two kinds of bacteria. A difference in LET dependence is also predicted in equation (2) by the simpler picture above with only one type of molecular lesion. In sensitive bacteria, radiosensitivity would tend to be proportional to 1/L except at very low values of LET but in resistant bacteria, where u is supposed to be quite small, radiosensitivity would be proportional to uK/L. This quality could represent the observed maximum of radiosensitivity around 30 keV/μm^2 [2, 14] if K increased more rapidly than the first power of the LET, which seems theoretically possible for certain kinds of compound lesion in DNA.

An alternative explanation of the LET dependence in resistant bacteria could be an increase of u with LET, as suggested in general terms long ago [1]. In the present analysis no variation of u with LET or dose has been assumed. Therefore no possibility of a shoulder on a log-survival curve due to decrease in repair capacity with increasing dose is allowed for [7]. The small shoulder for *E.coli* B/r cultured in minimal medium and irradiated in log phase by gamma rays has been attributed to a multi-target situation, since the average number of chromatids per nucleus would be 1.44 [13]. In our experiments summarized in Fig. 2 the bacteria were cultured in rich medium; in those conditions there are multiple replication forks and a considerably increased mean number of chromatids per nucleus, which might explain the large extrapolation number for the proton irradiation of *E.coli* B/r. This possibility would not account for the absence of a shoulder with the soft X-rays, nor for B_{s-1} with either

radiation. Moreover, we have found a synergistic interaction of the two radiations in B/r but not with B_{s-1}
[19]. With B/r, pretreatment with protons to a survival
level at about the end of the shoulder increases the sensitivity of the survivors to soft X-rays by a factor of
two; after pretreatment with soft X-rays to the same survival level, the survivors show no shoulder for proton
irradiation. These preliminary results are analogous to
the interactions found between hard X-rays and UV or
chemical agents [6] and they suggest that the explanation
of the shoulder region may be complex, and that such interaction experiments in a variety of cells might throw
light on the relation between sublethal and potentially
lethal damage and the associated repair systems. It is
of interest that ∟ pair of related yeast cell types, the
haploid SC7 and the corresponding resistant diploid SC6
are quite analogous to the sensitive and resistant bacteria respectively, both in the relative radiosensitivity
to soft X-rays and protons and in the interaction of the
two radiations [20].

     In seeking mechanisms for cell killing, it is im-
portant to remember that the modes of death appear to be
different in sensitive and resistant bacteria; in the
former, several divisions may occur before the cells die,
whereas in the latter the killed cells have not usually
divided after irradiation [5, 11]. It is not clear
whether these facts imply a difference between the two
types of bacteria at the level of the primary radiation
damage or at some subsequent level of its development;
data at a variety of LET values are not available. It
has been suggested that the principal site of primary
damage in sensitive bacteria is the DNA (type N damage)
but that in resistant bacteria damage to a membrane (type
O damage) is important, possibly a localized region such
as the point of replication of the DNA [3]. The observed
equality of effectiveness of soft X-rays and protons of
equivalent LET in resistant bacteria would be compatible
with this model since unlike the extended DNA target, a
small region of a membrane would not be subjected to multiple intersections (and lesions) by a proton track.

     To sum up, the influence of radiation quality on

cellular effects, specifically cell killing, may be only
a very indirect reflection of the radiation quality dependence of the individual molecular lesions, owing to
the possibility of multiple molecular lesions in the extended DNA by a single track and the determination of the
cellular consequences by the repair or by-pass characteristics of the cells. On this basis it may be possible to
reconcile the continuous increase in effectiveness for
chemical effects in various molecules with increase in
LET and the fact that effectiveness for cellular effects
in all cases decreases at sufficiently high LET. An explanation is also provided for the relative effectiveness
of soft X-rays and protons of equivalent LET in closely-
related cells of different repair capacity. Here, the
important aspects of radiation quality appears to be the
short track length of the electrons generated by the soft
X-rays. The implication that there is 'overkill' in sensitive cells by radiations such as protons at the not very
high LET of about 20 keV/μ is somewhat suprising, but it
is 'overkill' on the cellular scale and not at the molecular level. It is of interest that in some cases the
critical volumes deduced by the methods of microdosimetry
[23] are of cellular rather than molecular dimensions.
Because of the indirectness of the relation between initial molecular lesions and their cellular consequences
there is still uncertainty about the nature and in some
cases even the site or sites of the molecular lesions responsible for particular cellular effects at different
radiation qualities.

ACKNOWLEDGEMENT

    I am indebted to my collaborator Mr. R.J. Preston
for permission to quote results from some of our unpublished work.

SUMMARY

    A single track which crosses a cell may make poten-
tially lethal lesions at several places in the cell and

even at several places in the same macromolecular target
such as the DNA. This fact may account for some of the
features of the dependence of cellular effects on radiation quality, but in general the identification of the
molecular lesions responsible for the effects remains
uncertain.

REFERENCES

1.   ALPER, T., *Radiat. Res. 5*, 573, 1965.

2.   ALPER, T., MOORE, J.L. and BEWLEY, D.K., *Radiat. Res.
     32*, 277, 1967.

3.   ALPER, T., *Proc. 2nd Symp. Microdosimetry*, ed. H.G.
     Ebert, (Brussels, EURATOM), 5, 1969.

4.   BURNS, W.G., MARSH, W.R. and REED, C.R.V., *Nature
     (Lond.) 218*, 867, 1968.

5.   HAEFNER, K. and STRIEBECK, U., *Mutation Research, 4*,
     399, 1967.

6.   HAYNES, R.H., *Photochem. Photobiol., 3*, 429, 1964.

7.   HAYNES, R.H., in: *Physical Process s in Radiation
     Biology*, eds. L. Augenstein, R. Mason and B. Rosen-
     berg (New York and London, Academic Press), 51, 1964.

8.   HAYNES, R.H., *Radiat. Res. Suppl. 6*, 1, 1966.

9.   HUTCHINSON, F., *Cancer Res., 26 Part 1*, 2045, 1966.

10. KAPLAN, H.S., *Actions chim. biol. Radiat., 12*, 69,
     1968.

11. KOROGODIN, V.I., KOROGODINA, YU.V. and MYASNIK, M.N.,
     Studia biophysica, 15-16, 127, 1969.

12. LANDSMAN, D.A. and BUTTERFIELD, J.E., *UKAEA Rep.
     AERE R-3625*, 1961.

13. MUNSON, R.J. and BRIDGES, B.A., *Nature (Lond.)*, *210*, 922, 1966.

14. MUNSON, R.J., NEARY, G.J., BRIDGES, B.A. and PRESTON, R.J., *Int. J. Radiat. Biol.*, *13*, 205, 1967.

15. NEARY, G.J., *Int. J. Radiat. Biol.*, *9*, 477, 1965.

16. NEARY, G.J., *Studia biophysica*, *18*, 11, 1969.

17. NEARY, G.J., *Proc. 2nd L.H. Gray Mem. Conf.*, Cambridge, April, 1969, eds. G.E. Adams, D.K. Bewley, J.W. Boag, (London Inst. of Physics and The Physical Society) p. 120-126, 1970.

18. NEARY, G.J., *Proc. Symp. Neutrons in Radiobiology*, Oak Ridge National Laboratory and University of Tennessee, CONF-691106, (TID 4500), p. 153-173, 1970.

19. NEARY, G.J. and PRESTON, R.J., unpublished work.

20. NEARY, G.J. and PRESTON, R.J., unpublished work.

21. NEARY, G.J., SIMPSON-GILDEMEISTER, V.F.J. and PEACOCKE, A.R., *Int. J. Radiat. Biol.*, *18*, 25-40, 1970.

22. PLATZMAN, R.L., in: *Radiation Research*, ed. G. Silini, (Amsterdam, North Holland Publ. Co.), 20, 1967.

23. ROSSI, H.H., *Advanc. biol. med. Phys.*, *11*, 27, 1967.

THE DEPENDENCE OF DAMAGE IN MAMMALIAN CELLS ON RADIATION QUALITY

G.W. BARENDSEN

Radiobiological Institute TNO, 151 Lange Kleiweg, Rijswijk Z.H., The Netherlands

1. GENERAL ASPECTS OF DIFFERENCES IN DOSE-EFFECT RELATIONS

Most biological effects of ionizing radiations in cells are observed only as final results of sequences of events, initiated by the absorption of energy in cellular material, followed by biophysical, biochemical and biological changes, which finally cause the end-point observed. In studies of effects produced by radiations of different quality, variations in effectiveness for producing the final response arise from differences in the first stage of the sequence of events, namely from differences in the spatial distribution of the absorption of energy. In this respect such studies differ from investigations of other factors capable of modifying the effectiveness of a dose of radiation, e.g., dose rate, temperature or chemical agents, because these latter factors can influence several stages in the sequence from the molecular up to the biological level [3].

Interest in the comparison of dose-effect relations for radiations of different quality is based on the well-known fact that radiations which differ with respect to the distribution of locally absorbed energy, may also differ considerably in their effectiveness for producing biological damage. For various types of damage in mammalian cells, quantitatively equal effects can be produced by doses of radiations which may differ by factors of more than 10 [4].

    In order to assess quantitatively the influence of
radiation quality on dose-effect relaticns, it is important to obtain data with radiations characterized by relatively narrow distributions cf local energy density. Such
distributions can be attained by the use of mono-energetic
ions, employed in conditions whereby their passage through
the sample causes only a small change in their velocity.
A quantity which for these irradiations can be used as a
first approximation for the description of the pattern
of energy deposition is the rate of energy loss or the
linear energy transfer (LET_∞)*, usually expressed in
keV/μ of unit density tissue or MeV·gm^{-1}·cm^2. It is
important to note however that even in the most favour-
able conditions of exposures of cells to heavy charged
particles, the energy deposited locally in small volumes
exhibits wide variations, due to statistical fluctuations
in the distances between individual energy dissipation
events along the tracks of the ions and to the production of δ-rays of different energies. In order to interpret quantitatively the relation between radiation quality and biological damage it is necessary to know the
distribution of local energy density for the relevant
sizes and shapes of the critical target volumes in cells
[12]. Because sufficient information about these distributions is not yet available, as a first approximation
the pattern of energy deposition by mono-energetic ions
traversing single cells will be characterized by the LET_∞
This is a mean value which provides a useful characteristic only if the distribution of dose in LET_∞ is relatively narrow, as can be achieved for instance by irradiation conditions whereby energy is deposited in cells
by short track segments of heavy ions [4].

    In Fig.1 a few dose survival curves are presented,
measured by the clone technique for cultured cells of
human kidney origin, after irradiation with deuterons
and α-particles of different energies [7]. These curves
illustrate some of the differences which can be observed
as a result of variation of the LET_∞. It can be concluded

_____

    *The subscript ∞ indicates that energy losses due to
    all δ-rays are included.

that with increasing LET_∞, the dose required to produce a given end-point, e.g., impairment of the capacity for unlimited proliferation in 50 per cent of the cells, decreases between 10 and 100 keV/μ, passes through a minimum and subsequently increases again. This implies that the relative biological effectiveness (RBE), defined as the ratio of doses of 200 kV X-rays and of the radiation considered respectively, which are required to produce equal effects, increases to a maximum and subsequently decreases.

Fig. 1 shows further that with mono-energetic ions, having an LET_∞ in excess of 60 keV/μ, the survival curves are within experimental errors indistinguishable from exponential curves. As lower LET_∞ values, the curves are not exponential but exhibit significant curvature in the low dose region, followed at larger doses by a part with less pronounced and frequently insignificant curvature. With deuterons at an LET_∞ of less than 10 keV/μ, the shape of the survival curve is very similar to that obtained with 200 kV X-rays, which is usually taken as a standard of reference for the calculation of RBE-values.

As a consequence of the observed differences in the shapes of survival curves measured with mono-energetic ions of various LET_∞ with X-rays, the relative biological effectiveness of a given type of densely ionizing radiation is not a single value, but depends on the level of damage. The largest values correspond to low doses. This is illustrated by curves 1 and 2 of Fig. 2, which represent RBE versus LET_∞ relations corresponding to doses required to obtain fractions of surviving cells of 50 per cent and 1 per cent respectively, as derived from the curves of Fig. 1.

The observation that experimental data with respect to survival of mammalian cells after different doses of densely ionizing radiations do not show significant deviations from an exponential curve, cannot be considered as direct evidence that cell reproductive death results from the passage of a single particle through some critical site or structure in the cell. If an irradiated population consists of cells with a wide distribution of

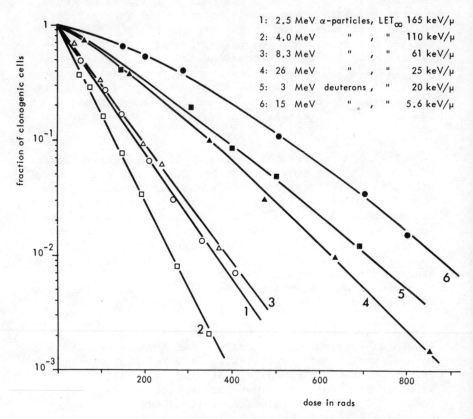

1: 2.5 MeV α-particles, LET$_\infty$ 165 keV/μ
2: 4.0 MeV   "   , "   110 keV/μ
3: 8.3 MeV   "   , "   61 keV/μ
4: 26 MeV   "   , "   25 keV/μ
5: 3 MeV deuterons , "   20 keV/μ
6: 15 MeV   "   , "   5.6 keV/μ

Fig. 1. Dose-survival curves of cultured cells of human kidney origin,
irradiated by the track-segment method with α-particles and
deuterons of different energies.

radio-sensitivities, then a composite survival curve may
be obtained, which is experimentally indistinguishable
from an exponential curve although the survival curves
of the sub-populations are not all exponential [15].
Various types of experimental evidence indicate however
that ionizing particles with LET$_\infty$ values in excess of
about 100 kev/μ cause reproductive death in mammalian cells
mainly by individual passages of the particles.

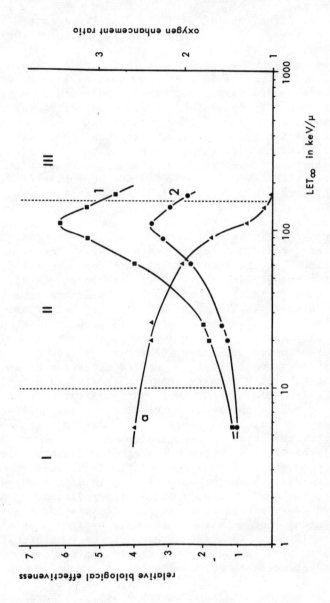

Fig. 2. RBE and OER as a function of the LET_∞ of α-particles and deuterons, measured for damage to the reproductive capacity of cultured cells of human kidney origin. The RBE curves 1 and 2 correspond to 50 percent and 1 percent survival respectively. Curve a represents the OER.

The first type of evidence is related to the phenomenon of repair of sub-lethal damage. As noted earlier
the shapes of survival curves obtained with radiations
of low LET_∞ show generally a significant curvature in the
low dose region. This indicates that cell reproductive
death is caused mainly through accumulation of a type of
damage which is not lethal unless a certain total amount
of damage is exceeded. Experiments with split doses,
first carried out by Elkind, have shown that in appropriate conditions sub-lethal damage can be repaired in intervals of a few hours [10]. For α-particles with an LET_∞
of about 140 keV/μ, we have demonstrated that fractionation of the dose does not reduce the effectiveness of a
given total dose [4]. In addition, at this LET_∞, changes
in dose rate do not cause variations in effectiveness of
a given total dose. It can be concluded that with this
high LET_∞ radiation repairable sub-lethal damage does not
contribute to the induction of cell reproductive death,
but the possibility that non-repairable sub-lethal damage
is produced cannot be excluded. In order to investigate
this latter possibility we have carried out experiments
in which a population of cells was first irradiated with
α-particles at an LET_∞ of 140 keV/μ and subsequently with
different doses of X-rays. The results showed that cells
surviving a conditioning dose of α-radiation at an LET_∞
of 140 keV/μ are equally sensitive to X-rays as unirradiated cells, i.e., their X-ray survival curve is indistinguishable from the X-ray survival curve for untreated cells.
This result shows that cells which survive after moderate
doses of this type of α-radiation have not accumulated
sub-lethal damage, which by interaction with sub-lethal
damage caused by X-rays can contribute to cell reproductive death. Furthermore, if a dose of X-rays is given
first, followed by graded doses of α-radiation at an LET_∞
of 140 keV/μ, it is observed that the pre-irradiation with
X-rays does not make the cells more sensitive to subsequent
α-irradiation. This indicates that the sub-lethal damage
produced by X-rays does not enhance the induction of cell
reproductive death by α-particles [8].

It can be concluded that the available evidence indicates that particles of sufficiently high LET_∞ can cause
reproductive death of mammalian cells by traversals of

of single particles. This does not imply that cell reproductive death is due to damage caused in a single
structure or macromolecule. It is possible that damage
caused by different parts of the track of a particle in
different molecules or structures in a cell, can interact and thereby initiate impairment of the reproductive
capacity. A simple calculation shows that in traversing
a mammalian cell nucleus, a particle may pass about 50
to 100 times through a DNA molecule.

2. MODIFICATION OF DAMAGE IN RELATION TO RADIATION QUALITY

In addition to the factors mentioned, damage produced
by radiation of high LET_∞ differs also from damage by radiations of a low LET_∞ with respect to variations in effectiveness which can be caused by dose-modifying agents,
e.g., oxygen, cysteamine, 5-BUdR, or which are due to cell
conditions, e.g., cell age. An example of the relation
between the effect of a dose-modifying agent and the LET_∞
is presented by curve a of Fig. 2. The presence of oxygen
in cells causes for deuterons at an LET_∞ of about 10
keV/μ and less, an increase in the radiosensitivity by a
factor of about 2.5 as compared with cells equilibrated
with pure nitrogen. This oxygen enhancement ratio (OER)
decreases with increasing LET_∞ and is indistinguishable
from 1.0 at LET_∞ values in excess of 165 keV/μ [6]. For
many other sensitizing and protecting compounds it has
been observed that in general the effectiveness of radiations of low LET_∞ for producing biological damage can
be affected to a much greater extent than the effectiveness of densely ionizing radiations [2].

On the bases of the experimental data discussed, it
is possible to make an approximate division of LET regions, as presented in Fig. 2. In LET region I, below
10 keV/μ, cell reproductive death is produced predominantly through accumulation of damage, corresponding to
survival curves with a pronounced shoulder. For this
region, the effectiveness of a given dose is strongly
dependent on dose fractionation and dose rate and may
be modified considerably by various cell conditions. In
region III, corresponding to LET_∞ values in excess of

150 keV/μ, cell reproductive death can be produced by
single traversals of particles, resulting in exponential
survival curves with little or no effect of dose fractionation, dose rate or cell conditions. Between these
two regions, region II can be considered as a transition
region. This is the most interesting region for studies
of changes in radiobiological parameters [4].

3. THE INFLUENCE OF RADIATION QUALITY ON THE INDUCTION OF NON-LETHAL DAMAGE AND MITOTIC DELAY

In measurements of fractions of cells which after
irradiation have retained the capacity for unlimited proliferation, a very specific end-point is assessed, whereby the complexities of the sequences of events which can
result in cell reproductive death are not considered [4].
Many investigations have shown however that cell reproductive death can be caused in various ways. In an irradiated population, a proportion of the cells may stop
dividing immediately, but another proportion may continue
to divide a few times before division ceases. Furthermore cells which have retained the capacity for unlimited proliferation may show a rate of increase of the number of viable off-spring which is much smaller than that
of unirradiated cells. This decreased rate of production
of viable cells may be due to a longer cell cycle or to
death of part of the progeny [13]. This phenomenon,
assayed as a decrease in the growth rate of the developing clones, is denoted "non-lethal damage". As a consequence of the variation in this damage between cells,
clones developing from irradiated cells in culture show
in general a wider spectrum of the number of cells per
clone as compared with clones arising from unirradiated
cells. Experimental data have been obtained indicating
that after irradiation with densely ionizing α-particles,
this type of non-lethal damage is produced with approximately the same RBE as the RBE for cell reproductive
death. This is shown in Fig. 3 [16]. With fast neutrons
similar results have been obtained recently [11].

It is important to note that this result was not expected on the basis of the data presented in the first

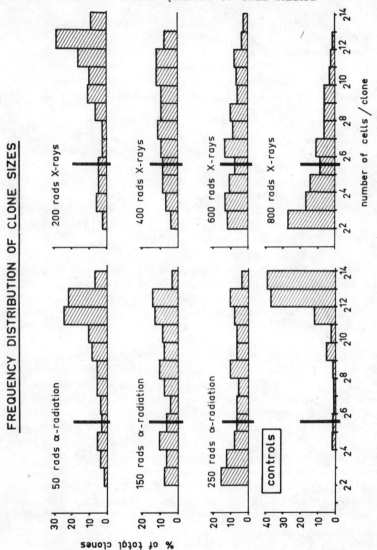

Fig. 3. Histograms of frequency distributions of clone sizes of cultured cells of human kidney origin, obtained 14 days after plating and irradiation of the cells with various doses of 250 kVp X-rays and 3.2 MeV α-particles. From Westra and Barendsen [16].

two sections, which indicate that at high LET_∞ cell reproductive death is predominantly produced by traversals
of single densely ionizing particles and that this damage
is to a large extent independent of dose fractionation,
dose rate and cell conditions. From these results it
might be deduced that damage by particles of high LET_∞
is an all-or-nothing effect and that consequently the
type of damage resulting in a reduced rate of production
of viable progeny would not be expected to be produced at
all. The experimental data obtained demonstrate however
that non-lethal damage is produced by high LET_∞ particles
with about the same RBE as derived from cell survival curves.
Since both types of effects must be assumed to be related
to damage to the cell genome, it must be concluded that
two different types of damage are involved or two different parts of the same critical structure.

Another type of effect which is produced with a high
efficiency by densely ionizing radiations is mitotic delay. Relatively few experimental data are available however on the dependence of this effect on radiation quality [1, 14]. Mitotic delay has usually been measured as
the time after irradiation when the mitotic frequency
after an initial decrease to very low values has increased
again to 50 per cent of the control value. RBE values
for mitotic delay, determined from the doses required to
effect a 10-hour delay in Chinese hamster cells after
heavy ion and X-irradiation showed a broad maximum between
100 and 500 keV/μ [14]. Studies with α-particles at an
LET_∞ of 140 keV/μ and with X-rays have shown that in cultured cells of human kidney origin (T-1g cells) the RBE
of α-irradiation for delays between 1 and 4 hours is 4.7
[1]. In further experiments with α-particles only, the
fractions of cells in G_2, which were delayed for at least
two hours, was measured. By comparison of curves relating
the fractions of cells in G_2 which were not delayed as a
function of the dose for different sub-lines of T-1 cells,
it could be shown that for 50 per cent effect cells with a
small nucleus require larger doses than cells with a large
nucleus. It might be inferred that damage to nuclear mem-
branes is primarily involved in mitotic delay.

4. BIOLOGICAL EFFECTS OF RADIATIONS WITH A WIDE DISTRIBUTION OF DOSE IN LET

The track segment method for heavy charged particles, which provides relatively narrow distributions of dose in LET, cannot be used for the irradiation of multi-cellular organisms with particles at an LET_∞ in excess of 100 keV/μ because with the heavy ions at energies presently available for radiobiological experiments, the LET of these particles changes considerably over a distance along the particle track of 1 mm or more. Consequently the influence of radiation quality on damage in multi-cellular organisms can only be investigated with radiations of high penetrating power, which produce in tissue secondary particles with a high mean LET, e.g., fast neutrons and pi$^-$-mesons. A disadvantage of such studies with respect to interpretation of the results, is that with these radiations the distribution of dose in LET is very complex and extends over a wide range of LET. Therefore it is very important that a few cellular systems have been investigated with mono-energetic ions as well as with fast neutrons of different energies, because this provides a basis for the interpretation of further data to be obtained with fast neutrons [4]. Such series of experimental data have been obtained for impairment of the capacity for unlimited proliferation by cultured cells of human kidney origin and various authors have used these data for further analysis.

The survival curves obtained with fast neutrons of different energies have shown that broadly speaking their characteristics reflect the complex distribution of dose in LET. In the low dose region the survival curves exhibit less curvature as compared with X- or γ-rays, while the effect of dose fractionation is also smaller. The OER has in general a value which is considerably lower than that for X-rays but is significantly larger than one [5]. A demonstration of the contributions of different fractions of the total energy dissipated at different ionization densities to the total damage in a cell population, has been obtained in experiments with fast neutrons in which secondary particle equilibrium was provided or deliberately perturbed [9]. Energy dissipation by fast neutrons in soft tissue is mainly due to interactions with

nuclei of H, C, N and O. The fraction of the energy dissipated through interactions of the neutrons with hydrogen
nuclei, can be characterized by a dose in LET which extends from a few keV/μ to a maximum value of 96 keV/μ at
the Bragg peak of the protons. With 15 MeV neutrons, most
protons have ranges which are large compared to the diameter of an individual mammalian cell [9]. The fraction
of the energy dissipated through interactions of fast neutrons with nuclei of C, O and N can be characterized by a
distribution of dose in LET which extends from about 100
to 1000 keV/μ. The heavy recoils have maximum ranges of
only a few microns in tissue. The difference between the
ranges of the protons and the heavy recoils can be ex-
ploited to evaluate to a first approximation the relative
contributions of the two components. This was accomplished by mounting under the 6μ thick Melinex bottoms
of the culture dishes, 3 mm thick disks of either tissue
equivalent plastic or of pure carbon. With tissue equivalent plastic, secondary particle equilibrium is provided
but with carbon adjacent to the thin bottom of the dish
the number of protons entering the cells is greatly reduced and most of the energy absorbed in the cells is dissipated by low energy protons, heavy ions and α-particles
produced by interactions of neutrons with nuclei of H, C,
N and O in the 6μ thick bottom of the dishes and in the
cells. In Fig. 4 survival curves of cultured T-1g cells
of human kidney origin are presented, obtained with 15
MeV neutrons in different exposure conditions. Comparison of curves 1 and 3 shows that for the same neutron influence the biological effects differ for irradiations
with and without proton equilibrium respectively. The
damage registered without proton equilibrium must be due
for a large part to heavy recoils. This is in agreement
with the observation that the curve 3 is exponential within experimental errors and that the OER of this part of
the damage is only 1.1. Curves 1 and 2 for cells irradiated with proton equilibrium show that the OER is 1.4.
This factor is somewhat, but not significantly, lower
than the value of 1.6 reported earlier [5]. By subtraction of the effects contributed by the high LET component
from the effect of the total energy deposited in the case
of proton equilibrium, it is possible to make an approx-
mate estimate of the OER of the proton component. This

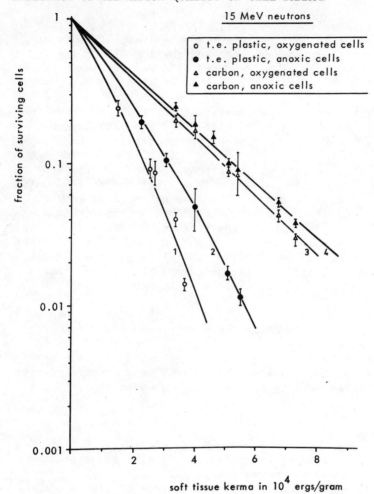

Fig. 4. Survival curves of cultured cells of human kidney origin in equilibrium with air or nitrogen, exposed to 15 MeV neutrons in experimental conditions whereby secondary particle equilibrium was
provided or deliberately perturbed to eliminate the largest part
of the proton component. For irradiations on tissue equivalent
plastic, curves 1 and 2 were obtained for cells equilibrated with
air and nitrogen respectively. The OER in this experimental arrangement with secondary particle equilibrium is 1.4. For irradiations on carbon, curves 3 and 4 were found for oxygenated
and hypoxic cells respectively. The OER in this experimental arrangement is 1.1. From Broerse, Barendsen and van Kersen [9].

value is equal to about 2.1. It can be concluded that in
the case of 15 MeV neutrons the relatively high OER of
2.1 for the proton component and the low OER of 1.1 for
the damage produced by heavy recoils results in an OER of
about 1.6 for the total energy dissipated.

From similar experiments with fission spectrum neutrons it can be concluded that the OER of 1.5 is due to
the low energy of the protons produced [9].

X-rays, γ-rays and electrons are characterized by an
energy disposition pattern with a distribution of dose in
LET which extends up to LET values of about 30 keV/μ.
From Fig. 2 it can be concluded that, although this spectrum is complex, mose of the cell reproductive death will
be due to accumulation of damage and the effectiveness of
a given dose can be modified considerably by dose fractionation, by variation of the dose rate and by experimental
conditions, e.g., the presence of oxygen.

These examples illustrate that if sufficient knowledge is available about the energy deposition pattern
of a type of radiation, its effectiveness and the possi-
bilities of modification can be predicted at least qualitatively on the basis of data on the dependence of damage
on radiation quality obtained with mono-energetic ions.

SUMMARY

The dependence on ionization density of several
types of damage in mammalian cells, namely cell reproductive death, reduction in growth rate of clones and
mitotic delay, was discussed. Damage induced by densely
ionizing radiations is less modified by dose fractionation, sensitizing and protecting agents and is less dependent on cell age as compared with X-rays. Effects of
fast neutrons of different energies can be interpreted
qualitatively by consideration of dose-effect relations
obtained with mono-energetic ions.

REFERENCES

1.   BARENDSEN, G.W., unpublished data.

2.   BARENDSEN, G.W., *Ann. N.Y. Acad. Sci.*, *114*, 96, 1964.

3.   BARENDSEN, G.W., In: *Advances in Theoretical and Experimental Biophysics* (Ed. A. Cole), Marcel Dekker Inc., New York, 167, 1967.

4.   BARENDSEN, G.W., In: *Current Topics in Radiation Research* (Eds. M. Ebert and A. Howard), North-Holland Publ. Co., Amsterdam, 293, 1968.

5.   BARENDSEN, G.W. and BROERSE, J.J., *Nature*, *212*, 722, 1966.

6.   BARENDSEN, G.W., KOOT, C.J., KERSEN, G.R., VAN, BEWLEY, D.K., FIELD, S.B. and PARNELL, C.J., *Int. J. Radiat. Biol.*, *10*, 317, 1966.

7.   BARENDSEN, G.W., WALTER, H.M.D., FOWLER, J.F. and BEWLEY, D.K., *Radiat. Res.*, *18*, 106, 1963.

8.   BARENDSEN, G.W., BEUSKER, T.L.J., VERGROESEN, A.J. and BUDKE, L., *Radiat. Res.*, *13*, 841, 1960.

9.   BROERSE, J.J., BARENDSEN, G.W. and KERSEN, G.R. VAN,, *Int. J. Radiat. Biol.*, *12*, 387, 1967.

10. ELKIND, M.M. and SINCLAIR, W.K., In: *Current Topics in Radiation Research* (Eds. M. Ebert and A. Howard), North-Holland Publ. Co., Amsterdam, Vil. I, 165, 1965.

11. NIAS, A.H.W., *Cell Tissue Kinet.*, *1*, 153, 1968.

12. ROSSI, H.H., In: *Advances in Biological and Medical Physics* (Eds. J.H. Lawrence and J.W. Gofman) Academic Press, New York, *11*, 27, 1967.

13. SINCLAIR, W.K., *Radiat. Res.*, *21*, 584, 1964.

14. SKARSGARD, L.D., *Radiat. Res.*, *22*, 235, 1964.

15. TERASIMA, T. and TOLMACH, L.J., *Biophys. J.*, *3*, 11, 1963.

16. WESTRA, A. and BARENDSEN, G.W., *Int. J. Radiat. Biol.*, *11*, 477, 1966.

INTRODUCTORY REMARKS

M. EBERT

*Paterson Laboratories, Christie Hospital
and Holt Radium Institute, Manchester M20, England*

The history of neutron radiobiology follows the standard path of any discipline. First is the period which lays the foundations with many qualitative observations; probably several thousand publications are available. Now we see the more quantitative approach and with it the formulation of the real questions and the difficulties in interpretation. The help of physicists and chemists is required for the understanding of the biological effects. Physics has provided the technique of track segment experiments which have pointed to the importance of the detailed knowledge of the LET of different neutron energies. Already the Harrogate Congress contained papers [11,16] which demonstrated this particular point. The physical dosimetry is a difficult problem for non monoenergetic neutron beams as are likely to be found in any irradiated material of several centimetres thickness, and the methods used for the measurement of neutron dose are fundamentally not fully understood as yet [14]. Only little radiation chemistry using high LET irradiations has been carried out. The effects observed on solutions can be explained by the very high radical concentration produced in the track of the particles. This leads to radical-radical interaction and only a few radicals diffuse out of the track to interact with substrates dissolved in the solvent. A notable contribution in summarising these problems appeared a few years ago [6]. Observations in the solid state demonstrate, so far mainly qualitatively, the microscopic damage produced by high LET particles in glasses and plastics.

The biologist is left to measure some endpoint, often
cell killing, after irradiation of biological material.
This type of experimentation is unsatisfactory even for
low LET radiations when questions are asked about the mode
of action of the radiation. Its limitation is inherent
in its low resolution at the molecular level. One of the
few parameters related to the LET of fast neutrons which
have been measured is the RBE for different biological
endpoints in different biological materials. The RBE varies from material to material and frequently is different
for different biological endpoints in the same material.
It therefore is at best only a vague indication of some
property of the radiation used and is strongly influenced
by biological factors of the system under investigation.

Since the Puck technique became available and Elkind's
detailed investigations of some recovery phenomena were
published, there is no justification to use a single and
non qualified value of RBE in any system investigated [8,
9]. It is well known that single cell survival after α-
irradiation is usually a pure exponential function of
dose. Single cell survival curves for low LET radiation
usually show a shoulder in the low dose range which is
often an expression of the ability of the cells to recover from sublethal damage. Single cells irradiated
with neutrons show usually only a small shoulder and their
D_0's are often lower than for low LET irradiations. Since
the shape of the survival curves change from low LET irradiations to neutron irradiations it becomes obvious that
for low total doses the RBE values tend to be high. In
some systems high LET irradiations show only an effect on
the shoulder of the curve and very little effect on the
D_0. Others show large changes in D_0. Rossi [15] reported last week that the logarithm of RBE could be plotted
against the logarithm of dose of neutron irradiation. If
this is done a more unified picture appears in that the
graphs of RBE versus dose appear linear for part of the
function. The slopes are slightly different for different
organs or different mammalian tissues and they tend to a
limiting slope of $-\frac{1}{2}$. It is remarkable that RBE values
for irradiated skin from different mammals, including human skin, fall on the same line [10] as will be mentioned

by Field et al later in this Symposium. Such plots of
RBE versus neutron dose were used by Rossi [15] to estimate formally the size of the important structure within the living cell which is responsible for biological
damage. It is encouraging to see that this novel approach
arrives at a figure of about 20 - 30 Å in diameter, a figure which is in fair agreement with many estimates of target size for biological materials derived in the past bio-
physically and chemically.

One unifying aspect of the papers to be read today
seems to be the use of neutron beams as a powerful tool
for the eradication of malignant tissues. Already by
the end of the last war Stone performed a neutron therapy
clinical trial [17]. Stone was discouraged by severe late
effects in some of the 40 patients treated. This disap-
pointment prevented the use of neutrons clinically for
many years. Today we believe to understand the reason.
for Stone's difficulties [12]. The repair capacity of
tissues is very much smaller after high LET irradiation
than after low LET irradiation. Stone's fractionation
schedules were based on the commonly used conventional
X-ray radiotherapy. This led to over-dosing of normal
tissues in Stone's fractionation schedules and resulted
in unfavourable late effects. A number of experiments
are being reported at this Symposium in which fractionation schedules of neutron and X-irradiations are tested
on experimental tumours as well as on healthy tissues.

The attraction of neutrons as a tool for radiotherapy
increased since it was realised that some human and animal
tumours contain a fair proportion of anoxic cells [3,12,
13]. Since the OER oxygen enhancement ratio for low LET
irradiation is high, the anoxic tumour cells are more likely to escape damage than normal tissue cells which are
well oxygenated. The OER is normally about 3 for low LET
irradiations and drops to the values of 1.2 to 1.6 for
fast neutron exposures. Later in this Symposium a number
of such estimates are given but no final agreement has
yet been reached on how constant the OER is for neutron
energies from 3 MeV to 20 MeV [1,2]. Barendsen et al as
well as Berry et al will be discussing some of their work
which they performed in the last few years on these par-

ticular questions. Some of this kind of experimentation
is difficult because recovery from sub lethal damage often depends on the presence of oxygen. The dose rates
normally used for high LET experiments are low and recovery during exposure can falsify the true oxygen enhancement ratios when oxic and anoxic conditions are
compared.

A point to remember in biological experiments with
fast neutrons was demonstrated last year when two groups
of workers, one at the Christie Hospital in England [7]
and the group at Rijiswijk in the Netherlands[4], investigated independently the survival of colony forming
cells in the bone marrow of the femur of mice. Both experiments were carried out with 14 - 15 MeV fast neutrons
and the assay methods used were essentially identical.
The RBE results differed by about 30%. This difference
caused the two groups of workers to intercompare the dosimetry. Part of the discrepancy could be resolved this
way and points to the need for internationally co-ordin-
ated standards for neutron dosimetry [5]. This need was
also recognised at last week's meeting in Rijswijk [15].

Rather than give a review of the literature on the
radiobiology of fast neutrons, I have attempted to point
out a few difficulties in the hope that by the end of the
day we will have come closer to some of the outstanding
answers.

REFERENCES

1. BARENDSEN, G.W. and BROERSE, J.J., *Nature (Lond.) 212*,
    722, 1966.

2. BERRY, R.J., Meeting on Fundamental and Practical As-
    pects of the Application of Fast Neutrons in Clinical
    Radiotherapy, Rijswijk, 1970.

3. BEWLEY, D.K., in: *Current Topics in Radiation Research*,
    ed. M. Ebert and A. Howard, North Holland Publishing
    Co. *6*, 249, 1970.

4. BROERSE, J.J., van PUTTEN, L.M. and LELIEVELD, P.,

Int. J. Rad. Biol., 16, 77, 1969.

5. BROERSE, J.J. et al., in preparation.

6. BURNS, W.G. and BARKER, R., in: *Progress in Reaction Kinetics,* ed. G. Porter, Pergamon Press, *3,* 303, 1965.

7. DUNCAN, W., GREENE, D., HOWARD, A. and MASSEY, J.B., *Int. J. Rad. Biol., 15,* 397, 1969.

8. ELKIND, M.M. and SINCLAIR, W.K., in: *Current Topics in Radiation Research,* ed. M. Ebert and A. Howard, North Holland Publishing Co., *1,* 165, 1965.

9. ELKIND, M.M., in *Current Topics in Radiation Research,* ed. M. Ebert and A. Howard, North Holland Publishing Co. In Press.

10. FIELD, S.B. et al., Meeting on Fundamental and Practical Aspects of the Application of Fast Neutrons in Clinical Radiotherapy, Rijswijk, 1970.

11. FOWLER, J.F., BEWLEY, D.K., BARENDSEN, G.W. and WALTER, H.M.D., in *Radiation Effects in Physics, Chemistry and Biology,* ed. M. Ebert and A. Howard, North Holland Publishing Co., p.4, 1963.

12. FOWLER, J.F., in: *Current Topics in Radiation Research,* ed. M. Ebert and A. Howard, North Holland Publishing Co., *2,* 303, 1966.

13. GRAY, L.H., *Amer. J. Roentgenol, 85,* 803, 1961.

14. ROSSI, H.H. and LUBERT, M., *Health Phys., 1,* 46, 1958.

15. ROSSI, H.H. Reported at the Meeting of Fundamental and Practical Aspects of the Application of Fast Neutrons in Clinical Radiotherapy, Rijswijk, 1970.

16. SKARSGARD, L.D., in: *Radiation Effects in Physics, Chemistry and Biology,* ed. M. Ebert and A. Howard, North Holland Publishing Co., p.4, 1963.

17. STONE, R.S., *Amer. J. Roentgenol., 59,* 771, 1948.

THE EFFECT OF 14 MeV NEUTRONS ON MAMMALIAN CELLS IN VITRO

R.E. ELLIS, J.D. LEWIS and PATRICIA J. LINDOP

Departments of Physics and Radiobiology,
The Medical College of St. Bartholomew's Hospital,
Charterhouse Square, London, E.C.1, England

If full advantage is to be gained from the use of fast neutrons in radiotherapy, more quantitative data are needed on relevant factors affecting cell survival, such as the effect of the dose rate, the R.B.E. at different levels of damage, and intracellular recovery. This we have tried to do, in the absence of knowing the under-lying mechanism leading to cell death and its modifications.

Cells have been irradiated *in vitro* from a low and a high dose rate neutron source.

A Sames 14 MeV neutron generator was used with a beam current of 400-500 µamps of deuterons accelerated by a 150 kV generator. The tritiated titanium-copper target (9.3 Ci) gave a dose rate at 3.5 cm of 10 rads/min in-itially, decreasing with a half-life of 1½ hours to give 1 rad/min after 8 hours.

For the high dose rate a 14 MeV neutron generator at A.W.R.E. Aldermaston was used, where the high deuteron currents available, bombarding a tritiated target, gave dose rates at 25 cm of 50 rads/min. Dose rates up to 1200 rads/min were obtained closer to the target.

The cells were Hela (Oxf-s) subcloned, and grown in Eagles with penicillin and streptomycin, and 2.5 mg/cm^3

501

Fungizone. These cells have a doubling time of about 30–38 hours.

For the low dose rate experiments, the cells were irradiated in suspension in polystyrene cylinders approx. 1 cm by 2.5 cm length. For hypoxic exposures a sintered glass microbubbler was cemented into the bottom of the cylinder through which nitrogen (B.O.C. < 1 part per 10^6 O_2) was bubbled.

All the cell suspension samples were kept for the same length of time at room temperature. After irradiation, the suspensions were diluted, cells counted, plated out on to polystyrene Petri dishes, and then incubated for 14–18 days for clone scoring of survival.

For the higher dose rate experiments the cells were plated in polystyrene dishes, incubated overnight, prior to being taken to Aldermaston the following morning (60 miles by road). On arrival, they were incubated for at least 3 hours at 37°C before exposure. In all but the lowest dose rate (2.5 rads/min), the medium was removed before irradiation and fresh medium replaced after exposure.

The plates were clamped in almost vertical positions at different distances from the target depending on the required dose rate, except for the 2.5 rads/min plates which were irradiated horizontally through the medium. In the first two experiments, the plates remained under incubation at Aldermaston for 18 days. In the third experiment the cells were returned, after overnight incubation on site, for their remaining incubation at Barts before scoring.

RESULTS

Low Dose Rate and the Effect of Hypoxia

Fig. 1 shows the cell survival curves for the dose rate 1–10 rads/min 14 MeV neutrons compared with 250 kV X-rays at 200 rads/min, given under oxygenated or hypoxic

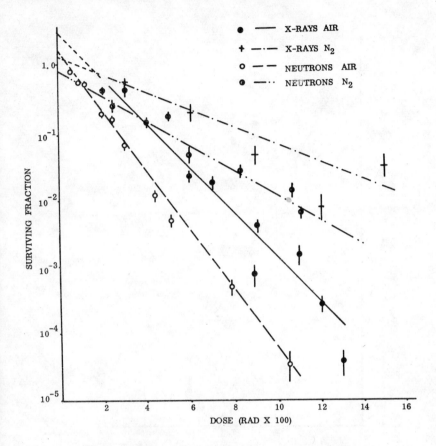

Fig. 1. Survival curves for Hela (Oxf-s) cells irradiated under oxygenated or hypoxic conditions with 250 kV X-rays compared with 14 MeV neutrons at 1-10 rads/min.

conditions. From these there is an R.B.E. in air of 1.7, and under hypoxia of 1.7 at the 10^{-2} level of survival.

Higher Dose Rates

Fig. 2 shows three single dose survival experiments for a dose rate of 50-100 rads/min. The response is a straight exponential decrease after a small shoulder, in

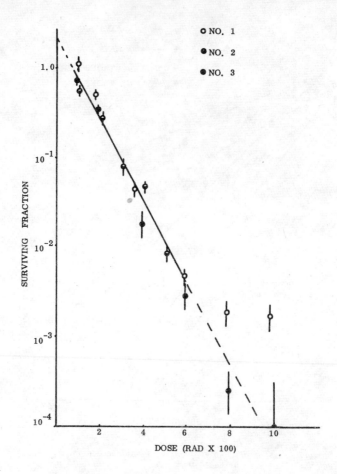

Fig. 2. Survival data for Hela (Oxf-s) cells irradiated with 14 MeV neutrons at 50-100 rads/min. Regression line fitted to data from experiment 2 ◕.

contrast to the continuously curving lines of Broerse, Barendsen and Kersen [3] for 15 MeV neutrons. There is good agreement between the three experiments except for the highest dose points of the first experiment. It was because of this apparent break in the dose response curve that the experiments were repeated several times, but it did not recur.

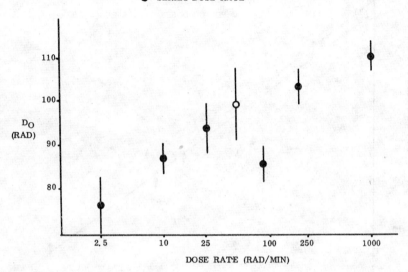

Fig. 3. The effect of dose rate of 14 MeV neutrons on cell survival *in vitro* expressed as D_0.

Effect of Dose Rate

Since a break to decreased effectiveness at approx. 10^{-2} level of survival resembled that found for high dose rate electrons by Town [6], survival curves were obtained from 2.5 rads/min up to 1000 rads/min. Since all curves were exponential after a small shoulder, Fig. 3 shows the comparative effectiveness of different dose rates, using the D_0. There is a trend to a higher D_0 at the higher dose rates, which may imply some temporal or spatial interaction occurring at high dose rates, with loss of effectiveness of the radiation due to disruption of the early initial reactions normally leading to biological damage.

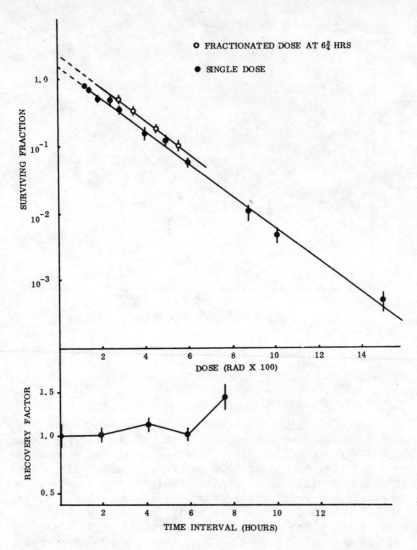

Fig. 4.   The effect of an initial dose of 70 rads on survival after a second
          dose given at different times. (a) cell survival curve at $6^3/4$
          hours after first dose. (b) recovery factor in split dose experi-
          ment.

Effect of Dose Fractionation

Intracellular recovery was measured by split dose experiments on asynchronous populations on both machines, and by a survival curve following an initial dose of 70 rads 63/4 hours previously, at the low dose rate (Sames) exposure only.

In the first series, at 1-10 rads/min, Fig. 4 shows that there was some recovery shown by split doses at 6 hours, and significant at 8 hours. The survival curve 6 3/4 hours after 70 rads showed an increased extrapolation number, but no significant change in slope, giving a D_q value of 42 rads, i.e. approx. 50% recovery from the first dose.

The amount of recovery may, however, depend on the size of the first dose, as seen in tissue irradiation [4], as well as on dose rate. Split dose experiments for the higher dose rate of 250 rads/min were done using initial doses of 70, 100 or 600 rads, followed at different times up to 24 hours by an equal dose. These preliminary data would confirm that recovery does occur after 70 rads first dose, but it was not seen in two repeat experiments after 100 rads first dose followed up to 14 hours. These cannot be interpreted yet as loss of recovery after a large first dose, because the one experiment using 600 rads + 600 rads, compared with a 1200 rads single dose survival level of 10^{-5}, shows increased survival. However, at this level of survival many repeat experiments are needed to obtain any statistical validity.

DISCUSSION

The R.B.E. for Hela cells irradiated with 14 MeV neutrons compared with 250 kV X-rays is greater for hypoxic than oxygenated conditions. The ratio of these R.B.E.'s, which is a measure of the relative gain by using neutrons to damage hypoxic cells, called the Therapeutic Gain Factor [1] was found to be 1.1 at 37% survival in comparison with 1.5 [2] and 1.6 [5].

At low dose rates there may be significant recovery which is delayed up to 6 hours in contrast to recovery following X irradiation. The amount of the recovery may depend, however, on the size of the first dose, being abolished by the first dose which results in a survival level of 10^{-2}.

CONCLUSION

These data, in conjunction with tissue data for effectiveness of the same neutron sources indicate clearly that there are many variables of relevance to the use of neutrons in therapy which need to be quantitated before a valid prediction of their relative effectiveness can be made, or until such time as the mechanism of damage is known.

ACKNOWLEDGMENTS

We are most grateful to Mr. D. Smith, A.W.R.E. Aldermaston for his continuous participation and contribution to these experiments; and to the Ministry of Health, and the C.R.C. for financial support of the project. We would also like to record our thanks to Jean Brims and Dr. C.D. Town who determined the X-ray and neutron hypoxic survival curves quoted in this communication.

SUMMARY

Hela cells have been irradiated under oxygenated and hypoxic conditions, *in vitro*, with 14 MeV neutrons at a dose rate between 1-10 rads/min. The oxygenated data are compared with those from 2.5 rads/min up to 1000 rads/min. An increase in D_0 was seen with increasing dose rate. Intracellular recovery was significant at 6-8 hours after a first dose of 70 rads, but was not seen after 100 rads. The possible effect of the size of first dose is to be tested.

REFERENCES

1. ALPER, T., *Br. J. Radiol.*, *36*, 97, 1963.

2. BROERSE, J. and BARENDSEN, G., *Nature*, *206*, 208 1965.

3. BROERSE, J., BARENDSEN, G. and van KERSEN, G., *Int. J. Radiat. Biol.*, *13*, 559, 1968.

4. LINDOP, Patricia J., ELLIS, R.E., PROUKAKIS, C. and SHEWELL, Jennifer, *Br. J. Radiol.*, *Proceedings of Annual Congress (Abstract)*, 44, 235, 1971.

5. NIAS, A., (personal communication), 1966.

6. TOWN, C.D., *Nature*, *215*, 847, 1967.

SOME ASPECTS OF THE RBE FOR FAST NEUTRONS

S.B. FIELD

M.R.C. Cyclotron Unit, Hammersmith Hospital, Ducane Road, London, W. 12, England

SHIRLEY HORNSEY

M.R.C. Experimental Radiopathology Unit, Hammersmith Hospital, Ducane Road, London, W. 12, England

The RBE (Relative biological effectiveness) is defined as the ratio of the dose of fast neutrons to that
of X-rays needed to produce the same level of damage.
Because the oxygen enhancement ratio is less for neutrons
than for X-rays, the RBE will be larger for a hypoxic
than for a well oxygenated system. Also because of the
different shapes of survival curves produced by radiations
of different LET [1], the RBE will depend on the dose
level, increasing with decreasing dose [13].

For treatment with any new radiation, the RBE, as a
function of dose, must be accurately known. Since the
absolute dosimetry of fast neutrons is not yet precise,
and since the quality of beams produced at different
centres may differ, the following analysis of RBE will
include only tissues irradiated on the M.R.C. cyclotron
at the Hammersmith Hospital. These neutrons are produced by 16 MeV deuterons on beryllium and have a mean
energy of 8 MeV.

Figure 1 shows a plot of the RBE obtained for the
visual observations of skin damage as a function of the

RBE for fast neutrons
relative to 250 kVp x-rays

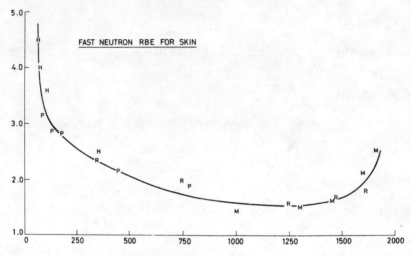

Dose per fraction of neutrons (rads)

Fig. 1.   The RBE for skin irradiated with fast neutrons from the Hammer-
          smith cyclotron, as a function of dose per fraction of neutrons.
          H   human skin [18]
          P   pig skin [3]
          R   rat skin [10, 11]
          M   mouse skin [5]

(Courtesy of D.K. Bewley in "Current Topics in Radiation
Research, North Holland, Amsterdam.)
dose per fraction of fast neutrons. Data for both single
and fractionated exposures are included, a valid comparison, since the rate of repopulation has often been
shown to be the same after X-rays or fast neutrons,[10,
11, 12, 23], and will therefore not affect the RBE. The
RBE for skin is independent of species Fig. 1, and increases with decreasing dose as expected from the differences in the shapes of survival curves [1]. The
small increase in RBE seen for doses greater than about
1500 rads of neutrons may be due to a small proportion
of hypoxic cells in the skin.

     Rossi [19] has suggested a method of plotting these
results as the logarithm of the dose of X-rays against
the logarithm of the dose of neutrons. The skin results

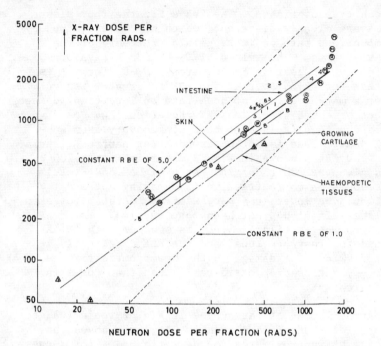

Fig. 2. Dose of X-rays as a function of the dose of neutrons to produce
the same effect.

△A mouse lymphocytes [17]
△T weight loss in mouse thymus [24]
△S mouse-haemopoetic cells, spleen colonies assay [17]
△D 30 day death in mice
▣ stunting of the tail growth in 1 day-old rats [6]
Ⓗ human skin [18]
Ⓟ pig skin reactions [3]
Ⓡ rat skin reactions [10, 11]
Ⓜ mouse skin reactions [5]
Ⓒ clones in mouse skin [8, 9]

6   5 day death in T O mice (1965) [21]
1   5 day death in T O mice (1969) [22]
3   5 day death in C₃H mice [22]
4   Survival of mouse colonies in the jejunum [16]
5   Reduction of crypts in the jejunum [22]
6   Reduction of crypts in the ileum [16]

are presented in this way in Fig. 2, together with the
data for damage to the haemopoetic system, growing cartilage and the intestinal system. Within the experimental
errors, straight lines may be drawn through the points

for each type of tissue. The RBE's for the four tissue
systems are clearly different, which may be explained by
the amount and rate of intracellular recovery of the
various systems. The values of D_2-D_1 for X-rays are similar for gut and skin. For neutrons, D_2-D_1 for gut is
less than for skin, so that the RBE is greater for gut.
However a marked effect of dose-rate on intestinal damage
has been observed after low LET radiation [14, 15].
This is due to a·rapid component of recovery from sub-
lethal damage, and is not observed after neutron irradiation. The RBE's shown in Fig. 2 are relative to 200 kV
X-rays given at 200 rads/min. At a higher dose-rate,
X-rays would be more effective in damaging gut and the
RBE's would be lower, and very similar to those for skin,
where this effect has not been observed [4]. For damage
to the growing cartilage, D_2-D_1 is smaller both for X-
rays and for fast neutrons, and the RBE is slightly less
than for skin. For damage to the heamopoetic tissues,
both D_2-D_1 ratios are considerably less than for skin,
and so with RBE.

Extrapolation of the curves in Fig. 2 would lead to
a theoretical RBE of less than 1. At large doses, however, the RBE approximates to the ratio of D_0 for X-rays
to that for neutrons. This ratio has been measured in
many mammalian systems, and has never been found to be
less than 1, implying that the curves in Fig. 2 cannot
be extrapolated, but might all lend towards constant
values of RBE.

In clinical terms, the variation of RBE from tissue
to tissue may be illustrated by the following comparison.
A single treatment of 120 rads of neutrons is equivalent
to 280 rads of X-rays to the haemopoetic tissue, 350 to
growing cartilage, 390 to skin and about 470 rads to gut.
The estimate for gut however requires an extrapolation
of the data, and is therefore less certain.

The damage to normal tissues will determine the
maximum dose which can be tolerated in radiotherapy.
With presently available neutrons sources it seems
likely that skin damage will be the limiting factor,
however it may in some cases be gut where it is included
in the field.

It has also been possible [20] to use the RBE data
to estimate the equivalent doses of X-rays given by Stone
and Larkin [21] in their early clinical trial of fast
neutrons. For each patient, each dose delivered to the
skin, on each occasion was converted to an equivalent
dose of X-rays, account having been taken of back-
scattered radiation and exit doses. The Ellis formula
[8] relating total dose of X-rays, number of fractions
and overall treatment time was then applied, so that all
treatments could be reduced to an effective single number
(the N.S.D.). Also, from the carefully kept patient
records and photographs it was possible to score both the
early and late skin reactions for each field and to relate these scores to the N.S.D. From this analysis, the
average dose to produce a tolerance skin reaction was
equivalent to about 6000 rads of Co^{60} γ-rays given in 30
treatments in 6 weeks. Since this is in accord with
present radiotherapy practice it confirmed the validity
of the mathematical procedures employed. It was concluded that the late reactions seen were generally consistent both with the early reactions, and the effective
doses given. The severe late reactions reported by
Stone [21] were the result of overdoses of radiation for
the following reasons:

(1) The variation of RBE with size of dose per
    fraction was not appreciated.
(2) No account was taken of exit doses.
(3) No account was taken of overall treatment
    time and number of fractions.
(4) Areas were treated which had previously been
    irradiated with X-rays, often to high doses.

Two other factors which must have played a part, are the
effect of field size and of increased absorption of fast
neutrons in fat [2]. If the range of the recoil protons
is long, relative to the diameters of capillaries, then
the dose to vessels in fatty tissues would be greater
than in non-fatty tissues. The prostate fields treated
by Stone developed severe telangiectasia and marked
atrophy, which may have been due to the layers of subcutaneous fat in these areas.

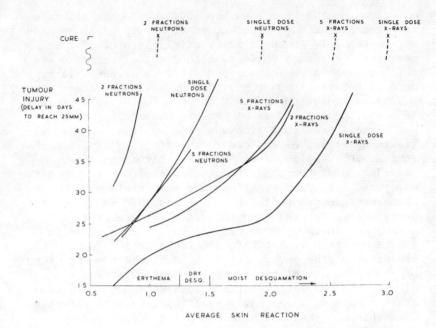

Fig. 3.   Tumour injury as a function of skin injury for various schemes
of fractionation with X rays and fast neutrons [10, 11].

(Courtesy of S.B. Field, T. Jones and R.H. Thomlinson,
Brit. J. Rad., Ref. 11.)

It seems likely that for single doses, the RBE for
damage to most tumours will be greater than for any of
the normal tissues. Whether such a therapeutic advantage is maintained for a fractionated course of treatment will depend on many factors, but particularly on
the kinetics of reoxygenation of the particular tumour.
Any gain with fast neutrons could be completely lost
in a tumour which reoxygenates rapidly and extensively,
but such information can ultimately only be determined
by a clinical trial. However, confirmation is being
obtained from experiments on animal tumours and normal
tissues. One such experiment has been done by Field,
Jones and Thomlinson [10, 11] who have irradiated the
sarcoma RIB$_5$ and the skin of rats with single, two and
five fractions of X-rays and fast neutrons. The results of these experiments are summarized in Fig. 3,

where the injury to the tumour is plotted as a function
of the injury to the skin for each of the six types of
treatment given. Clearly the aim is to find the treatment giving the curve nearest to the upper left hand
corner, i.e. as much damage to the tumour and little to
the normal tissue as possible. The least effective form
of treatment was the single dose of X-rays. Two and five
fractions of X-rays were more effective, probably resulting from improved oxygenation of the tumour between fractions. However, in this tumour, with the fractionation
schemes employed, the hypoxic cells still appear to affect
the overall response, and a single dose of neutrons was
more effective than any of the schemes of X-ray treatment.
There was also an optimum treatment, in these experiments,
of two fractions of neutrons. This rather unexpected
result should serve to emphasize that the oxygen effect
is only one of the factors involved. Other tumours will
almost certainly respond differently, so that a great
deal more knowledge of the processes underlying the radiation response of both normal and neoplastic tissues is
needed in order to optimize radiotherapy.

SUMMARY

The RBE for different normal tissue endpoints is
presented and shown to vary with size of dose, and with
the differential amount and rate of intracellular repair
of each tissue. RBE data has been used to estimate the
equivalent doses of X-rays given by Stone in a re-evalua-
tion of the early therapeutic trial of fast neutrons.

The possible advantages of fast neutrons in human
therapy are illustrated by the results of experiments
on animal normal and neoplastic tissues.

REFERENCES

1.   BARENDSEN, G.W., BEUSKER, T.L., VERGROESSEN, A.J.
     and BUDKE, L., *Radiation Res.*, *13*, 841, 1960.

2.   BEWLEY, D.K., *Brit. J. Radiol.*, *36*, 81, 1963.

3.   BEWLEY, D.K., FIELD, S.B., MORGAN, R.L., PAGE, B.C.
     and PARNELL, C.J., *Brit. J. Radiol.*, *40*, 765, 1967.

4.   DENEKAMP, J. and FOWLER, J.F., *Int. J. Radiation
     Biol.*, *10*, 435, 1966.

5.   DENEKAMP, J., FOWLER, J.F., KRAGT, K., PARNELL, C.J.
     and FIELD, S.B., *Radiation Res.*, *29*, 71, 1966.

6.   DENEKAMP, J., EMERY, E.W. and FIELD, S.B., *Radiation
     Res. 45*, 80, 1971.

7.   DIXON, B., *Int. J. Radiat. Biol.*, *15*, 541, 1969.

8.   ELLIS, F., In: *Current Topics in Radiation Research,
     4*, Editors: Ebert & Howard, North Holland Publish-
     ing Co., 357, 1968.

9.   EMERY, E.W., DENEKAMP, J., BALL, M.M. and FIELD,
     S.B., *Radiation Res.*, *41*, 450, 1970.

10. FIELD, S.B., JONES, T. and THOMLINSON, R.H., *Br. J.
     Radiol.*, *40*, 834, 1967.

11. FIELD, S.B., JONES, T. and THOMLINSON, R.H., *Br. J.
     Radiol.*, *41*, 597, 1968.

12. FOWLER, J.F., *Radiation Res. Suppl.*, *7*, 276, 1967.

13. FOWLER, J.F. and MORGAN, R.L., *Br. J. Radiol.*, *36*,
     115, 1963.

14. HORNSEY, S., Radiology 97,   *Radiology 97*, 649, 1970

15. HORNSEY, S. and ALPER, T., *Nature*, *210*, 212, 1966.

16. HORNSEY, S., VATISTAS, S., BEWLEY, D.K. and PARNELL,
     C.J., *Br. J. Radiol.*, *38*, 878, 1965.

17. HORNSEY, S., Personal communication.

18. MORGAN, R.L., In: *Modern Trends in Radiotherapy*,
     Editors: Deeley and Wood, Butterworths, London,
     p. 171, 1967.

19. ROSSI, H.H., *Phys. Med. Biol.*, *15*, 255, 1970.

20. SHELINE, G.E., PHILLIPS, T.L., FIELD, S.B., BRENNAN, J.T. and RAVENTOS, A., *Amer. J. Roentgen., Rad. Ther. and Nucl. Med.*, *111*, 31, 1971.

21. STONE, R.S., *Amer. J. Roentgen., Rad. Ther. and Nucl. Med.*, *59*, 771, 1948.

22. THOMLINSON, R.H., *Time and Dose Relationships in Radiation Biology as Applied to Radio Therapy*, p. 242.

23. WITHERS, H.R., BRENNAN, J.T. and ELKIND, M.M., *Brit. J. Radiol.*, *43*, 796.

24. WRIGHT, E.A., BEWLEY, D.K. and PARNELL, C.J., *Brit. J. Radiol.*, *39*, 551, 1966.

CHANGES IN THE BIOLOGICAL PARAMETERS FOR MAMMALIAN CELLS AS A FUNCTION OF POSITION IN A 14 MeV NEUTRON FIELD

A.H.W. NIAS and D. GREENE

Paterson Laboratories and Physics Department, Christie Hospital and Holt Radium Institute, Manchester M20 9BX, England

Fast neutron sources are now available for clinical use and sufficient radiobiology has been performed to explain the severe late effects experienced by the patients who survived the original trial of fast neutrons from the Berkeley cyclotron [3]. Overdosage was mainly attributable to the "fractionation trap" which results from the fact that RBE values are significantly larger with smaller fraction doses [6]. This relationship follows from the fact that single dose cell survival curves have much smaller shoulders after high LET irradiation than after X- or γ-irradiation. With 14 MeV monoenergetic neutrons, for example, the extrapolation number of the HeLa cell survival curves was 1.58, compared with 3.22 after X-irradiation [10]. This difference in shoulder size was associated with a two-fold range in values for Relative Biological Efficiency (RBE) from 3.8 at the 80% cell survival level (single doses of 115 and 30 rads of X-rays and neutrons, respectively) down to 1.9 at survival levels lower than 0.1%. With present radiotherapeutic fractionation schedules, doses between 100 and 300 rads of X-rays are used and this is the range over which there is the greatest variation in RBE values (2.8 - 3.8). The Neutron Therapist will need to know the precise values for the normal tissue in the treatment field before deciding what is the

biologically equivalent neutron dosage that is safe to
use in a particular fractionation regime.

The difference in shoulder size between neutron and
X-ray survival curves is attributable to a reduction in
the amount of recovery from sublethal damage after neutrons. Using the split-dose regime to treat HeLa cells
the recovery ratio after 300 kV X-rays rises to a maximum value of 2.19 after two hours [7]. The recovery
ratio after neutrons does not rise significantly above
unity up to four hours after the first dose (Table 1).
Although recovery from sublethal damage might occur more
slowly after neutron irradiation there is no evidence for
this from earlier studies. Broerse and Barendsen [4], using human kidney cells, showed the first rise in both their
X-ray and neutron two-dose fractionation curves to be complete four hours after the first dose. (Increasing multiplicity is a complication over longer periods). The
data in Table 1 show no significant recovery at two dose
levels of 100 and 200 rads. At the higher dosage, each
fraction of 100 rads is sufficient to reduce the level of
cell survival to a point on the survival curve where it
has become exponential. In fact, the recovery ratios with
this higher dosage are no higher than those after the lower dosage where the first dose only reduces survival to
a point which is still on the small shoulder of the curve.
Compared with the recovery ratio of 2.19 after X-irradiation of HeLa cells, this ratio of unity after neutron irradiation represents, at least, a significant reduction
in recovery from sublethal damage.

Qualitatively, these data confirm the previous findings of Broerse and Barendsen [4] who found a recovery
factor of 2 for 15 MeV neutrons and 9 for 250 kV X-rays;
an even larger reduction in the amount of recovery. Although their single dose survival curves were not drawn
with an exponential portion it was obvious that the
"shoulder" of their neutron curves is much smaller than
that of their X-ray curves. Again, this is the portion
of the survival curve most relevant to clinical radiotherapy and for which most radiobiological data are required, not only on changing values of RBE, but also on
the Oxygen Enhancement Ratio (OER). The lower OER with

TABLE 1. Split-Dose Treatments of HeLa Cells with Neutrons

Single Dose (rads)	Single Dose Survival %	Divided Doses (rads)	Recovery Ratios when Doses Divided by Time Interval (Hours)			
			1	2	3	4
100	42.1	50 + 50	1.02 ±0.11	0.90 ±0.07	0.87 ±0.01	0.88 ±0.12
200	11.8	100 + 100	1.065 ±0.025	0.90 ±0.01	0.945 ±0.005	0.99 ±0.05

neutrons relative to X-rays is the primary reason for developing a fast neutron source for radiotherapy [3].   Any
change in either of the biological parameters (RBE or OER)
which may occur under clinical conditions, should be pre-
dictable by physical and radiobiological experiments.

The physical variations in the field of a 14 MeV
monoenergetic beam have been described previously [8].
With suitable collimation the isodose charts are not
grossly different from those obtainable with medium voltage X-rays.   This means that at 10 cm. depth the dose
is 50% that of the surface at 75 cm. S.S.D., and therefore that the dose-rate is reduced to half.   It is just
conceivable that such a change in dose-rate might be accompanied by a change in RBE, but our HeLa cell survival
data have never shown any difference over the larger range
of dose-rates 10 - 30 rads/minute.

It is more likely that a change in RBE might follow
any change in the quality of the neutron beam at a depth
in tissue and in the penumbra.   The γ-ray contamination
of the 14 MeV beam was shown [8] to be 8% in the central
axis in air and 13% at 10 cm. deep in water (used as tissue equivalent material in their studies).   The difference
between these figures was not considered to be significant.   The proportion in the penumbra was similar.   A
significant degree of γ-ray contamination would be expected to influence cell survival data towards X-ray values, i.e. RBE values would fall and OER values would rise

Another change in the quality of the neutron beam
which might influence the radiobiological parameters,
would be the proportion of slow neutrons.   With mono-
energetic neutrons the mean energy would be expected to
fall due to scattering in the tissues at depth and a
higher LET would result.   The effect of such high LET
radiation is towards an increase in the RBE value and a
decrease in OER.   Although slow neutrons are less penetrating than fast neutrons and γ-rays, a significant
proportion in the effective beam would tend to cancel
out the effect of γ-ray contamination.   Quantitative information about the relative proportions of primary neutrons, scattered neutrons and γ-radiation, as a function

of position in a scattering medium is not available. The
most useful information about these effects is to be obtained by looking directly at the biological consequences.

The problem has been reviewed by Bewley [1] with
particular reference to the neutron beam obtained from
the Hammersmith cyclotron. With this beam, no change
was found in LET spectrum at 10 cm. deep in tissue equivalent material and McNally and Bewley [9] found no significant change in the value for OER between cells irradiated in air and those at 8.7 cm. deep in a phantom. By
contrast, Berry (reported by Brennan [3]) found a significant fall in OER levels between cells irradiated in air
and those irradiated at 10 cm. depth, both from cyclotron
neutrons and D-T neutrons.

For X-rays, the biological parameters (RBE and OER)
are constant within the radiation field, and an isodose
chart can therefore be regarded as an isobiological effect chart. It cannot be assumed that this is also true
for a neutron isodose chart. Figure 1 shows an isodose
chart for 14 MeV monoenergetic neutrons at 50 cm. S.S.D.
Ideally we should like to investigate the biological parameters at a large number of points in the field. The
present preliminary experiments have been confined to the
representative points illustrated in Figure 1. These are
the central axis and the 50% level in the penumbra in air,
and a point in the central axis at 10 cm. deep in water.

The method of neutron dosimetry has already been described [10]. Dose-rates varied between 10 and 30 rads/
min. and, as already stated, it has been confirmed that
the biological parameters are independent of these dose-
rates.

HeLa cells were grown in monolayer culture using
methods previously described [10]. Cells in the logarithmic growth phase were suspended in tris-buffered
saline plus 10% pooled human serum and irradiated [1]
for oxygenated samples, at a concentration of 3,000
cells in 1 ml. in polythene ampoules [2], and for hypoxic
samples, at a concentration of 300,000 cells in 0.05 ml.
in polypropylene disposable needle guards. After irradiation each cell sample was suitably diluted and aliquots

were plated to assay survival of their colony-forming a-
bility.

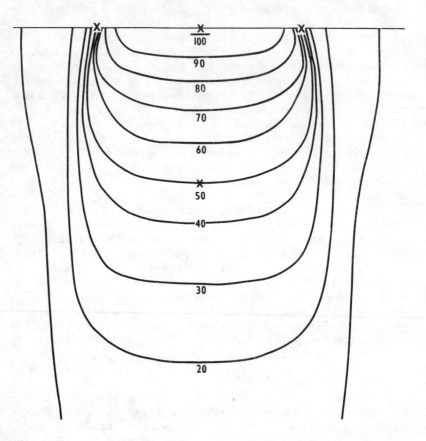

Fig. 1.   Isodose chart for 14 MeV monoenergetic neutrons at 50 cm. S.S.D.
          X marks points in the central axis at the surface and at 10 cm.
          depth, and in the penumbra at the 50% level on either side.

        This technique for comparing oxygenated and hypoxic
cells is different from the one previously used for our
neutron experiments [10] where hypoxia was achieved by
continuous gassing of cells suspended in glass test tubes
and the oxygen tension of the effluent gas was continu-

ously monitored through a Hersch cell. For the present
experiments plastic containers were necessary for dosimetry reasons, but simple gassing does not render cells
hypoxic when they are suspended in such containers. This
is because plastics, like polystyrene, contain a high
concentration of dissolved oxygen [5]. The present technique makes use of the fact that when cells are suspended
at a very high concentration (6×10^6 cells/ml. in this
case) cellular respiration rapidly reduces the oxygen
tension to a relatively low level [2]. This technique
has been used for radiobiological studies with 10 MeV
electrons from a linear accelerator at very high dose-
rates [11]. Under those conditions the OER was 3.2, a
higher figure than our previous determination using 300
kV X-rays where the OER was 2.4. The higher OER observed
with this technique is a direct demonstration that hypoxia was established.

For each experimental series, aliquots from the same
population of HeLa cells were compared under the two or
more conditions of the experiment using three dosage levels of neutrons; 150, 250 and 350 rads. These dose levels were chosen to obtain the widest range of survival
levels at the one cell dilution when plating for colony
formation. Smaller differences between survival curves
can be resolved when data points extend over a wider
range, but these preliminary studies were primarily concerned with radiobiological effects at dose levels likely
to be used in clinical neutron therapy. If these determinations did not indicate significant differences then
any differences obtainable from more extensive observations would be likely to be small.

The data are presented in Table 11 which summerises
the whole series of experiments. The figures are the
mean survival at each dose pooled from all the observations made under each experimental condition, together
with the standard error of the mean. As the study progressed more data were obtained for the initial conditions in the columns to the left of the table, but at
least two comparisons were made for the right hand columns.

TABLE 11. % Survival of HeLa Cells Irradiated at Different Positions in a Neutron Beam

Dose (rads)	Oxygenated Cells		Hypoxic Cells		Penumbra	
	in Air	10 cm. Water	in Air	10 cm. Water	Oxygenated	Hypoxic
150	35.4 ± 0.7	39.2 ± 1.2	40.6 ± 2.6.	49.9 ± 0.1	38.2 ± 3.3	43.8 ± 2.5
250	11.04 ± 0.71	13.97 ± 1.40	17.15 ± 0.55	24.35 ± 2.05	12.70 ± 0.77	19.7 ± 2.2
350	2.71 +0.40	3.58 +0.43	7.7 +0.1	9.93 +1.16	3.28 +0.71	9.35 +2.51

The second and third column shows data from the first
series of experiments. These invloved comparisons in the
central axis of the beam in air with those in the central
axis at 10 cm. depth of water. The cells irradiated at
10 cms. in water show a small increase in percentage survival of colony-forming ability. The difference is of
doubtful significance.

The next series of experiments involved a comparison of survival levels of oxygenated and hypoxic cells
irradiated under the same conditions; in air and at 10
cm. depth in water in the central axis. The fourth and
fifth columns in Table 11 show the data for the irradiation of hypoxic cells. Again, the cells irradiated at
10 cm. depth of water show a small increase in survival
compared with those irradiated at the surface.

Comparison of the data in columns two and four, and
those in columns three and five enables an estimate of
OER to be derived in air and at 10 cm. depth in water.
Estimates of OER require comparison of the D_O values of
the relevent survival curves. With only three dose
points the survival curves can not be drawn with complete
precision but, if an exponential curve is fitted by eye to
each set of points, D_O values are obtained for the data in
columns two to five as follows: – oxygenated cells irradiated in air, 80 rads; oxygenated cells irradiated at 10 cm.
depth in water, 90 rads; hypoxic cells irradiated in air,
115 rads; hypoxic cells irradiated at 10 cm. depth in
water, 130 rads. From these figures the OER for cells
irradiated in air is 1.45; the OER for cells irradiated
at 10 cm. depth in water is also 1.45.

Comparisons were then made between cells irradiated
in the central axis in air and those irradiated at the
50% level in the penumbra, also in air. Column six in
Table 11 shows the percentage survival levels for oxygenated cells irradiated in the penumbra. These values
should be compared with those in column two (oxygenated
cells irradiated in the central axis in air). They show
that there is an increase in survival when cells are irradiated at the penumbra instead of the central axis.

The seventh and last column in Table 11 shows sur-

vival levels for hypoxic cells irradiated in the penumbra.
These values can be compared with those in column six to
provide an estimate of OER for cells irradiated in the
penumbra by fitting exponential curves to the two sets
of survival data.   These curves have D_O values of 85 rads
for oxygenated cells and 123 rads for hypoxic cells indicating an OER value of 1.45.

As far as the parameter OER is concerned, these preliminary investigations have not shown any significant
difference between cells irradiated in the central axis
in air or at 10 cm. depth in water or in the penumbra in
air.   The values for OER are all smaller than the value
of 1.5 previously published [10], but the difference is
not significant.   The only valid conclusion from these
experiments is that OER did not change under the conditions examined.

As far as the parameter RBE is concerned, small
changes were observed; always towards lower values (e.g.
from 2.1 to 1.95 at the 20% survival level when comparing
the central axis in air with 10 cm. depth of water).   There
was more difference between the central axis comparisons,
in air and in water, than between the central axis and
penumbra comparisons in air; but none of these differences
was large.   It is reasonable to conclude that RBE values
certainly do not rise under the conditions of these experiments; if anything they tend to fall.

If these radiobiological observations with HeLa cells
can be applied to the clinical situation then the Neutron
Therapist can be assured that however the proportions of
primary neutrons, scattered neutrons and γ-irradiation
may vary at different positions in a 14 MeV monoenergetic
neutron beam, variations in the biological parameters are
small.   The effects that have been detected provide, if
anything, for greater clinical safety in that the RBE
value tends to fall in a scattering medium so that there
should be no unexpectedly high values.

SUMMARY

The biological parameters for HeLa cells have been
determined along the depth and at the periphery of a 14
MeV neutron beam. Preliminary results indicate a minimal
decrease in RBE values for cells irradiated at 10 cm.
depth in water in the central axis and in the penumbra
in air. No significant difference was found in the values for OER.

REFERENCES

1.   BEWLEY, D.K., *Current Topics in Radiation Research*,
     edited by M. Ebert and A. Howard (North-Holland
     Publishing Co., Amsterdam), Vol. 6, p.249, 1970.

2.   BOAG, J.W., *Current Topics in Radiation Research*,
     edited by M. Ebert and A. Howard (North-Holland
     Publishing Co., Amsterdam), Vol. 5, p.141, 1969.

3.   BRENNAN, J.T., *Radiologic Clinics of North America*,
     7, 365, 1969.

4.   BROERSE, J.J. and BARENDSEN, G.W., *Int. J. Radiat.
     Biol., 15*, 335, 1969.

5.   CHAPMAN, J.D., STURROCK, J., BOAG, J.W.and CROOKALL,
     J.O., *Int. J. Radiat. Biol., 17*, 305, 1970.

6.   FIELD, S.B., *Radiology, 93*, 915, 1969.

7.   FOX, M. and NIAS, A.H.W., *Europ. J. Cancer, 4*,
     325, 1968.

8.   GREENE, D. and THOMAS, R.L., *Brit. J. Radiol., 41*,
     455, 1968.

9.   McNALLY, N.J. and BEWLEY, D.K., *Brit. J. Radiol.,
     42*, 289, 1969.

10. NIAS, A.H.W., GREENE, D., FOX, M. and THOMAS, R.L.,
     Int. J. Radiat. Biol. 13, 449, 1967.

11. NIAS, A.H.W., SWALLOW, A.J., KEENE, J.P. and HODG-
     SON, B.W., *Int. J. Radiat. Biol. 17*, 595, 1970.,
     1970.

THE OXYGEN ENHANCEMENT RATIO FOR CALIFORNIUM-252*

R.G. FAIRCHILD, R.M. DREW, H.L. ATKINS and J.S. ROBERTSON

Medical Research Center, Brookhaven National Laboratory, Upton, L.I., N.Y., U.S.A.

Californium-252 has recently become available in forms suitable for use as implants in the therapy of tumors [2]. Such use has been suggested because ^{252}Cf emits neutrons by spontaneous fission, and because neutrons may have an advantage over gamma rays in the therapy of tumors having anoxic areas [1, 5, 8]. This expected advantage arises from the facts that anoxic cells are less sensitive than oxygenated cells to X or gamma radiation, but these cells are about equally sensitive to high LET (linear energy transfer) radiations such as neutrons. This effect is expressed as the oxygen enhancement ratio (OER), defined as the ratio of the doses required to produce equivalent effects in the absence and in the presence of oxygen. ^{252}Cf emits both gamma rays and neutrons, so its effective OER will be the resultant of the combined effects of these two kinds of radiation. OER measurements for ^{252}Cf have been made with bean roots [6], but have not been reported for mammalian cells.

In the studies reported here, tissue culture cells (Hela S3) were irradiated with an array of ^{252}Cf sources at a dose rate of about 15 rads/hr. This dose rate corresponds to that contemplated for use in clinical trials. At this dose rate the RBE for ^{252}Cf is about 2.8 relative

*Research supported by the U.S. Atomic Energy Commission.

to ^{226}Ra [3] and thus the effective dose rate corresponds
to about 40 rads/hour with radium.

Details of the tissue culture methods used have been
described elsewhere [4]. In brief, the cells were cultured in Puck's N16 medium. In the first experiments
polystyrene flasks were used, but these gave difficulty
in achieving anoxia, so later experiments were done using
glass flasks. Irradiation with ^{252}Cf was achieved using
about 70 μg of ^{252}Cf in a 36-needle array in a plane parallel to the cell plane and 1.75 cm distant. Similar
preparations were irradiated with acute X-ray exposure
which gave an OER of about 3 with the cultures in glass.
These results served to establish that adequately anoxic
conditions were achieved.

The radiation dose rates were determined both by
measurement and by calculation. The measurements were
made using a combination of silicon diode fast neutron
detectors, TLD extruded rods and ribbons and a tissue-
equivalent ionization chamber. Dose rate calculations
were made with a computer code, CALDOS [7], which com-
bines the calculations for neutron and gamma radiation
from encapsulated linear sources. In this code the inte-
gral $\int_{x_1}^{x_2} e^{-\mu\rho}/\rho^2 \, dx$, where x is measured along the source,
ρ is the slant distance to the point in question and μ is
the absorption coefficient, is evaluated by use of the
Gauss integration formula. This is equivalent to using
the Sievert integrals and shortens the computation time.
Using a factor of 2.9 rads/hour for 1 μg of ^{252}Cf in a
point source, and using absorption factors corresponding
to 0.25 mm of platinum-iridium to correct for gamma filtration in the encapsulating wall, there was close agreement between computed and measured dose rates for distances up to 5 cm.

Fig. 1 shows the survival curves obtained by irradiation with X-rays in glass and in plastic flasks.
Comparison of the oxygenated and anoxic curves in the
glass flasks shows an OER of about 3. The survival rates
in the glass flasks are lower than those in the plastic

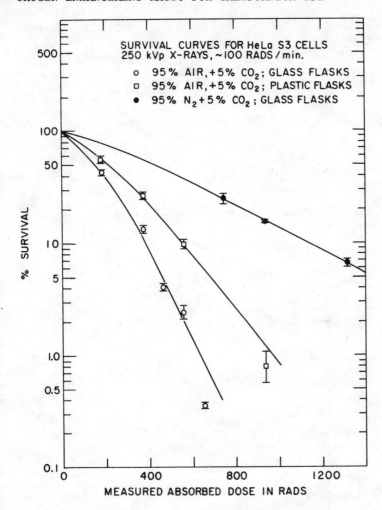

Fig. 1.   Survival curves for acute X-ray exposures.

flasks for the same measured dose because of additional backscatter of X-rays in the glass flasks.

Fig. 2 compares the oxygenated and anoxic survival curves obtained with ^{252}Cf irradiation.   The D_0 for

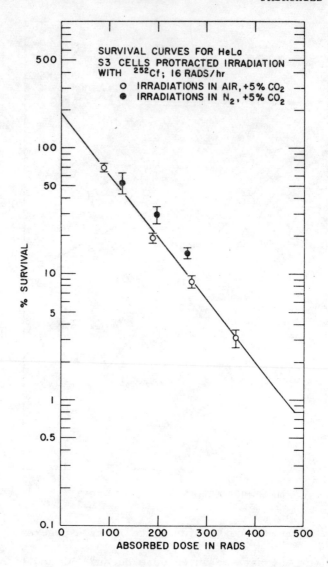

Fig. 2.   Survival curves for irradiation with ^{252}Cf.

oxygenated irradiations is 87 rads, and the OER, obtained
by comparing the doses for equal survivals, is about 1.2.

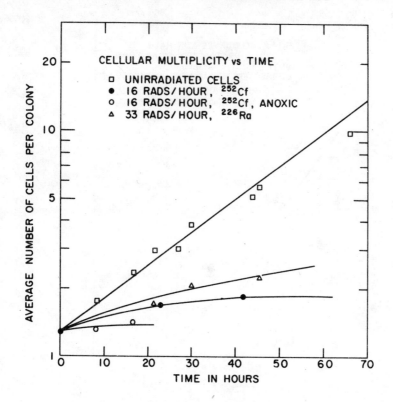

Fig. 3.   Cellular multiplicity.

The radiosensitivity of colony-forming units may change during protracted irradiation because cell replication increases the cellular multiplicity.

Fig. 3 presents the results of studies of the multiplicity for unirradiated cells, cells irradiated with ^{252}Cf under oxygenated and anoxic conditions and with ^{226}Ra. The results indicate that under the anoxic conditions cell replication is strongly inhibited.

Fig. 4 shows the results of correcting the data shows in Fig. 2 for multiplicity. The effect on the OER is very slight, changing it to about 1.3.

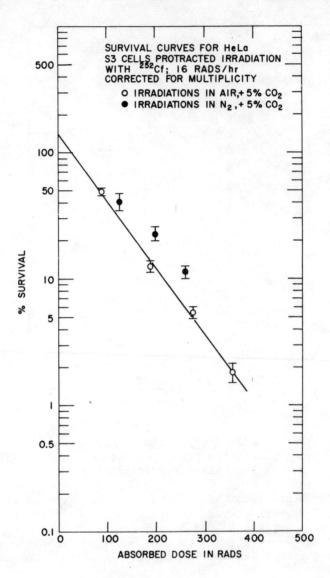

Fig. 4. Survival curve data from Fig. 2 corrected
         for cellular multiplicity.

SUMMARY

    HeLa S3 cells were irradiated in tissue cultures in glass flasks under oxygenated and anoxic conditions. The results indicate that the OER for ^{252}Cf is about 1.3 for a dose rate of 15 rads/hour.

REFERENCES

1. ATKINS, H., *Brookhaven National Laboratory Report No. BNL 12409*, February 1969.

2. BOULOGNE, A. and EVANS, A., *Int. J. Appl. Rad. and Isotopes, 20*, 453, 1969.

3. FAIRCHILD, R., DREW, R. and ATKINS, H., *Radiology, 93*, 1187, 1969.

4. FAIRCHILD, R., DREW, R. and ATKINS, H., *Radiology 96*, 171-174, 1970.

5. FOWLER, J. *et al., Brit. J. Radiol., 36*, 77, 1963.

6. HALL, E. and FAIRCHILD, R., *Brit. J. Radiol., 43*, 263, 1970.

7. ROBERTSON, J., FAIRCHILD, R. and ATKINS, H., 18th Annual Meeting Radiation Research Soc., Dallas, Texas, March 1-5, 1970.

8. SCHLEA, C. and STODDARD, D., *Nature, 206*, 1058, 1965.

CONSIDERATIONS RELATING TO FAST NEUTRON THERAPY

D.K. BEWLEY

MCR Cyclotron Unit, Hammersmith Hospital, Ducane Road, London, G.B.

The preliminary clinical trial of fast neutron therapy at Hammersmith Hospital has not yet shown any significant advantage or disadvantage of fast neutrons compared with X-rays or γ-rays. Neutrons may be advantageous in certain cases but the advantage is unlikely to be dramatic, and it is vital to ensure that it is not obscured by unfavourable physical factors or failure to exploit the biological properties of neutrons to the best advantage.

DEPTH DOSE AND SKIN SPARING

The most important physical property of a radiation used for beam therapy is its penetration in tissue. Figure 1 summarizes some data for a 5 × 5 cm field mostly at 125 cm fsd. Neutrons of mean energy 7.5 MeV and those of 14 MeV at 50 cm fsd give depth dose curves intermediate between 250 kVp X-rays and ^{60}Co γ-rays. Lower energy neutrons are less penetrating and are unsuitable despite a possibly lower Oxygen Enhancement Ratio (OER). To obtain penetration as good as that from ^{60}Co γ-rays it is necessary to use 14-15 MeV neutrons at 125 cm fsd or to use deuterons of at least 30 MeV on a beryllium target.

The build-up of dose under the skin due to onset of secondary charged-particle equilibrium is another

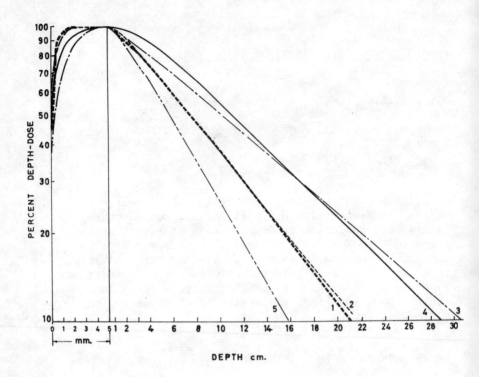

Fig. 1. Depth-dose and build-up curves for various neutron sources and ^{60}Co
γ-rays. All for 5 × 5 cm field. The first 5 mm is on an expanded
scale to show the build-up zone. 15 MeV neutrons at 125 cm fsd
give a curve similar to that for 30 MeV deuterons on a thin Be target. The curves are as follows:

(1) $\bar{E}_n$ = 8 MeV, 120 cm f.s.d. Bewley and Parnell (1969).

(2) E_n = 14 MeV, 50 cm f.s.d. Greene and Thomas (1969).

(3) ^{60}Co γ-rays at 80 cm SSD.

(4) 30 MeV d on thin Be target (0.81 mm) at 125 f.s.d.
Goodman et al. (1969).

important property of the beam. This is also shown in
Fig. 1. The skin-sparing obtained in clinical practice
with neutrons of 7.5 MeV mean energy can easily be demonstrated by covering half the field with tissue-equivalent
plastic, but skin reactions in the absence of bolus are
still severe. A similar state of affairs is likely to
hold with 14 MeV neutrons. Sacrifices of the skin-sparing
conferred by ^{60}Co γ-rays or megavoltage X-rays may not be
worth while if balanced against only a slight biological
advantage conferred by neutrons.

The curves of Fig. 1 represent in the main the
total dose of neutrons and γ-rays. As the RBE for γ-rays
with respect to neutrons is about 1/3 at the dose levels
used in therapy, the γ-component should be assessed separately. For a 14 × 14 cm field at 75 cm fsd, with
neutrons of mean energy 8 MeV, we have found [8] that the
dose due to γ-radiation represents a steadily rising
proportion of the total dose with increasing depth. Thus
a measurement with a chamber responding equally to neutrons and γ-rays will significantly overestimate the
percentage depth dose of neutrons.

USE OF A BIOLOGICAL DOSIMETER

Other factors besides γ-rays may disturb the relationship between biological effect and absorbed dose as
a function of depth. A change of neutron spectrum with
depth could result in a change in RBE. A build-up of
thermal and epithermal neutrons at a depth could produce
biological effects but remain undetected by physical
instruments. McNally and Bewley [8] checked the physical depth dose measurements using a biological dosimeter. A suspension of mouse ascites cells in perspex
tubes was bubbled slowly by air or nitrogen and then
irradiated either in air or at various depths in the
phantom. The biological results using air bubbling were
slightly higher than the values measured by a chamber
responding to neutrons alone, but agreed with the latter
when the γ-dose (divided by the RBE) was added. There
is therefore no indication of a change of RBE with depth
or of any significant effect from thermal or epithermal
neutrons.

DEFORMITY AT
23 WEEKS

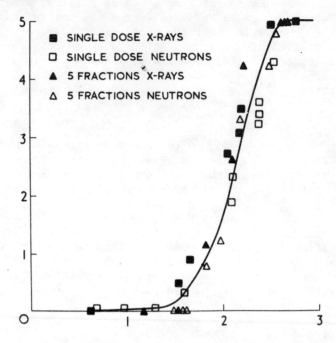

MEAN EARLY SKIN REACTION (7-30 DAYS)

Fig. 2. Deformity as a function of early skin reaction after various
treatments. S.B. Field (1969).

It has been suggested [2] that the OER may be less
at a depth in the phantom than in air. Our results
using this system are shown in Table 1 and do not confirm this finding. Our method ensured that the geometry
of irradiation was the same under aerobic and anaerobic
conditions; the differing geometries used by Berry et
al. [2] may have affected the dose actually absorbed by
the cells.

TABLE 1.

Neutron energy	Field size	In air OER (confidence limits)	Depth cm	In phantom OER (confidence limits)
8 MeV mean	14 × 14	1.80 (1.70-1.91)	8.7	1.71 (1.59-1.86)
	10 × 10	1.75 (1.55-1.98)	8.7	1.82 (1.77-1.98)
	20 × 20		8.7	1.83 (1.73-1.93)
14 MeV	10 × 10	1.64 (1.43-1.87)	9	1.76 (1.55-2.00)
	10 × 10	2.07 (1.85-2.31)		

LATE REACTIONS

A serious finding of the early trial of fast neutron
therapy was the appearance of severe late reactions [9].
To investigate this question we have kept 2 pigs for 6½
years after single and fractionated treatments by X-rays
and neutrons. All fields showed similar initial reactions but there is no indication of undesirable late
sequelae on neutron irradiated fields. All fields now
show some subcutaneous fibrosis and thickening of the
skin, and neutron and X-ray fields are indistinguishable.

Field [5] has compared early and late reactions in
the skin of rats after irradiation with X-rays and neutrons. He plotted late reaction (5-23 weeks) or deformity at 23 weeks against early reaction (7-30 days), and
found that the same curve described the results of all
forms of treatment used, namely X-rays or neutrons in
single treatments or 5 fractions in 5 days (Fig. 2).
Thus the RBE is the same for early and late reactions.
There seems to be no reason to fear specially severe
late reactions after neutron therapy provided the early
skin reactions are within the normal range accepted by
radiotherapists.

FRACTIONATION AND HYPOXIA

In any trial of fast neutron therapy the first task
is to discover how to use the new quality of radiation.
There are many differences between the response of
tissues to neutrons and γ-rays, and two of the most important are the differing effects of oxygen and differing capacities for recovery from sub-lethal damage.

The smaller protective effect of hypoxia is the
main rationale for neutron therapy. Berry et al. have
discussed this in detail [2]. In a fractionated course
of treatment the full Gain Factor of about 1.6 will not
be realized owing to changes in the number of hypoxic
cells, as discussed below. With regard to recovery from
sublethal damage, Table 2 gives some information on the

TABLE 2.

System	Author	D_2-D_1 (rad) at 24 hours	
		X-rays	Neutrons
Pig skin (early and medium term reactions)	Bewley et al. (1967) [3]	600	120
Mouse gut (LD_{50} at 4 days)	Hornsey (personal communication)	270*	40*
Mouse skin (early reaction)	Denekamp et al. (1966)	500	160
Rat skin (early reaction)	Field et al. (1968) [4]	900	180
Rat skin (late reaction)	Field et al. (1968) [4]	500	120
Clones in mouse skin	Emery (personal communication)	570	140
Clones in rat cartilage	Kember (1969)	400	100
Stunting in baby rat tails	Dixon (1968)	450	0
Tumour RIB_5	Field et al. (1968 [4]; and personal communication	400 (anoxic divided by 3)	0
Spleen nodules	Hornsey (personal communication)	100	20

*Measured at 2 hours

sparing effect of split-dose irradiation with X-rays and
neutrons. $(D_2 - D_1)_{24}$ represents the additional dose
required for a given effect when the irradiation is given
in two equal fractions separated by 24 hours. $(D_2 - D_1)$
is always less for neutrons than it is for X-rays, and
this is still true when allowance is made for RBE. In
the case of tumours containing hypoxic cells, a meaningful value of $(D_2 - D_1)$ is obtained only if the tumour is
irradiated while anoxic, owing to the likelihood of reoxygenation between treatments. The particular tumour
included in the table shows no sparing effect of fractionation with neutrons. If some human tumours behave
in the same way a large number of small fractions of
neutrons would be a good method of treatment.

Some experiments of Barendsen et al. [1] on the
treatment of a rhabdomyosarcoma in rats containing 10-
15% of hypoxic cells may also serve as a guide for
radiotherapy. He found that cells surviving a single
dose of irradiation remained approximately constant in
number for a week and then multiplied at a much greater
rate than before treatment, repopulating the tumour to
its original size after a further two weeks. If this
is also true in some human tumours, a short total treatment time, of one or two weeks, would be called for.
This however would not be effective with X-rays because
of the hypoxic component, but could be useful with neutrons since hypoxia is less important. This idea is
supported by the results of Field, Jones and Thomlinson
[4] who found, using neutrons, that two fractions in two
days was a better way of treating the rat tumour than
5 fractions in 5 days, whereas with X-rays the two regimes of treatment gave the same result.

The important point here is that neutrons are so
different from X-rays that the best way of using them
is of likely to be different. Before a decision can
be reached as to whether neutrons can give any therapeutic advantage compared to X-rays, much more information is needed on the best way of using neutrons.

CONCLUSION

Neutron beams of up to 14 MeV have inferior physical characteristics when compared with ^{60}Co γ-rays or mega-voltage X-rays, both with respect to penetration and build-up under the skin. Use of treatment regimes customary with X-ray and γ-rays may not represent the best way of using neutrons. To determine the value of fast neutron therapy it is necessary to use a beam of good physical characteristics and to find the regimes of treatment best suited to neutrons.

REFERENCES

1. BARENDSEN, G.W. and BROERSE, J.J., *Europ. J. Cancer*, *5*, 373, 1969.

2. BERRY et al., this book.

3. BEWLEY, D.K. and PARNELL, C.J., *Brit. J. Radiol.*, *42*, 281, 1969.

4. FIELD, S.B., JONES, T. and THOMLINSON, R.H., *Brit. J. Radiol.*, *41*, 597, 1968.

5. FIELD, S.B., *Radiology*, *92*, 381, 1969.

6. GOODMAN, L.J., MARINO, S.A., BRENNAN, J.T. and WILSON, M.J., *Minimum cyclotron size for radiation therapy*, Symposium on cyclotrons, Oxford, 1969.

7. GREENE, D. and THOMAS, R.L., *Brit. J. Radiol.*, *41*, 455, 1968.

8. McNALLY, N.J. and BEWLEY, D.K., *Brit. J. Radiol.*, *42*, 289, 1969.

9. STONE, R.S., *Am. J. Ront.*, *59*, 771, 1947.

EFFECTS OF 15 MeV NEUTRONS ON TUMOURS AND NORMAL TISSUES IN EXPERIMENTAL ANIMALS

J.J. BROERSE, G.W. BARENDSEN and L.M. van PUTTEN

Radiobiological Institute TNO, 151 Lange Kleiweg, Rijswijk Z.H., The Netherlands

INTRODUCTION

Studies of the effects of different types of ioniz-ing radiation on cell culture systems have greatly in-creased the insight in cellular aspects of the radio-therapy of neoplasms. In particular the investigation of the differences between dose-effect relations, with re-spect to impairment of the reproductive capacity of mam-malian cells, for low-LET and high-LET radiation have induced a renewed interest in the use of fast neutrons for radiotherapy. It has been shown that the influence of dose-modifying factors, notably oxygen, is much smaller for high-LET radiation, e.g. fast neutrons, than for low-LET radiation, e.g. X-rays [1]. On the basis of these experiments it was concluded that fast neutron beams might provide a significant advantage for the treatment of tumours containing fractions of anoxic cells.

In view of this possible application it is important to evaluate the responses of various types of normal tis-sue in comparison with responses of experimental tumours after fast neutron- and X-irradiation. In the present paper, the RBE values of 15 MeV neutrons for effects on normal rodent tissues, notably mouse bone marrow, mouse intestine and rat skin, will be compared with the effec-tiveness of these neutrons for responses of a rat rhabdomyosarcoma and a mouse osteosarcoma. For both

types of tumours it has been shown that a fraction between 10 and 20% of the cells is severely hypoxic.

MATERIALS AND METHODS

a.   *Irradiation*

Mono-energetic neutrons of 15 MeV energy were produced through the D-T reaction using a Van de Graaff accelerator (400 kV, 250 μA of deuterons). Details about
the neutron dosimetry with sulphur activation detectors
and tissue equivalent ionization chambers are given elsewhere [5]. The X-irradiations were carried out with a
General Electric Maxitron generator (250 kVp, 30 mA,
HVL 2.1 mm Cu) and a Philips-Müller X-ray generator (300
kV, 10 mA, HVL 2.5 mm Cu).

b.   *Mouse bone marrow and mouse intestine*

Bone marrow death has been taken as the final end-
point resulting from radiation effects in the haemopoietic
cells. $LD_{50/30d}$ values have been determined for neutron-
and X-irradiations of (CBA/Rij × C57BL/Rij)F_1 hybrid mice.

Proliferation of the haemopoietic stem cells in
these hybrid mice was investigated with the spleen colony
technique for single and fractionated exposures [9].
Technical details of the stem cell assay will be published in the near future [7]. The donor cells were irradiated either *in vitro* or *in vivo*.

In the same animal strain the $LD_{50/5d}$ values for the
intestinal syndrome have been determined. The survival
of intestinal crypt cells has been investigated with the
microcolony method of Withers and Elkind [12].

c.   *Rat skin*

A transplantation technique was employed to study
radiation-induced damage to the skin of rats [6]. Circu-
lar pieces of skin were cut from the backs of white
WAG/Rij rats after irradiation with 300 kV X-rays or

15 MeV neutrons. These pieces of skin were transplanted onto the backs of brown (WAG/Rij × BN/Bi)F₁ hybrid rats. The remaining area of grafted skin was measured three months after transplantation and the ratio of treated and untreated areas has been used as a parameter for skin damage.

d.   Rat rhabdomyosarcoma

The origin and growth characteristics of the rhabdomyosarcoma transplantable in the inbred strain of WAG/Rij rats have been described elsewhere [2, 3]. This tumour obtained by a special selection procedure, consists of cells which after excision of the tumour and application of a cell dispersion technique, can be cultured directly *in vitro*. The plating technique provides the possibility to assay changes in the fractions of clonogenic cells in tumours during and after fractionated treatments.

e.   Mouse osteosarcoma

The experiments with a transplantable osteosarcoma were carried out with (CBA/Rij × C57BL/Rij)F₁ hybrid mice. Tumour cell survival was estimated by an end-point dilution assay after suspending the tumour cells by a dispersion technique. It has been shown that this tumour has a lower capacity for reoxygenation of its anoxic cells than generally observed in subcutaneous sarcomas [10].

RESULTS

a.   Mouse bone marrow and mouse intestine

Death due to the haemopoietic syndrome occurred mainly between 8 and 14 days after exposure, whereas a mean survival time of 4.5 days was found for the intestinal syndrome. The 5-day mortality and 30-day mortality were investigated for different radiations and exposure periods [4]. In Fig. 1 the dose-mortality curves are given for 15 MeV neutron irradiation with an exposure time of 2 hours. RBE values of 1.12 and 1.42 with

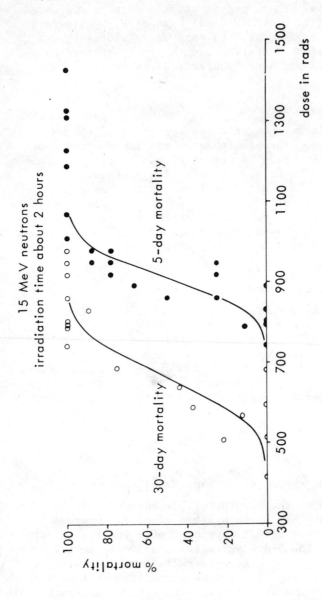

Fig. 1. Dose-mortality curves for the haemopoietic and the intestinal
syndrome in mice for 2-hour exposures to 15 MeV neutrons.
From Broerse [4].

respect to X-irradiation under comparable exposure conditions, were obtained for haemopoietic death and intestinal death, respectively.

From a comparison of the LD_{50} values for 2-hour and
8-hour exposures it may be concluded that protraction
produces comparable effects for neutron- and gamma-
irradiations as far as the haemopoietic syndrome is concerned. The intestinal cells show a higher degree of
recovery of damage after gamma-irradiations than after
15 MeV neutron irradiations. Nevertheless recovery from
sub-lethal damage produced by 15 MeV neutrons occurs to
a significant extent [4].

The results for the effects on the intact animal
have been compared with the effects at the cellular
level. Survival data of the haemopoietic stem cells have
been obtained after neutron- and X-irradiations. The two
survival curves of the colony forming units (CFU) after
in vitro irradiation of the bone marrow cell suspensions
have a similar slope. The difference in effectiveness is
mainly associated with the lower extrapolation number for
the neutron curve. For the neutron- and X-irradiations
D_0 values of 66 and 62 rads and extrapolation numbers of
1.3 and 4.0 were found respectively. For 0.1% survival
an RBE of 1.10 has been obtained.

The survival curves for the *in vivo* irradiations
have slopes which also differ only slightly and again the
extrapolation numbers differ significantly. D_0 values of
78 rads and 73 rads and extrapolation numbers of 1.2 and
2.5 were found for neutron- and X-irradiations respectively. For 0.1% survival the RBE is equal to 1.03.

For a valid comparison of the effects of neutron-
and X-irradiation on the intact animal and the effects on
the haemopoietic stem cells comparable survival levels
should be considered. Doses in the $LD_{50/30d}$ range correspond to surviving fractions between 10^{-3} and 10^{-4}. It
should be emphasized that the RBE values for CFU survival
levels are based on extrapolation estimates which gave a
low accuracy. Taking this into account, it can be con-

cluded that the RBE for the $LD_{50}/30d$ is in good agreement
with the RBE values for the CFU survival at a surviving
fraction of 0.1%.

With regard to the effects on the gastro-intestinal
tract in the mouse, only preliminary results are available at present on the survival of jejunal crypt cells
after 15 MeV neutron- and X-irradiation. Measurements of
the number of microcolonies in transverse sections of irradiated mouse jejunum indicate an RBE value between 1.4
and 1.5 [6]. This value is also in good agreement with
the RBE for 5-day mortality.

b.   Rat skin

During the first 14 days after transplantation of
the skin graft, little difference between irradiated and
non-irradiated skin is observed macroscopically and
microscopically with respect to the healing of the graft.
After about 14 days however, the irradiated skin grafts
start to decrease in area. The ratio of the remaining
areas of the irradiated skin graft relative to the area
of unirradiated grafts approaches a constant value after
about 8 weeks. This ratio depends on the dose and can be
used as a measure of the skin damage produced by the irradiation. Dose effect curves can be made for the area
of remaining skin as a function of the dose of 15 MeV
neutrons and 300 kV X-rays [6]. Both curves show a considerable shoulder and consequently at low doses of up to
600 rads an RBE value cannot be estimated. At single
doses in excess of about 1200 rads of 15 MeV neutrons and
in excess of 1600 rads of 300 kV X-rays, very small areas
of grafted skin remain, which cannot be measured accurately. An estimate of the RBE of 15 MeV neutrons can
only be made with sufficient accuracy for the dose region
where the relative area of remaining skin is equal to a
factor of 0.6 to 0.2. For this region the RBE of 15 MeV
neutrons after single irradiations can be calculated to
be equal to 1.45 ± 0.2. For two daily fractions an RBE
of 1.65 ± 0.2 has been obtained, whereas for five daily
fractions an RBE in excess of 2.0 can be estimated.

c.   *Rat rhabdomyosarcoma*

Various responses of the rhabdomyosarcoma have been
investigated including variations of the fractions of
cells capable of unlimited proliferation, tumour volume
changes and proportions of tumours cured after single and
fractionated doses of 300 kV X-rays and 15 MeV neutrons
[2, 3]. In the present paper only the survival curves
obtained by the cloning technique will be discussed. In
Fig. 2 survival curves are presented for cells from tumours irradiated in the flanks of rats, which were either
alive during irradiation or had been killed ten minutes
prior to irradiation. This latter condition produces
severe hypoxia of the cells. After preparation of a cell
suspension the cells were plated. Clones were scored
after 12 days of incubation and the fraction of surviving
cells was calculated from the mean number of clones per
dish, relative to the numbers of cells plated.

Curve 6 of Fig. 2 has been obtained with 300 kV X-
rays for cells from tumours irradiated in dead animals.
The shape of the curve is not significantly different
from the curve for cultured cells, irradiated in equilibrium with nitrogen. It can be concluded that rhabdomyosarcoma cells grown in culture and in the tumour respectively, exhibit closely similar sensitivities to X-rays if
they are irradiated in severely hypoxic conditions.
Curve 5 of Fig. 2 for cells irradiated in tumours in
living animals has a shape which is characteristic for a
population of cells consisting of a large fraction of
oxygenated cells and a smaller fraction of hypoxic cells.
The dotted curve 4, included for comparison, represents
the survival of cultured rhabdomyosarcoma cells irradiated in equilibrium with air. Curve 3, obtained with 15
MeV neutrons for cells from tumours irradiated in dead
rats, has a shape which does not differ from the corresponding curve for cultured cells equilibrated with nitrogen. Curve 2 has been obtained with 15 MeV neutrons
for cells from tumours irradiated in the living animals.
The survival curve for cells irradiated in equilibrium
with air (curve 1), has been included for comparison.
Relatively large RBE values are obtained for single doses
of 15 MeV neutrons compared to 300 kV X-rays with respect

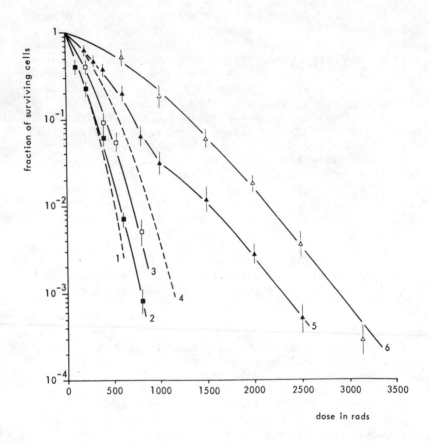

Fig. 2.   Survival curves obtained by the clone technique for cells from a
          rhabdomyosarcoma in the rat, irradiated in different conditions.
          Curves 2 and 3 were obtained for tumours irradiated with 15 MeV
          neutrons in living anaesthetized and dead rats, respectively.
          Curves 5 and 6 were obtained for tumours irradiated with 300 kV
          X-rays in living anaesthetized and dead rats, respectively.
          Curves 1 and 4, included for comparison, represent the survival
          curves for cultured tumour cells, in equilibrium with air, ir-
          radiated with 15 MeV neutrons and 300 kV X-rays, respectively.
          From Barendsen and Broerse [2].

to survival of cells in the tumour. For a surviving
level of 0.001 an RBE of 2.9 can be calculated. The
large RBE values at low doses are due to the reduced
shoulder of the survival curve obtained with 15 MeV neutrons as compared with X-rays, while at large doses these
large RBE values are caused by the presence of anoxic
cells and the fact that the OER values of 15 MeV neutrons
and 300 kV X-rays differ by a factor of about 1.6.

A complete report of the experimental results can be
found elsewhere [2, 3]. The studies of the response of
the tumour for different end-points have shown that the
phenomena occurring in the tumour after irradiation are
more complicated than have been demonstrated thus far,
especially with respect to a rapid repopulation of the
tumours by cells which have retained the capacity for unlimited proliferation. From the studies on the effects
of fractionated treatments it can be concluded that repair of sub-lethal damage, the presence of anoxic cells,
their changing oxygenation status during treatment and
proliferation of cells during the interval between subsequent irradiations, all influence the final result of
the treatment. The experimental results indicate that
reoxygenation of previously anoxic cells occurs to a
considerable extent in the rhabdomyosarcoma. For fractionated irradiations RBE values of about 3.0 are found,
as indicated in the table. These values are not significantly different from the value of 2.9 obtained for
single doses at the 0.001 level. For single doses the
relatively large value of 2.9 was due to the presence of
anoxic cells. In the fractionated treatments reoxygenation between fractions diminishes the importance of
hypoxia and consequently the RBE of 2.9 to 3.0 obtained
is due to differences in the repair of sub-lethal damage.

d. Mouse osteosarcoma

From studies of the effects of single and fractionated irradiations with X-rays, it had been concluded that
little or no reoxygenation of previously anoxic cells has
taken place in the tumour after the preferential elimination of oxygenated cells [10]. In view of the low rate
of reoxygenation the osteosarcoma can be classified as a

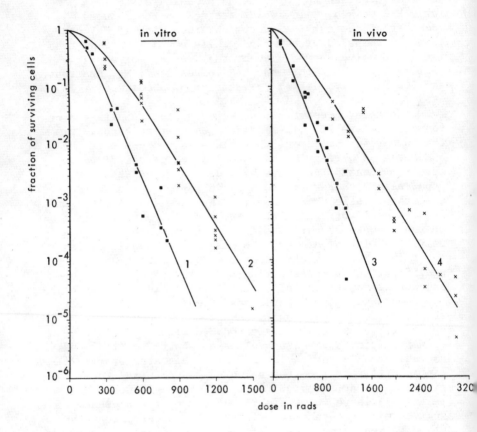

Fig. 3. Dose survival curves of cells from an osteosarcoma in the mouse for *in vitro* irradiations of the tumour cells with 15 MeV neutrons (curve 1) and 300 kV X-rays (curve 2) and *in situ* irradiations of the tumours with 15 MeV neutrons (curve 3) and 300 kV X-rays (curve 4).

poorly reoxygenating tumour. In Fig. 3 survival curves
are presented for *in vitro* and *in vivo* irradiations of
the osteosarcoma with single doses of 15 MeV neutrons and
300 kV X-rays.

At a surviving level of 0.001, RBE values of 1.6 and
1.8 can be calculated for *in vitro* and *in vivo* irradiations respectively. The results after fractionated
treatment which will be reported elsewhere [11] indicate
an RBE of 2.5 for the same level of survival. Contrary
to the phenomena found with the rat rhabdomyosarcoma, a
clear difference is obtained between the RBE values for
single and fractionated *in vivo* irradiations of the osteosarcoma. Studies of the survival of osteosarcoma
cells after *in vitro* irradiation in oxygenated and
hypoxic conditions have yielded a low factor of 1.2 for
the ratio of the OER values of 300 kV X-rays and 15 MeV
neutrons [11]. The relatively small difference between
the RBE values found after *in vitro* and *in vivo* irradiations for single treatments can be related to the low
gain factor of 1.2. The relatively high RBE value for
the fractionated treatments as compared with the value
for the single treatment might be explained by the absence of recovery from sub-lethal damage after fast neutron irradiation which is for this tumour not compensated
by an efficient reoxygenation process which increases for
most tumours the sensitivity for fractionated X-irradiation as compared with single doses.

DISCUSSION

The experimental results presented in this paper
have clearly demonstrated that a number of factors must
be considered in investigations of differences between
the effects of X-rays and fast neutrons. Because of the
differences between the shapes of the survival curves of
cells irradiated with fast neutrons and X-rays, the RBE
of fast neutrons increases with decreasing dose fractions.
Cells which after a given dose of radiation have retained
the capacity for unlimited proliferation sustain sub-
lethal damage which renders them more susceptible to subsequent irradiation than unirradiated cells. With fast

neutrons this effect is reduced relative to X-rays and
consequently the RBE depends on the size and number of
fractions and on the time intervals employed. The tumours described in this paper contain a proportion of
hypoxic cells, rendering them more resistant to X-rays
and gamma-rays as compared to well-oxygenated cells.
This dependence of radiosensitivity on the oxygen concentration is smaller for fast neutrons than for X-rays.
The situation may even be more complicated since it has
been shown that in a number of experimental tumours the
oxygenation status of cells may change during a course of
fractionated irradiation. Consequently, the effectiveness of fast neutrons for responses of tumours depends on
the fraction of anoxic cells, the rate of reoxygenation,
as well as on the dose of radiation employed. In general
it can be concluded that the RBE values for the effects
on tumours and normal tissues are determined by a combination of the factors mentioned earlier.

     For an assessment of the possible use of fast neu-
trons in radiotherapy the effects of 15 MeV neutrons on
experimental tumours have to be compared with the effects
on normal tissues. In the table a summary is given of
the RBE values for tumours and various types of normal
tissues. As far as the haemopoietic tissue in the mouse
is concerned it has been found that the RBE does not differ greatly from one for both single and fractionated
irradiations. For the other normal tissues, however,
higher RBE values have been found, which is in agreement
with the general observation of the different responses
of two distinct groups of tissues [8]. For these types
of normal tissues e.g. gastro-intestinal tract and skin,
very limited data are available. It has to be concluded
that more data have to be obtained for the effects of
normal tissues after fractionated irradiations with 15
MeV neutrons and X-rays. At present no definitive evaluation can be given with respect to a possible therapeutic
advantage of 15 MeV neutrons.

RBE-VALUES OF 15 MeV NEUTRONS RELATIVE TO 300 kV X-RAYS FOR
SINGLE AND FRACTIONATED IRRADIATIONS OF ANIMAL TUMOURS
AND NORMAL TISSUES

Biological system	Irradiation conditions	RBE
Haemopoietic tissue in the mouse (spleen colony assay*)	in vitro, single irr.	1.10
	in vivo, single irr.	1.03
	in vivo, 5 daily fractions	0.97
(haemopoietic syndrome)	single irr.	1.12
Gastro-intestinal tract in the mouse (G.I. syndrome)	single irr.	1.4
Skin of the rat	single irr.	1.45
	2 daily fractions	1.65
	5 daily fractions	>2.0
Rhabdomyosarcoma in the rat (cloning technique*)	in vitro, single irr.	1.6
	in vivo, single irr.	2.9
	in vivo, 10 daily fractions	3.0
	in vivo, 15 daily fractions	2.9
Osteosarcoma in the mouse (end-point dilution assay*)	in vitro, single irr.	1.6
	in vivo, single irr.	1.8
	in vivo, 5 daily fractions	2.5

*RBE-values for cell survival are calculated at surviving fractions of 0.001

In view of the possible application of fast neutrons in radiotherapy, it is important to assess the responses of various types of normal tissues and of experimental tumours after irradiations with X-rays and fast neutrons. In the present paper RBE studies of 15 MeV neutrons are reported for effects on normal rodent tissues, namely mouse bone marrow, mouse intestine and rat skin and for effects on a rat rhabdomyosarcoma and a mouse osteosarcoma. Due to the lack of data on the effects of normal tissues after fractionated irradiation, no definitive evaluation can be given at present with respect to a possible therapeutic advantage of 15 MeV neutrons.

REFERENCES

1. BARENDSEN, G.W. and BROERSE, J.J., *Nature*, *212*, 722, 1966.

2. BARENDSEN, G.W. and BROERSE, J.J., *Eur. J. Cancer*, *5*, 373, 1969.

3. BARENDSEN, G.W. and BROERSE, J.J., *Eur. J. Cancer*, *6*, 89, 1970.

4. BROERSE, J.J., *Int. J. Radiat. Biol.*, *15*, 115, 1969.

5. BROERSE, J.J. and AMMERS, H. VAN, *Int. J. Radiat. Biol.*, *10*, 417, 1966.

6. BROERSE, J.J., BARENDSEN, G.W., FRERIKS, G. and PUTTEN, L.M. VAN, *Eur. J. Cancer*, to be published.

7. BROERSE, J.J., ENGELS, A.C., LELIEVELD, P., PUTTEN, L.M. VAN, DUNCAN, W., GREENE, D., MASSEY, J.B., GILBERT, C.W., HENDRY, J.H. and HOWARD, A., *Int. J. Radiat. Biol.*, *19*, 101, 1971.

8. FIELD, S.B., *Radiology*, *93*, 915, 1969.

9. TILL, J.E. and McCULLOCH, E.A., *Radiat. Res.*, *14*, 213, 1961.

10. PUTTEN, L.M. VAN, *Eur. J. Cancer*, *4*, 173, 1968.

11. PUTTEN, L.M. VAN, LELIEVELD, P. and BROERSE, J.J., *Eur. J. Cancer*, *7*, 171, 1971.

12. WITHERS, H.R. and ELKIND, M.M., *Int. J. Radiat. Biol.*, *17*, 261, 1970.

ACUTE EFFECTS OF 1-MeV FAST NEUTRONS ON THE HAEMATO-POIETIC TISSUES, INTESTINAL EPITHELIUM AND GASTRIC EPITHELIUM IN MICE

J.A.G. DAVIDS

Reactor Centrum Nederland, Petten (N-H), The Netherlands

There is a rapid accumulation of experimental evidence which confirms that most of the complex radiation effects developing in mammals after whole-body exposure may be traced back to damage in the stem-cell populations of particular tissues. With two of these populations the dose-effect relationship for stem-cell damage has been studied quantitatively by direct means, the haematopoietic stem cells [10] and more recently the intestinal crypt stem cells [11].

A comparison of these results demonstrates that with the low-LET X-rays and γ-rays the crypt stem-cell population in mice is less radiosensitive than the haematopoietic stem cell population.

It is of interest to consider if a similar difference in radiosensitivity exists between stem cells when exposed to high-LET radiation. Therefore a comparative study of stem-cell damage was carried out with mice exposed to high-LET fast neutrons with a mean energy of 1 MeV. All results were collected with animals of the same inbred strain which were exposed to the same neutron spectrum. In order to compare the RBE values for stem-cell damage the effects of X-rays were studied at the same time.

CHARACTERISTICS OF FAST-NEUTRON EXPOSURE

The animals were exposed to fast neutrons from a
[235]U-converter in the Low Flux Reactor at Petten. The
design of the exposure facility, the tissue dosimetry and
neutron spectrometry have been described previously [6].
The mice were irradiated bilaterally at a fast-neutron
dose-rate equal to 10 rads/min in the centre-line of the
animals. The bilateral exposure reduces the maximum variation of the neutron dose in soft tissue over the animal to 15%. The absorbed dose due to γ-rays is 9% of the
total centre-line dose but its contribution to the biological effect will be less than 3.5% and consequently it
has been neglected

The measured fast-neutron spectrum has a mean energy of 1.0 MeV. It deposits more than 90% of the dose
in standard soft tissue by the production of densely-i-
ionizing recoil protons having a mean track-average LET_∞
of 57 keV per μm in water, which is near the maximum value (74 keV/ μm) obtainable with fast neutrons.

RESPONSE OF MICE TO WHOLE-BODY FAST-NEUTRON IRRADIATION

Male mice of the inbred CBA strain were chosen as
experimental animals because their response to fast neutrons and X-rays are qualitatively similar, i.e. in the
30-day lethal dose range the 8-15 day bone-marrow lethality prevails, wheras the 4-5 day intestinal death is
limited to higher doses. The LD50/30d and LD50/5d values
calculated from the combined data of several experiments
are equal to 351 ± 2 rads and 452 ± 4 rads respectively.
The identity of the bone marrow syndrome was proved by
the therapeutic effect of syngeneic bone-marrow transplantation. This treatment increases the LD50/30d to
395 ± 2 rads [5]. A further increase of the LD50/30d
up to 451 ± 3 rads is effected by combining bone-marrow
transplantation with a daily antibiotic treatment.

A comparison with the effects of 250-kVp X-rays

at a dose rate of 30 rads/min has shown that the neutron RBE factor for 5-day intestinal death is equal to 3.06 ± 0.05 (S.E.) whereas for the 30-day bone-marrow death it is equal to 1.89 ± 0.02 [4]. A more recent comparison with 300 kV X-rays (30 rads/min) gave the same value for the intestinal syndrome. The RBE value for the bone marrow syndrome however are slightly higher (between 2.0 and 2.1).

RESPONSE OF HAEMATOPOIETIC STEM CELLS TO FAST NEUTRONS AND X-RAYS.

Survival curves of haematopoietic stem cells in bone marrow and spleen were determined by irradiating the cells in the donors (*in vivo*) with either fast neutrons or 250-kVp X-rays and subsequent testing of bone-marrow and spleen cell suspensions for their capacity to protect lethally X-irradiated recipient mice of the same inbred strain [3]. The fraction of undamaged stem cells is inversely proportional to the number of viable cells' which has to be injected in the recipients in order to give a 50% chance to survive for 30 days: the 50% effective cell dose or ED50. The method which has been developed by McCulloch and Till [9] provides a good measure of the total proliferative potential of the surviving fraction of haematopoietic stem cells.

Figure 1 shows the dose-effect curves for both types of radiation. With fast neutrons the surviving fraction of bone-marrow stem cells decreases exponentially with dose over the whole range with a D_0 equal to 45 rads. The exponential relationship allows a reliable extrapolation to be made down to the LD50/30d of the bone-marrow syndrome. The surviving fraction at this point is equal to 0.0004. The X-ray curve has a shoulder which extends down to a surviving fraction of about 0.1. The extrapolation downwards was made by assuming an exponential decrease below this level. The RBE for a surviving fraction of 0.0004 is 2.1. This is close to the RBE factor measured for bone-marrow death and therefore it seems justified to conclude that the RBE factors for the beginning and terminal phase of the bone-marrow syndrome are equal.

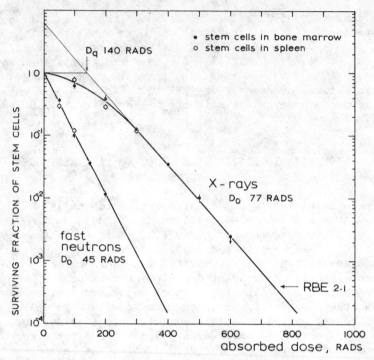

Fig. 1. Survival curves for haematopoietic stem cells irradiated *in vivo*
with either 1-MeV fast neutrons or 250 kVp X-rays.

The ED50 of spleen cells is about 60 times higher
than the ED50 of bone-marrow cells. Hence surviving
fractions could only be determined down to 0.1. The
available data reveal no difference between the dose-
effect curves for stem cells irradiated in bone marrow and spleen. This result demonstrates that with
fast neutrons of rather low mean energy the mean absorbed
dose in the bone marrow is not significantly modified by
perturbations at the bone-soft tissue interphase.

RESPONSE OF INTESTINAL-CRYPT STEM CELLS TO FAST NEUTRONS
AND X-RAYS

The second stem-cell compartment which was studied,

is located in the crypts of the small intestine. Recently Withers and Elkind [12] have described a method for studying quantitatively the damage to the stem-cell population in the intestinal crypts by counting the regenerating crypts in transverse histological sections of the small intestine.

The method is based on the assumption that one surviving cell within a crypt is sufficient for its regeneeration. Its use is limited to rather high doses which sterilize a certain fraction of crypts completely and in contrast to the method used for the haematopoietic stem cells it provides information about the lower part of the cell survival curve.

In our measurements we have used a slightly different technique by counting the regenerating crypts per cm in 5 μ-thick longitudinal sections of the jejunum. Groups of animals were irradiated with graded doses of fast neutrons and 300-kV X-rays. At 96 hours after irradiation the intestinal tract was removed, fixed in neutral formaline and processed·by standardized routine histological methods. Counts were made in longitudinal sections which were perpendicular to the surface.

The results are presented in Figure 2. The open symbols refer to the number of crypts per cm. The points are based on data for 3 animals with the exception of the highest X-ray dose point which is based on 2 animals. The indicated standard error refers to the total number of crypts counted. The variation between counts for separate animals of the same dose group is less than 2. In sections of unirradiated jejunum the number of crypts per cm is equal to 189 ± 6 (S.E.).

The closed symbols refer to the number of surviving stem cells per cm. It is calculated by assuming a Poisson distribution of the surviving cells over the irradiated crypts. Through these points the lower parts of the two survival curves were drawn by eye. At the

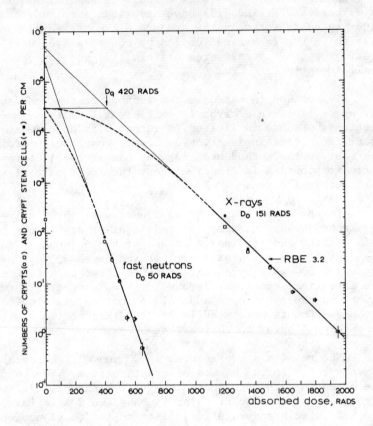

Fig. 2. Survival curves for intestinal stem
          cells irradiated *in vivo* with either
          1-MeV fast neutrons or 300 kV X-rays.

LD50/5d for neutrons only one stem cell survives per 7 irradiated crypts. The RBE for this level of damage to the stem-cell population is equal to 3.2. The results demonstrate that also for the intestinal syndrome the RBE values for the initial stem-cell damage and the terminal phase are equal.

The lower exponential parts of the neutron and X-rays curves have D_O values equal to 50 rads and 151 rads respectively. The upper parts have been extrapolated to zero dose with the assumption that a crypt contains, on average, 160 stem cells, a figure determined by Hagemann, Sigdestad and Lesher [7]. The resulting curve for X-rays has a pronounced shoulder and a quasi-threshold dose D_q equal to 420 rads which is similar to values determined with split-dose techniques by Hornsey and Vatistas [8] and Withers and Elkind [11]. The fast-neutron curve has a small shoulder and a D_q of 106 rads. A similar curvature was found for the dose-effect curve of cultured human cells exposed in the same neutron facility and studied by Broerse et al. [2].

COMPARISON OF RADIOSENSITIVITIES OF INTESTINAL AND HAEMATOPOIETIC STEM-CELL POPULATIONS.

In Figure 3 the survival curves for both groups of stem cells have been plotted on the same scale. It may be concluded that for both radiation qualities the radiosensitivity of the haematopoietic stem-cell population is significantly larger. The difference is most pronounced for the low LET-radiation where the D_O values differ by a factor of about 2 and the D_q values by a factor of 3. With the high-LET fast neutrons the D_O values are about equal and here the difference is mainly due to the presence of a small D_q equal to 106 rads. However owing to the steepness of the lines this relatively small difference causes the surviving fractions to differ by a factor of 20 in the lethal dose range. This large difference puts the LD50/30d below the LD50/5d in spite of the fact that the critical surviving fraction connected with 50%-survival is 4×10^{-3} with the intestinal stem cells. (Figure 3). It may be further concluded from the data collected in Figure 3 that the dif-

ference in neutron RBE values for the two radiation syndromes is reducible to an equal RBE difference for the
initial stem cell damage.

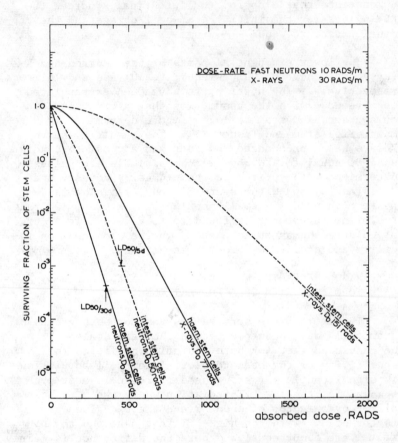

Fig. 3.   Survival curves for haematopoietic stem cells and intestinal-crypt
          stem cells after *in vivo* exposure to 1-MeV fast neutrons and X-Rays.

RESPONSE OF GASTRIC EPITHELUM

The difference in response of the blood-forming
tissues and the epithelium of the small intestine raises the question how other proliferating tissues in the

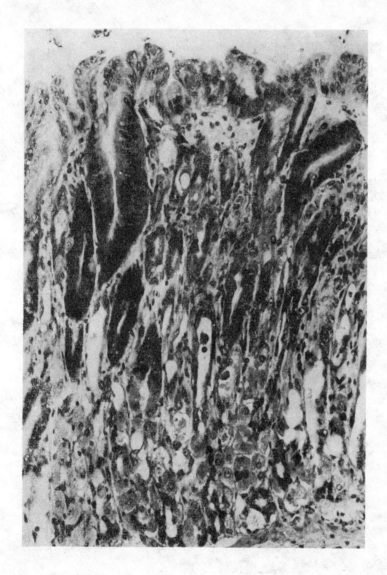

Fig. 4A.   Gastric mucosa with fundic glands of ♂ CBA
           mouse, sacrificed 12 days after exposure to
           fast neutrons (420 rads) (× 250).

574

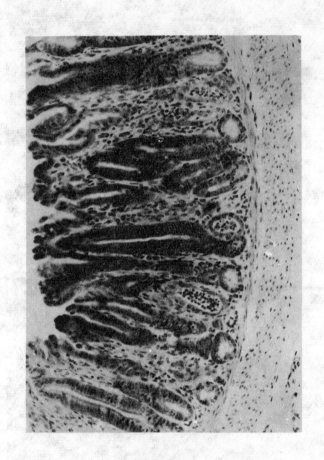

Fig. 4B. Gastric mucose with fundic glands of ♂ CBA mouse, sacrificed 16 days after exposure to fast neutrons (380 rads) (× 250).

body compare in this respect. With the CBA mice some
data have been collected regarding the response of the
epithelium which covers the glandular stomach. this tissue which lines the gastric pits and the gastric glands
is generally regarded as rather radioresistant because
it shows little damage after X-ray exposure in the lethal range [1]. However after fast-neutron exposure
in the lethal range severe damage develops in the glan-
ular stomach at the end of the second week involving extensive cellular necrosis in the gastric glands. At the
same time and more or less vigorously, depending on the
neutron dose, a new epithelial lining grows out of the
isthmus of the glands. First a new epithelial lining
of the gastric pits and surface is formed and subsequently'the proliferation is directed downwards to the bottom
of the glands (Figure 4). The proliferation starts first
in the pyloric region at about the 8th day. Similar processes were observed in X-irradiated and bone-marrow
treated animals but at X-ray doses which were about 3
times as high. Therefore the RBE for gastric damage appears to be similar to the RBE for intestinal damage.

SUMMARY

Survival curves of haematopoietic stem cells and intestinal stem cells of mice exposed to either high-LET fast
neutrons or X-rays were compared. With both types of
radiation the haematopoietic stem-cell population is the
most radiosensitive. The difference in RBE factors for
bone-marrow and intestinal lethality is reducible to an
equal RBE difference for the initial stem cell damage in
the two tissues. The RBE factors for damage to the gastric and intestinal epithelia appear to be similar.

REFERENCES

1. BRECHER, G., CRONKITE, E.P., CONARD, R.A. and
    SMITH, W.W., *Am. J. Pathol.*, *34*, 105, 1958.

2. BROERSE, J.J., BARENDSEN, G.W. and VAN KERSEN, G.R.,
    Int. J. Radiat. Biol., *13*, 559, 1967.

3. DAVIDS, J.A.G., *Int. J. Radiat. Biol.*, *10*, 299, 1966.

4. DAVIDS, J.A.G., *Int. J. Radiat. Biol.*, *13*, 377, 1967.

5. DAVIDS, J.A.G., *Int. J. Radiat. Biol.*, *17*, 173, 1970.

6. DAVIDS, J.A.G., MOS, A.P.J. and DE OUDE, A., *Phys.
    Med. Biol.*, *14*, 573, 1969.

7. HAGEMANN, R.F., SIGDESTAD, C.P. and LESHER, S.,
    Int. J. Radiat. Biol., *16*, 291, 1969.

8. HORNSEY, S. and VATISTAS, S., *Br. J. Radiol*, *36*,
    795, 1963.

9. McCULLOCH, E.A. and TILL, J.E., *Radiat. Res.*, *13*,
    115, 1960.

10. TILL, J.E. and McCULLOCH, E.A., *Radiat. Res.*, *14*,
    213, 1961.

11. WITHERS, H.R. and ELKIND, M.M., *Radiat. Res.*, *38*,
    598, 1969.

12. WITHERS, H.R. and ELKIND, M.M., *Int. J. Radiat.
    Biol*, *17*, 261, 1970.

HYPOXIC PROTECTION AGAINST LETHAL EFFECTS OF FAST NEUTRONS OF DIFFERENT ENERGIES, STUDIED IN A MURINE LEUKAEMIA USING COLLIMATED EXTERNAL NEUTRON BEAMS AND SIMULATED TISSUE IMPLANTS

R.J. BERRY, *Medical Research Council, External Scientific Staff, Radiobiology Laboratory, Churchill Hospital, Oxford, England.*

J.T. BRENNAN, *Department of Radiology, Hospital of the University of Pennsylvania, Philadelphia, Penn., U.S.A.*

L. GOODMAN, *Radiological Research Accelerator Facility, Columbia University, Upton, Long Island, N.Y., U.S.A.*

A.C. LUCAS and W. QUAM, *Edgerton, Germeshausen and Grier, Goleta, Calif., U.S.A.*

G.D. OLIVER, JR., *Physics Department, M.D. Anderson Hospital and Tumor Institute, Houston, Texas.*

It has been repeatedly shown that hypoxia offers only reduced protection against the cell-killing effects of irradiation with fast neutrons, when compared with the response of the same cells to irradiation under aerobic or hypoxic conditions with X- or gamma-radiation. Thus, radiotherapy with fast neutrons has been presumed to offer the promise of increased local control of human tumours containing hypoxic cells. The present study was designed to evaluate quantitatively the magnitude of the reduction in hypoxic protection (the *Therapeutic Gain Factor*) against irradiation with collimated beams of fast

577

neutrons of five different enegies when muring tumour
cells were irradiated at the surface or 10 cm deep in
a tissue-equivalent phantom. This simulation of the
geometrics of irradiation of superficial and deep human
tumours with external beams was complemented by irradiation of the same muring tumour cells in a tissue-
equivalent phantom at distances of 0.5 and 2.5 cm from
planar arrays of ^{226}Ra (gamma) or ^{252}Cf (neutron) sources
to simulate the geometry of interstitial implant or surface mould bracytherapy.

    The tumour used was the ascitic P-388 leukaemia of
the highly-inbred DBA/2J mouse. Cells of this tumour can
be held *in vitro* for at least 24 hours without affecting
their radiosensitivity, and survival of their reproductive capacity can be assessed by injecting serial dilutions of tumour cells into recipient animals of the
same strain [4]. If animals bearing 7-day tumour are irradiated prior to aspiration of the tumour cells, the
cells exhibit the radiosensitivity of a hypoxic population [3, 4]. For operational reasons, as the experiments were all performed at sites remote from our laboratories, all aerobic irradiations were *in vitro*, while
all irradiations under hypoxic conditions were *in vivo*
except the protracted irradiations simulating tissue implants. For *in vitro* irradiation, cells suspended in
Fischers medium plus 15% foetal calf serum were allowed
to settle on the surface of a tissue-equivalent plastic
chamber which was rotated during irradiation to ensure
equilibration of the cells and their supernatant medium
with air (or nitrogen); for *in vivo* irradiation, the
tumour-bearing mouse was held in a tissue-equivalent
plastic cylinder and rotated about its axis during irradiation to ensure uniform distribution within the animal. The experimental set-up is shown diagrammatically
in Fig. 1; the collimator was of Benelex, a wood composition material, and the phantom when filled contained
a glycerol-urea mixture which was tissue-equivalent in
its major elemental composition. The radiation sources
used, and the dose-rates obtained at the position of the
tumour cells are shown in Table I; where possible, a
higher dose-rate was used for irradiation of the cells
at 10 cm depth in the phantom so that the overall

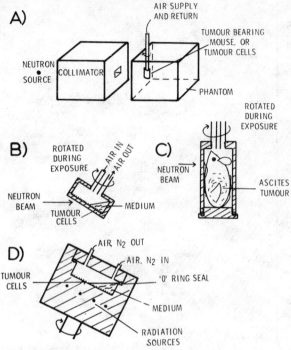

Fig. 1. a) Overall view of experimental set-up for irradiation with
            external beams of fast neutrons.

        b) Tissue-equivalent plastic holder for irradiation of P388
            leukaemia cells under aerobic conditions.

        c) Tissue-equivalent holder for irradiation of P-388 leukaemia
            cells *in situ* in the tumour bearing donor mouse. These
            cells respond as a hypoxic population [4].

        d) Experimental set-up for irradiation of P-388 leukaemia cells
            under aerobic or hypoxic conditions in a tissue-equivalent
            plastic holder simulating a planar brachytherapy implant.

exposure times were similar to those for irradiation of
the tumour cells at the surface of the phantom. Total
dose was measured using tissue-equivalent ionization
chambers, the proportion of the dose contributed by gamma
radiation was measured using thermoluminescent dosimeters.
In the case of the irradiations simulating tissue implants, the neutron dose was measured using silicon
diode detectors.

TABLE 1. Survival of Reproductive Capacity of P-388 Leukaemia Cells Irradiated with Fast Neutrons of Different Energies

Neutron Source and position of tumour cells during irradiation	Mean Neutron Energy (MeV)	Dose-rate (rads/min)	Extra-polation Number (n)	D_0 (rads) Aerobic	D_0 (rads) Hypoxic	OER	Thera-peutic Gain Factor*
A) EXTERNAL NEUTRON BEAMS							
1. Fission-Spectrum A.F.R.R.I. Bethesda 'TRIGA' reactor							
a) at surface	~1	40 – 60	0.9 (0.3-1.7)	91	102	1.1 (0.9-1.4)	2.8
b) 10 cm depth in T.E. phantom			2.8 (1.5-5.5)	96	119	1.2 (1.2-1.3)	2.6
2. M.R.C. Cyclotron, Hammersmith Hospital 16 MeV D-Be							
a) at surface	~6	15 – 40	1.9 (0.4-9.2)	77	125	1.6 (1.4-1.8)	1.9
b) 10 cm depth in T.E. Phantom			0.8	99	127	1.3	2.4

Figures in brackets represent 95% confidence intervals.
*Relative to OER = 3.1 for 250 KVP X-rays, (aerobic) irradiation *in vitro*, hypoxic irradiation *in vivo* [3].

TABLE 1. Continued

	(MeV)							
3. 14 MeV (D-T) neutrons Lawrence radiation lab. I.C.T.								
a) at surface	14	10 - 15	3.1 (1.0-9.9)	87	153	1.8 (1.6-2.0)	1.7	(1.2-1.3)
b) 10 cm depth in T.E. phantom			1.2 (0.2-6.5)	115	146	1.3 (1.1-1.5)	2.4	(0.5-1.3)
4. 14 MeV (D-T) neutrons, A.W.R.E., Aldersmaston I.C.T.								
a) at surface	14	5 - 15	0.8 (0.2-2.7)	76	139	1.8 (1.5-2.2)	1.7	
b) 10 cm depth in T.E. phantom			1.0 (0.05-21)	73	113	1.5 (0.5-4.3)	2.0	
5. Texas A&M variable energy cyclotron 30 MeV D-Be								
a) at surface	~15	10 - 15	2.2 (1.2-4.3)	94	168	1.8 (1.7-1.9)	1.7	
b) 10 cm depth in T.E. phantom			0.8 (0.3-2.6)	139	154	1.1 (0.9-1.3)	2.8	

TABLE 1. Continued

Neutron Source and position of tumour cells during irradiation	Mean Neutron Energy (MeV)	Dose-rate (rads/min)	Extra-polation Number (n)	D_0 (rads) Aero-bic	D_0 (rads) Hyp-oxic	OER	Thera-peutic Gain Factor
50 MeV D-Be							
a) at surface	~25	25	2.4 (1.0-6.0)	102	201	2.0 (1.8-2.2)	1.5
b) 10 cm depth in T.E. phantom			3.5 (0.9-14)	112	181	1.6 (1.4-1.9)	1.9
B) TISSUE IMPLANTS ^{252}Californium needles (fission-spectrum)							
a) at 0.5 cm	1 – 2	3 – 4	9.0 (4.2-19)	80	161	2.0 (1.8-2.2)	1.3**
b) at 2.5 cm		0.6	1.6 (0.2-16)	112	-	-	-

**Relative to OER = 2.7 for ^{226}Ra gamma rays, measured using the same implant geom-etry, and both aerobic and hypoxic irradiations *in vitro*.

The tumour cell survival data are summarised in Table I; survival curves were fitted to the several individual determinations of tumour cell reproductive capacity by the method of Pike and Alper [6]. In all cases the data for irradiation under aerobic and hypoxic conditions were satisfactorily fitted by curves with a common extrapolation number so that a single dose-modification factor, the Oxygen Enhancement Ratio (OER) represented the magnitude of the protection afforded by hypoxia. For P-388 leukaemia cells irradiated *at the surface*, the OER varied significantly, and inversely with the energy of the fast neutron beam. This was in contrast to the results obtained by Barendsen and Broerse with human kidney cells irradiated *in vitro* [1], where the OER was essentially independent of the energy of the fast neutrons studied over the range 1-14 MeV. In an attempt to explain this difference, the response of P-388 cells to irradiation *in vitro* under aerobic and hypoxic conditions was studied using track-segments of beams of deuterons and alpha-particles from the M.R.C. Cyclotron, Hammersmith Hospital, and the tandem Van de Graaff generator at A.E.R.E., Harwell. The data were treated similarly to the fast neutron survival curves, and the OER values at each value of radiation ionization density (LET) are plotted in Fig. 2, where they are compared with the data of Barendsen, *et al.* for human kidney cells [2]. This comparison appears to explain the difference between the fast neutron responses of the two cell lines, as Bewley has pointed out that for irradiation with fission-spectrum (*circa* 1 MeV) neutrons approximately one-third of ionizing events are of the 80-150 KeV/μm size [5] —events for which the response of the P-388 cells is oxygen-independent but against which hypoxia still gives a significant degree of protection in the human kidney cells.

The response of P-388 leukaemia cells irradiated with collimated neutron beams at 10 cm depth in a tissue-equivalent phantom is not so easily explained; for all except the highest neutron energy studied, the OER is relatively invariant and is lower than expected. For fission-spectrum neutrons, the OER at 10 cm depth is higher than for irradiation with the same neutrons at the

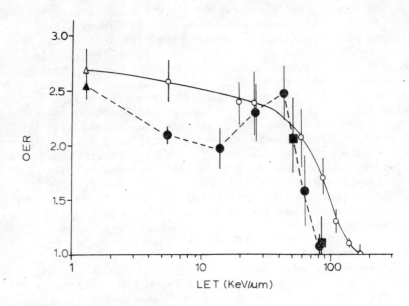

Fig. 2. Oxygen enhancement ratio (OER) as a function of the ionization
density (LET) of the radiation used.
○ Charged particle data for human kidney (T-1) cells from Barendsen,
et al. [2],   △ data for human T-1 cells from Barendsen, et al. for
250 kVp X-rays,   ▲ 250 kVp X-ray data for P-388 leukemia cells irradiated *in vitro*[3],   ● data for P-388 leukemia cells obtained using
deuteron and alpha-particle beams from the M.R.C. Cyclotron, Hammersmith Hospital,   ■ P-388 data obtained with the alpha-particle beam
from the tandem Van de Graaf generator at the A.E.R.E., Harwell,
| indicates standard error.

surface of the phantom due to the higher proportion of
the total dose delivered by gamma-rays. For other neutron energies, however, there is an apparent decrease in
OER at 10 cm depth compared with the OER at the surface,
in spite of an increase in the gamma dose and in spite
of the absence of any dramatic changes in the LET spectrum measured for each neutron energy at the two sites
with a Rossi-type spherical proportional counter [7].
If taken at face value, however, these results suggest
that for irradiation of a deep-seated human tumour with
fast neutrons, even higher Therapeutic Gain Factors may
be obtained than have been predicted from experiments
using cellular and animal radiobiological test systems

whose dimensions are small.

Experiments with P-388 leukaemia cells using ^{252}Cf
sources in a planar array simulating an interstitial or
surface implant have yielded a disappointingly low Therapeutic Gain Factor, when compared to those for collimated
external fast neutron beams. These data are also summarised in Table I. In a geometrical arrangement which re-
alistically represents those used in clinical brachytherr-
apy, a high proportion of the total dose delivered is due
to gamma rays and this in turn results in a relatively
high OER for radiation from the ^{252}Cf sources. The
effect of this mixed neutron-gamma irradiation is also
surprisingly dependent on dose-rate; the Relative Biological Effectiveness of the ^{252}Cf radiation in a geometrical arrangement simulating a tissue implant does not
increase as the dose-rate decreases.

SUMMARY

For murine tumour cells irradiated at the surface
of a tissue-equivalent phantom with collimated beams of
fast neutrons, the protection afforded against lethal
radiation damage by hypoxia varies inversely with the
neutron energy. The Oxygen Enhancement Ratio (OER)
ranges from 1.1 for fission-spectrum (*circa* 1 MeV) neutrons to 2.0 for cyclotron-produced neutrons of *circa*
25 MeV (50 MeV D-Be). This change in OER correlates well
with the response of the same cells to irradiation with
mono-energetic track segments of deuteron and alpha-
particle beams of known ionization density (LET). However, for irradiation of the tumour cells with collimated
beams of fast neutrons at 10 cm depth in a tissue-equivalent phantom, the OER is uniformly lower than predicted
by consideration of the average LET.

For irradiation from a planar array of neutron-
emitting ^{252}Cf sources in a tissue-equivalent holder
simulating a brachytherapy implant, the OER is disappointingly high (2.0), although still significantly lower than
for irradiation with ^{226}Ra gamma rays in the same geometry.

ACKNOWLEDGEMENTS

The work of the Radiobiology Laboratory, Churchill
Hospital, Oxford, is supported by the Medical Research
Council. This project was largely supported by U.S.
Public Health Service Planning Grant CA-10059 to Pro-
fessor J.T. Brennan.

The track-segment experiments at the M.R.C. Cyclotron, Hammersmith Hospital, were carried out with the
help of Dr. D.K. Bewley and Mr. C.J. Parnell, and those
at A.E.R.E., Harwell with Dr. G.J. Neary. Miss T. Alper
kindly provided access to the computer programme for calculation of survival curves.

REFERENCES

1.   BARENDSEN, G. and BROERSE, J., *Nature (Lond.), 212,*
     722, 1966.

2.   BARENDSEN, G., KOOT C., VAN KERSEN, G., BEWLEY, D.,
     FIELD, S. and PARNELL, C., *Int. J. Rad. Biol., 10,*
     317, 1966.

3.   BERRY, R., *Brit. J. Radiol., 41,* 921, 1968.

4.   BERRY, R. and ANDREWS, J., *Brit. J. Radiol., 36,*
     49, 1963.

5.   BEWLEY, D., In: *Biophysical Aspects of Radiation
     Quality*, Second Panel Report, pp. 65, I.A.E.A.,
     Vienna, 1968.

6.   PIKE, M. and ALPER, T., *Brit. J. Radiol., 37,* 458,
     1964.

7.   ROSSI, H., *Radiology, 78,* 530, 1962.

LENS OPACITY IN MOUSE AFTER RADIATION EXPOSURE; ROLE OF 1) RADIATION QUALITY AND DOSE, AND 2) TISSUE OXYGENATION AND DOSE RATE*

JOHN L. BATEMAN and VICTOR P. BOND

Lahey Clinic Foundation,
605 Commonwealth Avenue,
Boston, Mass. 02215, U.S.A.

INTRODUCTION

Opacification of the mammalian lens following exposure to ionizing radiation is of clinical interest in
hazard and protection considerations for man. Further,
in the experimental animal the lens has become a valuable
in vivo system for study of the influence of physical
factors upon radiation response. The early work of Evans
[8] established the sensitivity of the lens to radiation,
particularly to fast neutrons. The studies of Riley *et
al.* [13] and Upton *et al.* [15] further clarified the RBE
(relative biological effectiveness) of fast neutrons
relative to X-rays in a variety of mammalian species.
Merriam *et al.* [11] and Bateman and Snead [5] have investigated the RBE of monoenergetic neutrons in the 0.43-
14-MeV energy range, and the marked dependence of neutron
RBE upon dose. The implications of these findings for
hazard and protection considerations in man have been discussed by Bond [6].

---

*Research supported by the U.S. Atomic Energy Com-
mission, and in part by Grant RH 99, Division of Radiological Health, Bureau of State Services, U.S. Public
Health Service.

The purpose of this presentation is to 1) describe
the unique features of the mammalian optic lens as a
radiobiological system, 2) report an experiment utilizing
this system to evaluate the combined influence of radiation dose rate and tissue oxygenation, and 3) to consider
the net influence of radiation quality, dose, dose rate
and tissue oxygenation by a comparison of the findings in
normally hypoxic lens to those in experimentally oxygenated lens and several normally oxygenated plant and animal
systems.

DESCRIPTION OF THE LENS

The unique radiobiological test system represented
by the mammalian lens is shown in Fig. 1, which is a
schematic sagittal section of the adult organ. In es-
sence, the murine lens is a sphere enveloped by a thin
capsule which precludes cell penetration. The anterior
half of the lens is covered by an epithelium (lying be-
neath the capsule) which is comprised of a nondividing
central portion (but capable of wound repair) and a proliferative outer (germinal) zone, which is mitotically
active at a declining rate throughout the life span of
the animal. The daughter cells migrate to the vertical
equator, and there differentiate into mature fiber cells
and extend their cytoplasmic termini toward the anterior
and posterior poles. The continued apposition of new
fibers to the lens cortex causes growth of the lens cortex causes growth of the lens thoughout life, and the
weight increases with the logarithm of time. As the lens
fiber position becomes relatively deep in the cortex, the
fiber nucleus disappears. Considerably later the lens
fiber walls disappear and the contents of the fiber join
the crystalline lens "nucleus".

With aging alone or following irradiation, minute
scattered opacities within the posterior cortex become
visible with the slit-lamp biomicroscope, and from electron micrographic studies these appear to be defective
portions of single lens fiber cells. They are believed
to result from heritable defects in cytoplasmic protein
synthesis, and begin to occur in the mouse six to seven

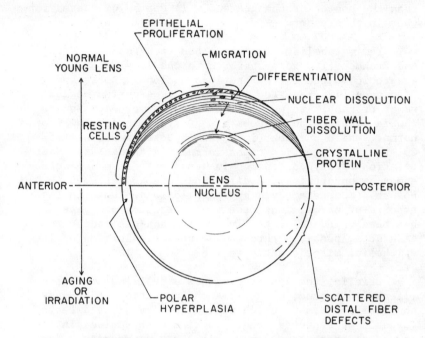

Fig. 1.   Schematic section along the axis of an adult mammalian lens.
          Epithelial zones and stages of lens fiber development are
          shown above the center. Changes which occur with aging
          irradiation are shown below the center.

weeks post-irradiation, which is the time interval from
desoxyribose nucleic acid (DNA) synthesis in the germinal
zone to fiber differentiation. The nature of this defect
appears identical whether found in a young irradiated or
an aged animal. In either case, the appearance of these
minute discrete opacities is followed by the development
of a confluent central posterior opacity of much larger
size.

     The anterior polar region of the lens also reveals a
lesion caused by either aging or irradiation. This consists of hyperplasia of the epithelium, with resultant
thickening and eventual rupture posteriorly into the cortex. This lesion is less easily produced by radiation

than the posterior changes and will not be discussed further in this paper.

The metabolism of glucose has been found by Kinsey and Frohman [10] to be aerobic in the lens epithelium and anaerobic in the cortex and lens nucleus. Pirie and Heyningen [12] reported the oxygen tension in the aqueous humor of rabbit to equal that of venous blood. Severe anoxia reduced the aqueous humor oxygen to one-third of normal, while one hour in an atmosphere of 95% O_2 - 5% CO_2 raised it to five times normal. Although the exact relation of oxygen tension in lens epithelium and aqueous humor is uncertain, the difference due to extremes in exposure atmosphere could approach 15-fold. Despite the hypoxia of normal lens, the administration of cysteine has been found to partially protect against radiation cataracts, possibly through the known inhibition of lens epithelial mitotic activity [16].

Briefly, the lens represents a cell-isolated proliferative tissue, with permanent retention of progeny, abnormal members of which will display visible defects (capable of repeated nondestructive observation) in marked contrast to the nonvisible normal progeny. Further, it appears that each viable (though injured) lens epithelial germinal cell may give rise to several abnormal offspring, thus providing further amplification to the manifestation of germinal cell injury. Finally, the normally hypoxic condition of the lens epithelium renders it less susceptible to the influence of dose rate with low LET radiations, by a probable reduction in the fraction of reparable damage, which facilitates the comparison of radiations on the basis of their linear energy transfer (LET).

MATERIAL AND METHODS

Exposure to 250 kVp X-rays utilized a G.E. Maxitron deep therapy unit with external filtration by 0.5 mm Cu and 1.0 mm Al, yielding a HVL = 1.25 mm Cu. All exposures were made within a variable atmosphere chamber, which provided an equilibration layer of 3.0 cm of Lucite and back-

scatter of 2.5 cm of Lucite plus 10.2 cm of compressed
fiberboard.

Exposures at 103.6 rads per minute involved a target-
to-mouse midline distance of 171 cm and operation of the
machine at 6 ma.

Hyperbaric exposures were carried out at three atmospheres of pressure with 100% O_2 flowing (after flushing)
at one liter per minute. Hypoxic exposures utilized a
mixture of 6% O_2 - 94% N_2 achieved by the use of flow
meters, and were performed at atmospheric pressure. To
obtain the maximum possible difference in tissue oxygen
concentration, the pressure and oxygen content were adjusted to produce a few deaths at each extreme. A five-
minute "soaking" period was allowed the animals before
each irradiation was begun. Unfortunately, the process
of adjusting the oxygen and pressure reduced the number
of animals available for the experiment, and therefore
comparison radiation exposures at room atmosphere could
not be accomplished.

Albino Swiss female mice, thirty per treatment group,
averaged 13 weeks of age at the time of the experiment.
Animal handling, serial slit-lamp examinations of their
lenses, and the observer-based scoring scale have been
previously described [3, 4].

The basic experimental plan involved the exposure of
animal groups to graded doses of X-rays delivered at two
or 100 rads per minute at each of the two atmospheric conditions. The doses were selected according to the anticipated radiation effectiveness at each of the four basic
experimental conditions.

RESULTS

Posterior lens opacity scores from serial examinations post-irradiation were tabulated as to the number
of lenses within each treatment group which had reached
or exceeded each of multiple (increasing) levels of
opacity severity. These values were then graphed against

a linear scale of time as illustrated in Fig. 2.   Each
curve represents the rising incidence (within a particular treatment group) of opacities equal to or greater
than the indicated level of opacity.   The coordinates

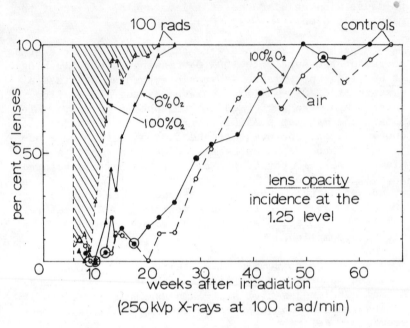

Fig. 2.   The increasing incidence with time of treated lenses exhibiting
         posterior opacification at or exceeding the 1.25 level.   The
         area above each curve was measured by planimeter, as shown by
         the shading above one curve.   (40 lenses = 100%).

were so ordered that the distance for one lens (of 40
scored per group) on the vertical scale equaled one week
of time on the horizontal scale.   The area above each
curve was then measured utilizing an engineering plani-
meter, and expressed in lens-weeks.   In these computations
the six-week interval post-irradiation was excluded because, as noted earlier, no changes are evident during
this period, even with the highest radiation exposures.
The magnitude of the term "lens-weeks" indicated the size
of the interval before the occurrence of opacity at each

of the multiple levels. In Fig. 2 are shown the incidence curves for one level of opacity obtained at 100
rads per minute with 100 rads oxygenated, 100 rads hypoxic, non-irradiated animals maintained in 100% O_2 at 3
atmospheres for $1\frac{1}{2}$ hours, and non-stressed control animals. It can be seen in the figure that the hyperbaric
exposure caused an earlier rise in incidence of opacity
(was more effective) than the hypoxic exposure to the
same dose at the same dose rate. Both of these were much
more effective than either control "treatment", the latter
two being approximately equal as judged from the inter-
weaving of their incidence curves.

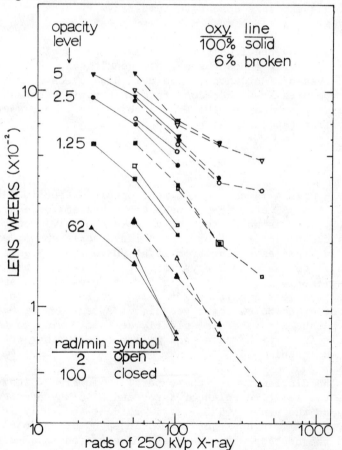

Fig. 3. Results of the lens experiment in dose rate and oxygenation.
Control values of lens-weeks ($\times 10^{-2}$) were: 0.62 level - 5.3,
1.25 level - 10.6, 2.5 level - 15.0, and 5.0 level - 18.1.
(These values represent averages of the 100% O_2 and air controls, which were similar at each level.)

In Fig. 3 are shown the results from all experimental groups, derived as discussed for the preceding
figure. The logarithm of lens-weeks has been graphed
against the logarithm of radiation dose to facilitate
comparison of radiation doses of the various treatments
necessary to produce the same effect. Inspection of the
figure reveals 1) the similarity of results with two or
100 rads per minute given under hypoxic conditions, 2)
the slightly greater effectiveness with hyperbaric oxygenation of exposures at 100 rads per minute compared with
those at 2 rads per minute, and 3) the almost two-fold increase in effectiveness of hyperbaric oxygenated exposures
at either exposure dose rate compared with hypoxic exposures.

As noted previously, it had not been possible to
carry out X-ray exposures at room conditions. However,
the curves of incidence at the multiple levels of opacity
for exposures at either dose rate in hypoxia were found
to be very similar to those obtained in previous experiments from exposures at room conditions.

DISCUSSION

In Fig. 4 is shown, for lens opacification in the
mouse, the RBE of 0.43-MeV neutrons compared to X-ray
dose, which has been previously presented [5]. Neutron
doses can be located from the inclined scale shown, with
isodose lines extending from it at 90°. Their magnitude
is equal to that for X-rays where they intersect the ab-
scissa (RBE = 1.0). The RBE's for neutrons of 1.8 and
14 MeV for lens opacification have been found [5] to lie
in that order below the regression for neutrons of 0.43
MeV, but have not been so clearly defined, owing to the
relative paucity of data, and will not be further considered in this paper.

The diagram toward the upper left in Fig. 4 indicates the relative roles of X-ray and 0.43-MeV neutron
OER upon the neutron RBE. It is evident that only if a
neutron RBE were constant (i.e., independent of dose)
would the neutron OER and X-ray OER exert an equal effect

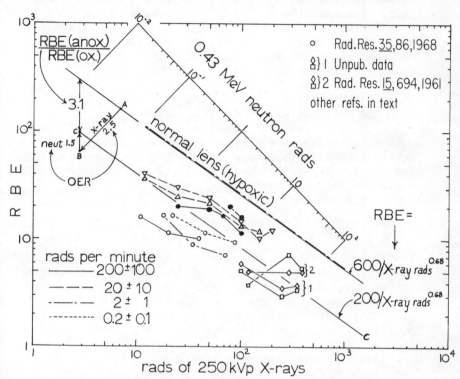

Fig. 4. A comparison of fast neutron maximal RBE experimentally obtained
in normally hypoxic mouse lens and an OER-derived oxygenated
minimal RBE with experimental data in other biological systems.
Symbol code is as follows: Somatic mutations in *Tradescantia*:
colorless ∇, pink Δ; lens opacification in oxygenated mouse ●;
cell loss in mouse: spermatogonia O, spleen weight loss □, thymus weight loss◇.

upon the RBE. The greater the dependence of neutron RBE
upon dose, the less will be the influence of the neutron
OER and the greater will be that of the X-ray OER.   In
the example shown, if the oxygenated dose of X-ray is
less by a factor of 2.5 (the OER) than the hypoxic dose
to produce an equal effect (measured along a neutron isodose), the influence on neutron RBE is by a factor of 4.8.
If a neutron OER of 1.5 pertains, the influence of this

value upon the neutron RBE will be by a factor of about
1.55. The net effect upon RBE would be a factor of 3.1,
even larger than the X-ray OER. The sequence of these
steps in the figure is: point "A" to point "B", to point
"C". An approximate mathematical expression is as follows:

$$\frac{\text{RBE (hypoxic)}}{\text{RBE (oxygenated)}} = 1.85 \frac{\text{OER (X-ray)}}{\text{OER (neutron)}}$$

To determine the maximum possible difference in 0.43-
MeV neutron RBE within one system, the OER values of 2.5
and 1.5 for X-rays and neutrons [2, 7], respectively, will
yield:

$$\frac{\text{RBE (hypoxic)}}{\text{RBE (oxygenated)}} = 1.85 \left(\frac{2.5}{1.5}\right) = 3.1$$

The above OER values, obtained for microorganisms and cell
cultures, have not been obtained in the whole animal who
cannot survive the extreme conditions. They can be employed, however, for the purpose of demonstrating that two
given biological systems may not involve the same radiobiological mechanism.

If the above mathematical steps are employed at intervals along the hypoxic RBE regression and both the
neutron and X-ray OER values can be considered constant
(i.e., dose-independent), the validity of line "C-C" as a
lower limit for "oxygenated RBE" is established. It is
then of interest to consider experimental data in oxygenated biological systems within this framework.

The curves for the different exposure conditions
shown in Fig. 3 were compared at frequent intervals of
dose and averaged at each dose for the five levels of
opacity utilized. Thus average dose-specific OER values
were obtained for the dose rates of 100 and 2 rads per
minute. These values were then entered in Fig. 4 to produce the curves shown for lens by utilization of the neutron isodose lines to connect each hypoxic X-ray dose on
the hypoxic lens RBE regression with the equally-effective
"oxygenated" X-ray dose.

A variety of other biological systems has also been entered on the graph, including two involving the production of nonlethal plant mutations, and three involving animal cell mortality. These systems are generally considered normally oxygenated, and it is likely that their regression of 0.43-MeV neutron RBE on X-ray dose would fall below the results obtained for hypoxic lens. The dose rates employed in the cited works are indicated in Fig. 4, and although the influence of X-ray dose rate cannot be quantified, the work of Hall [9] and the lens experiment reported herein show a decrease in dose rate effect with decreasing oxygen concentration.

Examination of the experimental evidence shown in Fig. 4 reveals that only those with *Tradescantia* could occur by the same mechanism as lens opacification. Additionally, it appears possible that spermatogonia depletion and spleen and thymus weight loss (lymphocyte death) could involve a common mechanism. Lastly, the bulk of the data implies a dose-dependence of net OER by the nonparallel relation of the experimental regressions to line "C-C". Alper and Moore [1] have postulated a linear relation between neutron and X-ray OER's which can neither be supported nor rejected on the basis of data presented in this paper.

In summary, the 0.43-MeV neutron RBE for opacification of the normally hypoxic mouse lens has been compared to experimental data in oxygenated lens and normally oxygenated biological systems, utilizing a maximum possible difference in RBE derived from limiting X-rays and fast neutron OER values from the literature.

REFERENCES

1. ALPER, T. and MOORE, J., *Br. J. Radiol.*, *40*, 843, 1967.

2. BARENDSON, G. and BROERSE, J., *Nature*, *212*, 722, 1966.

3. BATEMAN, J.L. and BOND, V.P., *Radiation Res. Supp.* *7*, 239, 1967.

4. BATEMAN, J.L., BOND, V.P. and ROSSI, H.H., In: *Biological Effects of Neutron and Proton Irradiations*, Vol. II, IAEA, Vienna, 1964.

5. BATEMAN, J.L. and SNEAD, M.R., *Proceedings of a symposium on neutrons in radiobiology, at Oak Ridge, Tenn., Nov. 11-14, 1969.* University of Tennessee, Oak Ridge National Laboratory and the U.S. A.E.C., p. 192, CONF-691106, 1970.

6. BOND, V.P., In: *Biophysical Aspects of Radiation Quality*, p. 149, IAEA Report, Vienna, 1968.

7. DENNIS, J. and BOOT, S., *Nature, 215*, 310, 1967.

8. EVANS, T.C., *Radiology, 50*, 811, 1948.

9. HALL, E. and CAVANAGH, J., *Br. J. Radiol., 40*, 128, 1967.

10. KINSEY, E.V. and FROHMAN, C.E., *Arcj. of Opthalmol., 46*, 536, 1951.

11. MERRIAM, G., Jr., BIAVATI, B., BATEMAN, J., ROSSI, H, BOND, V., GOODMAN, L. and FOCHT, E., *Radiation Res., 25*, 123, 1965.

12. PIRIE, A. and HEYNINGEN, R., Blackwell Scientific Publications, Oxford 1st publication, 1965.

13. RILEY, E.F., EVANS, T.C., RHODY, R.B., LEINFELDER, P.J. and RICHARDS, R.D., *Radiology, 67*, 673, 1965.

14. UNDERBRINK, A., SPARROW, R., SPARROW, A. and ROSSI, H., *Radiation Res.*, in press.

15. UPTON, A.C., CHRISTENBERRY, K.W., MELVILLE, G.S., FURTH, J. and HURST, G.S., *Radiology, 67*, 686, 1965.

16. VON SALLMANN, L., MUNOZ, C.M. and BARR, F., *A.M.A. Arch. Ophth., 47*, 305, 1952.

CELL LOSS RATE IN EXPERIMENTAL TUMORS FOLLOWING 14 MeV-NEUTRON IRRADIATION. IN VIVO EXPERIMENTS WITH LABELED IODODEOXYURIDINE

W. PORSCHEN and L.E. FEINENDEGEN

Institute of Medicine, Kernforschungsanlage Jülich GmbH, 517 Jülich, W. Germany

1. INTRODUCTION

The growth curve of an experimental tumor (volume as a function of time) is distinguished by three successive phases: exponential phase, slowing down phase and plateau. This curve results from the difference between cell production and cell loss. Estimates of cell loss rates are conventionally based on the difference between the true doubling time and the potential doubling time.

In this communication labeled iodo-deoxyuridine, as DNA-precursor analogue to thymidine, is shown to be useful for *in vivo* measuring cell loss rates in unirradiated and irradiated experimental tumors. Irradiation with 14 to 15 MeV-neutrons (LET 12 keV/μ; OER 1.6) [1, 2] is used in these experiments. The data indicate that useful dose effect curves may be obtained by *in vivo* measurements. They moreover show that the tumor cells are more sensitive to high energy neutrons during S-phase than during the other phases of the cell cycle.

II. MATERIALS AND METHODS

Sarcoma 180 transplanted in the right hind leg of white mice (male, NMRI) weighing 20 g at average was kindly supplied by the Research Laboratory of Chemie

Grünenthal, Stolberg*. The tumor volume was calculated
from three diameter measurements. The change of volume
as a function of time ($dV/dt = \dot{V}$) is the growth rate; the
volume doubling time T_2 is easily obtained from the volume curve.

The mitotic cycle of proliferating sarcoma 180 cells
in tumors 5 days old, was analyzed by Simpson-Herren,
Blow and Brown (1968) [7]: generation time (T_G) = 13.5 h;
S = 7.8 h; G_2 = 2.5 h; G_1 = 2.7 h; mitosis = 0.5 hours.

The change in the number of tumor cells per time
(dN/dt) is determined by cell production and cell loss
[8]:

$$dN/dt = \dot{N} = \mu N - \lambda N = (\mu - \lambda)\, N$$

where

   λ = cell loss rate in %/hour
   μ = cell production rate in %/hour
   N = number of cells in the tumor.

If cell density (N/V) is assumed here to be constant
throughout, the last equation may be transformed to

$$\dot{V} = (\mu - \lambda)\, V \text{ or } \dot{V}/V = \mu - \lambda$$

Since the cell loss factor $\phi = \lambda/\mu = 1 - T_G/T_2$, $\dot{V}/V$
and ϕ allow also estimating λ and μ.

Cell loss rate

For measuring cell loss rates from solid tumors *in
vivo*, labeled iododeoxyuridine (I^{125} - IUdR)**, a thy-

---

*The authors thank especially Dr. Mückter from
Chemie Grünenthal, Stolberg, Germany, for the generous
gift.

**I^{125} - IUdR was purchased from the Radiochemical
Centre, Amersham, (spec. act. 2 Ci/mMol).

midine analogue was used, because it is advantageous in
comparison with H^3-thymidine for it can easily be measured
externally, and reutilization is negligible [3, 5].

IUdR is specifically incorporated into DNA and remains bound within the cells until death. Following i.v.
injection of I^{125} - IUdR, the regression of tumor counting rate signals cell loss or cell death. The regression
constant α(= ln2/biological half-life) serves as index of
the cell loss rate.

Measuring device

The iodine-125 retained in the tumor was measured
with a crystal scintillation counter. The tumor bearing
mice were fixed above the crystal on a lead plate with a
hole in such a way, that the crystal only sees the tumor.
The counts were taken with a single channel analyzer combined with a precision rate meter (Telefunken MSPR 1001/2)
[6].

Normal cell loss rates

On day 3 or 4 after tumor transplantation the normal
drinking water was replaced by a 0.1% solution of sodium
iodide. On day 5 to 6 the tumor had grown to a volume of
about 300 mm^3. Then one single intravenous injection of
20 µCi (about 3 µg) in 0.1 ml normal saline was given per
mouse. The activity injected was controlled with a whole
body counter for laboratory animals.

Fig. 1 shows the tumor counting rate to fall rapidly
to a plateau region beginning at approximately 40 hours.
From approximately 70 hours on, the counting rate declines
exponentially, indicating random loss of cells from the
tumors.

The initial rapid loss of activity was paralled by
the rapid loss of sodium iodide-125 (0.05 ml) injected
directly into the tumor with a volume of 300 mm^3. The
data indicate the speed of exchange of inorganic soluble
iodine.

Three tumors in the plateau region of I^{125}-activity

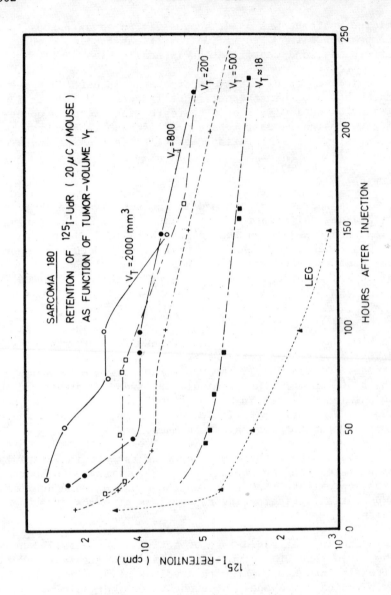

Fig. 1.   Retention of I^{125}-UdR in solid sarcoma 180 as function of
tumour volume.

were biochemically analyzed for labeling distribution.
The DNA contained 85%, the protein 10%, and acid-soluble
material 2.4%, the RNA 0.3% and the lipid fraction 0.4%
of the total I^{125}.

Fig. 1 indicates that the efficiency of labeling expressed by the I^{125}-retention in the plateau region, decreases with increasing volume. This may be the result
of either a decrease in the number of cells in S-phase,
i.e. a decrease in the growth fraction, or of a decrease
in the rate of IUdR incorporation per DNA-synthesizing
cell. The known diminution of the growth fraction with
increasing tumor size speaks in favor of the first interpretation.

Attention is drawn to the fact that with increasing
tumor volume, the rate of loss of I^{125} from the tumors
also increases. The highest rate of activity loss is observed in the tumors having a volume of about 2,000 mm^3.
Also included in Fig. 1 is the data obtained from the
healthy leg and indicates the contribution to the tumor
counting rate from I^{125} incorporated into the bone marrow
and skin of the leg. The tumor curves represent values
corrected for this contribution.

Irradiation and dosimetry

The tumors were irradiated with 14 to 15 MeV-neutrons produced with a Dynagen-Neutron-Generator, Type
Jülich*. The machine operates with a voltage of 300 kV
and the Duoplasmatron Ion Source delivers a mixed Deuteron
beam up to 8 mA on the target. The D-T reaction produces
10^{11} neutrons/sec per mA at the target**. The neutron
output was monitored by various methods. The neutron
fluence for short exposure times was measured via the activation of the teflon-spheres, containing 74% fluorine

---

*Manufactured by Radiation Dynamics Incorporated,
Westbury, Long Island, New York, USA.

**Rotating targets (1 turn/sec) with 60 Curie tritium
were purchased from Nukem, Hanau.

19, having dimensions similar to those of the tumors (diameter 10 mm, 1.2 g weight). For absolute dosimetry Silicon-Diodes (Type 5422) and the dosimeter reader 3806 were used.

Radiation - induced cell loss

In a first series of experiments the dose dependence of cell death after irradiation was analyzed in the dose range of 250 - 700 rad. Animals bearing tumors of 200 - 300 mm^3 volume were injected with I^{125}-UdR, and 28 hours later they were irradiated near the target. The dose rate at the tumor amounted to 150 rads/min. The body dose was 30% or less of the tumor dose. Fig. 2 demonstrates the relative tumor volumes as a function of time and dose. The upper part of the figure clearly shows the influence of dose on cell death rate. The regression curves are normalized to the value at 50 hours, the initial part of the plateau region.

Radiosensitivity during the cell cycle

In a second series of experiments the correlation between cell loss and timing of irradiation during various phases of the cell cycle was investigated. For that reason the time of irradiation was chosen at intervals following the injection of I^{125}-UdR. Thus, various groups of 5 animals each were irradiated with 450 rads at 7.5 hours after IUdR injection at a time, when most of the labeled cells have progressed from S-phase into the subsequent G_2 and G_1-phases. The next interval was 10 hours after I^{125}-UdR injection. At 13.5 hours after I^{125}-UdR injection most of the labeled cells have divided once and re-entered S-phase. Again 7 hours later, at 21 hours after IUdR-injection, most of the labeled cells are out of S-phase again. The control group received no irradiation. The data are listed in Fig. 4. Following the plateau region is an enhanced loss of radioactivity in all irradiated groups. Whereas the regression is very similar for those animals irradiated at 7.5 hours, 10 hours and 21 hours after I^{125}-UdR injection, the values for the animals irradiated at 13.5 hours show a significantly enhanced regression until approximately 150 hours after ir-

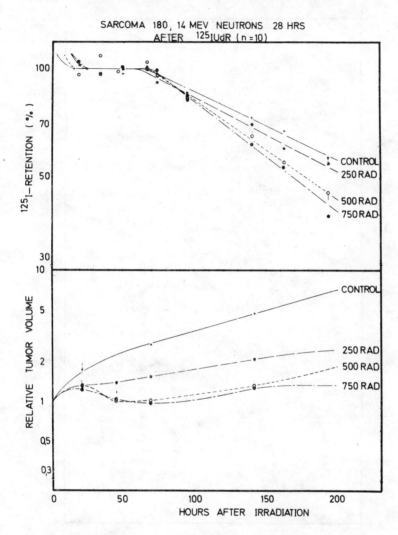

Fig. 2. Relative tumour volume and I^{125}-UdR retention for sarcoma 180 after 14 MeV-neutron irradiation.

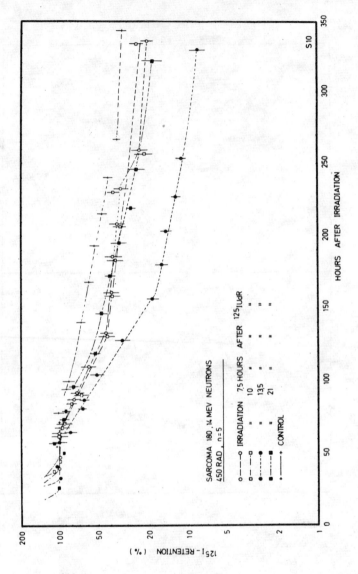

Fig. 3.   I^{125}-UdR retention for sarcoma 180 after irradiation with 450
          rad of 14 MeV-neutrons at different times (7.5, 10, 13.5 and 21
          hours) after I^{125}-UdR.

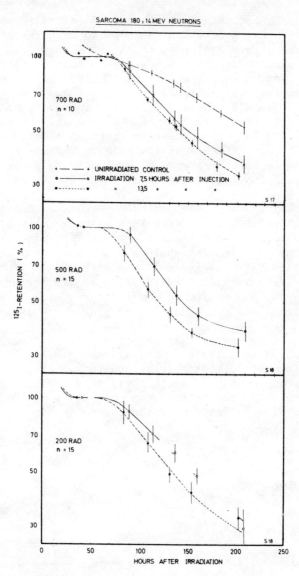

SARCOMA 180 , 14 MEV NEUTRONS

Fig. 4. I^{125}-UdR retention after irradiation with 14 MeV-neutrons (700, 500 and 200 rad) 7.5 or 13.5 hours after injection.

radiation.   From then on, all curves decline in parallel.
This indicates, that those cells which were irradiated
13.5 hours after labeling with I^{125}-UdR, the time when
they were again in DNA-synthesis, are most sensitive to
irradiation, whereas there is no significant difference
in radiosensitivity between cells which are out of S-
phase.   It is also obvious, that the induced enhancement
of activity from the tumors is observed only up to approximately 120 - 150 hours after irradiation; thereafter
regression curves behave in parallel.   Obviously the surviving cells have recovered sufficiently to exhibit a
life span indistinguishable from the control tumor cells.

An additional experiment was performed to study the
effect of radiation on cells in S-phase as a function of
dose.   Therefore 10 - 15 mice were irradiated either 7.5
or 13.5 hours after I^{125}-UdR labeling.   Whereas the latter
irradiation hits labeled cells in S-phase, 7½ hours after
I^{125}-UdR labeling all labeled cells should be out of S-
phase.   200, 500 or 700 rads were given.   The data are
again normalized to values at the plateau region.

Fig. 4 indicates that there is a significant increase
in radiation sensitivity after all dose levels used.   The
effect is most prominent after 500 rads.   It should be
noted, that the curves exhibit values pertaining to cells
that survived.   For this reason, analogous to the situation in Fig. 4, the regression curves decline rather in
parallel.

SUMMARY

Irradiation of Sarcoma 180 at different times after pulse-labeling with I^{125}-UdR allows determining cell loss rates from the tumor.

The efficiency of tumor labeling with I^{125}-UdR decreases with increasing tumor volume.

This technique of *in vivo* measuring cell loss rates led to the recognition that labeled cells in S-phase are more radiosensitive than those labeled cells out of S-phase.

REFERENCES

1. BARENDSEN, G.W., in: *Current Topics in Radiation Research*, Ebert and Howard, Eds., North-Holland, Amsterdam, vol. IV, pp. 295, 1968.

2. BROERSE, J.J., *Effects of Energy Dissipation by Monoenergetic Neutrons in Mammalian Cells and Tissues*, the University of Amsterdam, 1966.

3. FEINENDEGEN, L.E., BOND, V.P. and HUGHES, W.L., *Proc. Soc. Exptl. Med. Biol., 122*, 448, 1966.

4. FEINENDEGEN, L.E., *Tritium Labeled Molecules in Biology and Medicine*, Academic Press, New York/London, 1967.

5. HUGHES, W.L., COMMERFORD, S.L., GITLIN, D., KRUEGER, R.C., SCHULTZE, B., SHAH, V. and REILLY, P., *Federation Proc., 23*, 640, 1964.

6. PORSCHEN, W. and FEINENDEGEN, L.E., *Strahlentherapie, 137*, 718, 1969.

7. SIMPSON-HERREN, L., BLOW, I. and BROWN, P., *Cancer Res., 28*, 724, 1968.

8. STEEL, G., *Cell Tissue Kinetics, 1*, 193, 1968.

CHEMICAL PROTECTION AGAINST NEUTRON IRRADIATION

A.G. SVERDLOV, A.S. MOSJUCHIN, L.M. PAVLOVA,
N.G. NIKANOROVA, and L.N. POSTNIKOV

A.F. Ioffe Physico-Technical Institute,
Academy of Science of the U.S.S.R., Leningrad, U.S.S.R.

Chemical protection against neutron radiation is an important but slightly investigated problem. According to the works cysteine, sodium nitrite, AET Br HBr and its combinations with serotonine have revealed poor effectiveness (I, 3-6). In addition the investigations were not systematical and were limited by the few number of radioprotectors.

Chemical protection of mice against gamma-neutron radiation has been investigated by us by means of sulphur compounds: cystamine, cystaphose 2 -(aminoethyl)-phosphorothioate, AET Br HBr ethyronethylphosphinate (ethyrone) and one of indolilalcilamines-mexamine (5-metoxytryptamine) and also combinations of cystaphose with mexamine or ethyrone.

EXPERIMENTAL TECHNIQUE

(WWR-M) reactor has been a neutron source. Mice were irradiated in the vertical biochannel (dimensions 400 × 600 mm) placed in the concrete shielding within 1.5 m from the core of the reactor [2]. Lead shielding has provided gamma-component filtration up to 10 per cent and less in the total radiation dose. The gamma-neutron field of the biochannel was induced by the dispersed radiation of the horizontal beam placed tangentially to the vertical channel.

611

Mice have been irradiated in the duraluminic biochamber inserted into the channel by means of a crane.
Normal gas composition of air and temperature no higher
than 20°C have been provided during the time of irradiation by the ventilation system.

Inside the biochamber animals were placed in duraluminic cells with thin walls. These cells are divided
into 12 chambers. One mouse has been placed into each
chamber. Four such cells have been simultaneously inserted one above the other into the biochamber. The uniformity of neutron irradiation has been 3 - 7 per cent
along altitude of those cells. The cells with animals
have been installed on the rotational platform which provided uniform round irradiation of mice. Equal quantity
of protected and non-protected (control) mice has been
placed in each cell.

During the time of irradiation continuous control of
gamma-neutron field dose rate by tissue equivalent ionization chambers placed in the rotational irradiated volume
has been performed. Ionization currents have been permanently recorded.

Neutron dose rate of all the experiments has been
6 - 14 rad/min. The calculation of the absorbed dose was
performed taking into account the disturbance of the
gamma-neutron field in the biochannel due to biological
objects. Determining gamma-neutron radiation dose by
means of ionization chambers the standard error has been
found to be 6 - 8 per cent.

Fast neutron spectrum has been determined by recoil-
ing-protons in nuclear emulsion of BK - 400 type. Mean
energy of fast neutrons has been 2.0 Mev, their impact to
the total neutron radiation dose has been estimated by
the results of fast neutron flux measurements by means of
threshold detectors J_n and S.

Aqueous solutions of radioprotectors have been injected into mice intraperitoneally 20 minutes before irradiation in the following doses: cystamine-2mM/kg, cys-
taphose-2mM/kg, AET Br HBr-0.87mM/kg, ethyrone-0.23mM/kg,
mexamine-0.27mM/kg.

RESULTS

Obtained results are demonstrated in Table 1 and in Fig. 1. It is seen that at the exposure of control animals to 150 rad 84 per cent of mice survive at the average survival time 26.1 ± 5.0 days; with the irradiation dose increase up to 300 rad 100 per cent of tested animals die at the average survival time 4.9 ± 0.1 days.

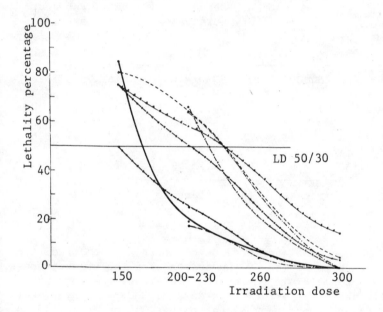

Fig. 1. Mouse survival after neutron irradiation.

cystaphose- - - - , cystamine-•-•-•-, AET-▲-▲-, mexamine-o-o-, ethyrone-ıı-ıı-ıı-, cystaphose combination with mexamine-x-x-x-, cystaphose combination with ethyrone- - -·-, irradiated control——— .

Data obtained demonstrate some sulphur compound effectiveness at neutron irradiation. Radioprotective effect has depended on radiation dose. Maximum effectiveness is observed at $LD_{50/30} - LD_{80/30}$. The most effective against neutron radiation has been cystaphose saving from death up to 45.3 per cent of animals (DRF 1.35). Cystamine and AET effectiveness has been no higher than

TABLE 1.   The Efficiency of The Radioprotectors Injected

Dose (rad)	Control irradiated		Cystaphose			AET Br	
	Total number of animals	Per cent survival	Total number of animals	Per cent survival	Effectiveness	Total number of animals	Per cent survival
150	60	84.0±4.7	25	80.0±8.0	0	16	75.0±35.4
200-300	209	19.0±2,7	120	64.3±4.4	45.3	50	58.0± 7.0
250-260	208	7.6±1.8	145	30.7±3.7	23.1	32	37.7± 6.6
300	133	0	105	4.2±1.9	4.2	72	13.9± 4.1

Note: Effectiveness is the difference on survival

31 - 39 per cents respectively (DRF 1.20 and 1.30).

The decrease and increase of neutron dose irradiation have been accompanied by the decrease of the effectiveness of radioprotectors.   The protective effect has been practically absent at irradiation dose of 300 rad ($LD_{100/30}$). Mexamine and ethyrone application has not notably told on the survival of protected animals.   The results tested on cystaphose combinations with mexamine or ethyrone have shown that these radioprotector combinations did not considerably increase the effectiveness of cystaphose itself.

To realize the possible mechanisms of radioprotector effect of the compounds under investigation against neutron radiation it is essential to analyse the lethality curve of protected and control mice since the lethality curve is known to reflect the syndromes of radiation sickness (Fig. 2).

Most of the control mice died within 3 - 6 days after

Intraperitoneally Before Neutron Irradiation

HBr	Cystamine			Mexamine			Ethyrone		
Effectiveness	Total number of animals	Per cent survival	Effectiveness	Total number of animals	Per cent survival	Effectiveness	Total number of animals	Per cent survival	Effectiveness
0	32	75.0±7.6	0	35	49.9±3.6	0			
39.0	109	50.4±9.5	31.4	75	25.0±5.6	6.0	58	17.2±4.6	0
30.1	111	23.6±4.2	16.0	77	6.7±2.8	0	54	3.7±2.5	0
13.9	115	3.5±1.7	3.5	62	0	0	24	0	0

of the protected and control mice.

neutron irradiation. Evidently the death of the main quantity of the animals exposed to neutron radiation corresponds to the acute gastrointestinal syndrome, which is also proved by autopsy.

The protected animals died within 3 - 6 days after radiation exposure as well, but the decrease of lethality peaks due to the injection of radioprotectors was evident. This statistically significant decrease of lethality is well observed on animals injected with cystamine, AET and particularly with cystaphose. Thus the radioprotection of exposed mice is due to diminishing intestinal damage.

In contrast to the substances mentioned above mexamine and ethyrone are not protectors against neutron radiation and they do not decrease the first lethality peak.

Regarding the reasons of mexamine and ethyrone ineffectiveness our suggestions are as follows. Many

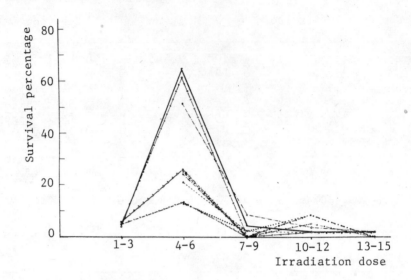

Fig. 2. Lethality of mice irradiated by a neutron dose of 230 rad.

cystaphose------, cystamine-•—•—•—, AET-▲-▲-▲-,
mexamine-₀-₀-₀-₀- , ethyrone-\-\-\-\-, cystaphose combination
with mexamine-x-x-x-x-, cystaphose combination with ethyrone
—.—.—.—, irradiated control ———

authors consider the radioprotective effect of these substances to be due to their hypoxic action. The role of
hypoxy in protection against neutron radiation being neg-
ligibly small, the substances active as hypoxic agents
appeared to be ineffective. Besides mexamine has shown
to protect poorly the intestine against ionizing radiation
if the animals were exposed to radiation for more than
\5 - 10 minutes. In our experiments radiation exposures
lasted 20 - 25 minutes so the protective effect of this
substance could not become apparent. Probably as a result
of this the combination of cystaphose with mexamine or
ethyrone failed to increase the efficiency of cystaphose.

SUMMARY

Some sulphur compound radioprotectors (cystaphose, AET Br HBr, cystamine) protect mice against neutron radiation. Analysis of the lethality of protected and control showed that the prophylaxis of intestinal damage was the principal mechanism of animal protection against neutron radiation. Mexamine and ethyrone application has not notably told on the survival of protected animals.

REFERENCES

1.   BOND, V.P., COLE, L.J. and CARTER, R.E., *Feder. Proc.*, *13*, 424, 1954.

2.   KAMINKER, D.M., MOSJUCHIN, A.S., SVERDLOV, A.G. and POSTNIKOV, L.N., *Radiobiologia (Acad. Sc. U.S.S.R.)*, *7* (3), 462, 1967.

3.   PATT, H.M., CLARK, J.W. and VOGEL, H.H., *Proc. Soc. exptl. Biol. and Med. 84* (9), 189, 1953.

4.   ROMANTSEV, E.M., *Radiation and Chemical Protection*, Moscow, 1963.

5.   SZTANYIK, L., *Studia biophysica*. Radiobiological Symposium and Fifth Annual Meeting of the European Society for Radiation Biology, Vienna, 219, 1967.

6.   VOGEL, H.H., FRIGERIO, N.A. and JORDAN, D.L., *Radiation Research*, *12*, 483, 1960.

OBSERVATIONS BY HUMAN SUBJECTS ON RADIATION-INDUCED LIGHT FLASHES IN FAST-NEUTRON, X-RAY, AND POSITIVE-PION BEAMS*

C.A. TOBIAS, T.F. BUDINGER and J.T. LYMAN

Lawrence Radiation Laboratory, University of California, Berkeley, California 94720, U.S.A.

ABSTRACT

In order to examine the hypothesis that light flashes seen by astronauts on lunar missions are the result of primary cosmic particles, two human subjects were exposed to a fast neutron beam (20 MeV to 640 MeV) at the Berkeley 184-inch cyclotron. Both subjects saw 25 to 50 discrete pinpoint bright momentary light flashes in response to a flux of 10^4 neutrons $cm^{-2}sec^{-1}$ (1 mrem dose). The star-like phosphene phenomenon in the neutron exposure is different from X-ray induced radiophosphenes and from electrically produced visual flashes. No visual phenomenon was noted on positive pi meson exposure at 200 neutrons cm^{-2} sec^{-1}. We believe that bright flashes seen by astronauts are from primary cosmic particles traversing the retina. The mechanism is probably ionization, although light from Cerenkov effect has not been ruled out.

During the space flights of 1969 that carried man to his first lunar landings, Edwin Aldrin and other astronauts on Apollo 11, 12, and 13 observed a series of light flashes and streaks when they were in darkness at great

---

*Work done under the auspices of the U.S. Atomic Energy Commission and NASA Biotechnology and Human Resource Division Agreement L-43541 (Langley).

distances from the earth [1]. It has been known for
many years that relatively low doses of X-rays impinging
on the retina can cause light sensation and alteration
of light sensitivity threshold [2]; however, the astronauts' descriptions of discrete flashes and streaks do
not conform to the homogeneous flood of light characteristic of X-ray phosphenes.

During surveys of the radiobiological hazards of
high-altitude flight and manned space exploration, one
of us suggested that heavy cosmic ray particles might
cause light sensations ("... it would seem that a dark
adapted person should be able to 'see' very heavily
ionizing single tracks as a small light flash, since
they would pass through several retinal receptors,
enough to correspond to a visual object of greater than
1' angular aperture. If a track travels within the
plane of the retina, several rods and cones may be inactivated...") [3, 4]. Although these suggestions were
made in 1952 and 1958, it was not until after light
flashes were seen by the astronouts that definitive experiments were commenced to elucidate the mechanism of
the phenomenon and the validity of the above hypothesis.

It is possible that these flashes were due to ionization or some other form of interaction of primary cosmic particles with tissues. The streaks might be principally due to heavy primaries, and double points could
be accounted for by one cosmic particle intersecting the
retina at two points. Energy transferred to tissue by
these particles is proportional to the square of their
atomic number, and it also depends on their velocity
($\approx 1/v^2$). It is important for the safety of long interplanetary flights to understand such effects and the
potential hazard they may cause. Further, knowledge
about induction of light sensation by charged particles
may also lead to a better understanding of the process
of vision.

Other studies that bear on these effects include
cosmic μ meson interactions, ionization from low energy
protons, and the Cerenkov effect. On the basis of
statistical analysis of coincidences in cosmic-ray counts
and light sensations reported by subjects, μ mesons have

been reported to cause light sensations [5]. According to a recent report, proton recoils from 3-MeV neutrons impinging on the human head during activation analysis can cause light flashes in the dark-adapted eye [6]. A suggestion was made by G. Fazio et al. [7] that the phenomenon observed in space may be due to light from the Cerenkov effect that accompanies fast particles.

In order to learn more about light sensation induced by fast atomic particles, we have made an initial exploration of visual phosphene phenomena due to a beam of fast neutrons at the Berkeley 184-inch cyclotron [8]. Subsequently, the tests were expanded to π^+ mesons from the Bevatron.

Very fast neutrons lose energy by elastic and non-elastic collisions with nuclei. These results in heavy ionizing nuclear recoils and in high speed nuclear spallation fragments. Although the range of these fragments is much less than that for primary cosmic ray particles, they might be able to cause qualitatively similar biological effects.

METHODS

Fast Neutron Exposure

A 0.64-GeV proton beam impinged on a 12-cm-thick beryllium target. Fast neutrons were collimated and channeled by a set of iron and lead apertures of total thickness of about 2 meters, shown in Fig. 1. Charged particles are either deflected away or absorbed by this arrangement, and the resulting beam consisted mainly of high energy neutrons in the domain of 20 to 640 MeV. The majority of the neutrons had energies near 300 MeV. Polaroid photographic paper was used with calcium tungstate intensifier to localize the beam and to monitor the overall exposures. The beam size was 6.5 by 5.2 cm.

Measurement of the neutron flux density for neutrons greater than 20 MeV in the beam was carried out

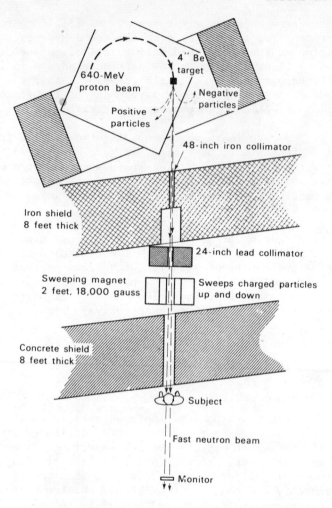

Fig. 1. Configuration used at the 184-inch cyclotron
         for fast neutron exposures in the region of
         the human eye.

by use of a plastic scintillator (4 in. diam., 1 in. thick), following prealignment of the beam and determination of its size. This previously calibrated instrument utilizes the production of radioactive ^{11}C by the (n, 2n) than 20 MeV for which the cross section is known as function of energy [9]. The scintillations are counted for ^{11}C decay immediately after neutron beam exposure. It yielded a maximum intensity of 1.04×10^6 neutrons cm^{-2} sec^{-1} when the primary proton beam intensity was maximized. The plastic scintillator was used to calibrate the beam monitor, which is a large scintillating crystal counter placed in the neutron beam downstream from the experiments. This monitor was used to lower the neutron-beam flux density by a factor of approximately 100; a level near 10^4 neutrons cm^{-2} sec^{-1} was used for the exposure of the subjects.

The ratio of slow to fast neutrons was measured by activated indium foils.

In addition, a tissue-equivalent liquid, simulating the human body in composition and shape, was also exposed to the neutron beam at high level (1.04×10^6 neutrons cm^{-2} sec^{-1}). By converting the ^{11}C counts obtained to dose in rem units, we obtained agreement within a factor of 2 with the plastic scintillator data. The conversion factor of 5.5×10^{-8} rem/neutron cm^2 was assumed. A separate determination of dose was made in a wood phantom having approximately the geometry of the head. Landsverk pocket electrometers (L-50) were used (full-scale deflection, 200 milliroentgens).

The subjects were dark-adapted by wearing a combination of green sunglasses and red X-ray dark-adapting glasses for more than 2 hours prior to exposure. During the last 15 minutes all light was excluded by a black hood which covered the entire head and neck region. This procedure is considered more than adequate for the usual dark adaptation and visual threshold experiments. The hood had four layers of black cloth. Both individuals wore film dosimeters near their eyes on both sides of their head for the duration of the tests. The subjects were exposed to the beam while in the dark-adapted state.

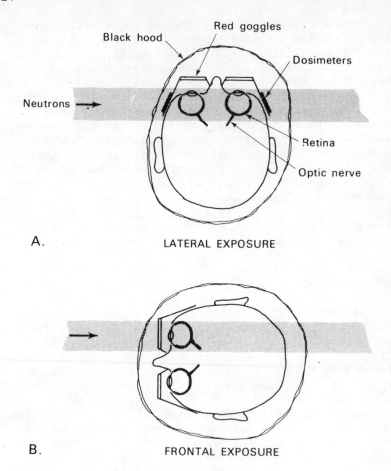

A.   LATERAL EXPOSURE

B.   FRONTAL EXPOSURE

Fig. 2. Subject head positions relative to the fast
         neutron beam.

Two different geometries were used for the exposures. These are shown, schematically, in Fig. 2. In setup A, the beam was allowed to go through both eyes; the subject was facing perpendicular to the beam. It was believed that more streaks might be observed in this position, and that there would be a greater chance for more than one retinal rod, or cone, to be penetrated by the same nuclear recoil. The spallation recoils would tend to move forward and more tangential to the retina than in setup B, where one eye of the subject was exposed, facing the beam. In setup B, a single particle might affect fewer rods than with laterally directed beams.

DESCRIPTION OF EXPERIMENT

Dose

A flux density of 1.4×10^4 fast neutrons cm^{-2} sec^{-1} was used and continuously monitored throughout the tests. The dose rate was measured by three independent techniques. Electrometer-type dosimeters at a position of the eyes in a phantom gave a dose rate of 0.1 mR/sec during a separate long exposure. There was a buildup of the dose in the phantom by a factor of two (compared with free air dose). The dose rate from the neutron flux measurements was calculated in rems by using the conversion factor of 5.5×10^{-8} rem/neutron. This calculated dose rate was 1.25 mrem/sec. The indium foil detectors yielded a dose rate of 0.78 mrem/sec. All three types of dose determinations are thus in reasonable agreement, if we assume a quality factor of 8 to 12.5.

The dose from slow neutrons was less than 2% of the fast neutron dose. Gamma rays from the beam cause less than a few percent of the dose.

The total dose received by both subjects together for the neutron experiment was less than 1 mR by pocket ion chamber determination. By the flux calculation method, CT received 8.5 mrem and TB 2.6 mrem. Standard film badge dosimeters worn near the eyes of the subjects showed no measurable exposure. This confirms that the dose was low and that there was negligible X-ray or thermal neutron exposure.

Summary of Observations

When the beam was "on" both subjects experienced clusters of star-like flashes over their entire visual field. This phenomenon was never experienced by the subjects previously or during the waiting period, and it disappeared promptly, in a fraction of a second, when the beam was turned off.

Detailed Protocols are as Follows:

Subject #1 (CT), June 19, 1970

Time: 1335 (hour) Sunglasses and red dark-adaptation goggles applied. A staging area for the neutron beam was prepared. The beam was centered in a 8-cm-diam metal pipe that was used as a positioning landmark for head alignment relative to the beam. The intensity was adjusted to 1.4×10^4 neutrons cm^{-2} sec^{-1}.

1613 Subject was enclosed in black cloth hood over goggles and sunglasses.

1630 The dark-adapted subject made observations of his pattern of visual sensations *prior to* exposure to any beam. With open or closed eyes he saw a very dark grey background with exceedingly faint blue-green light formations in slowly changing pattern. No light flashes or other rapidly changing light phenomena were seen.

1640 After 27 minutes under the black hood and more than 2 hours under dark-adaptation goggles, CT was positioned for exposure under a protocol that called for several small bursts of beam up to 200 seconds if necessary (maximum dose to be less than 10 millirads). Actually much less beam time was necessary to demonstrate the unequivocal effects.

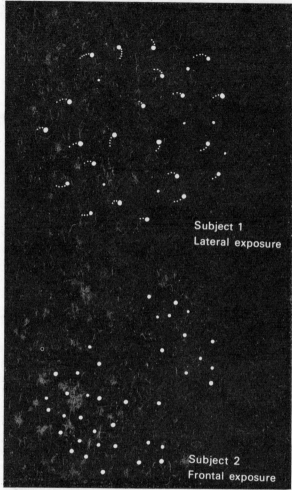

Fig. 3.   A-subject's representation of the relative size,
shape and abundance of white flashes represented
by black dots. Lateral exposure is position A
of Fig. 2. B-subject's representation of flash
phenomenon seen on exposure in position B of
Fig. 2.

Subject was positioned in Position A (Fig.2) for lateral passage of the neutron beam through both eyes.

First Exposure:

The beam was turned on for 1 sec and CT saw three or four star-like flashes. He had difficulty describing precisely the duration and color.

1645
Second Exposure:

The next exposure was for approximately 3 sec at 1.4×10^4 neutrons/sec. Unknown to the subject, but after the head was centered and all were ready, the beam was turned on. The subject immediately exclaimed that he saw flashes. The beam was left on for 3 sec, during which time the subject saw a cluster of small scintillations similar to luminous balls seen in fireworks with the initial tails fuzzy and the heads like tiny stars. His subsequent description and diagrams showed these to be comma-shaped (see Fig. 3A). More of these were seen in the peripheral than in the central fields of vision. They had subjectively brief lifetimes, and extinguished completely. Attempts to "focus" the eyes on them were futile but several different shapes and intensities seemed to be present. Perhaps these attempts to "look at" the scintillations resulted in the appearance of the comet-like tails. The total number in the visual field at any given time was 25 to 50. The luminous dots were about as bright as the average stars in the sky, and while the subject was visualizing them, the background seemed to have turned very black. The color of the scintillations seemed white, with possibly an occasional color tinge on a few, as one sees on the star Betelgeuse.

1650
Third Exposure:

> Subject was shifted to Position B, facing the
> beam path in such a way that the neutrons
> went through his left eye. The right eye re-
> mained unexposed. He saw flashes at both 1-
> sec and 3.5-sec exposures. They seemed
> somewhat harder to detect in this position
> than laterally and gave a dynamic picture of
> change, somewhat like a blinking, star-filled
> sky, or small tracks in a continuously ex-
> panding cloud chamber, with greatly acceler-
> ated sequences. The tests on CT were termin-
> ated after a total exposure time of about
> 9 sec.

> The appearance of the visual field returned
> to normal in the immediate postexposure
> period. There were no other subsequent sen-
> sations or sequelae from this exposure. For
> all exposures knowledge that the beam "on"
> came from visualizing flashes. This pheno-
> menon was markedly different from any pheno-
> mena ever seen by the subject in the dark.

Subject #2 (TB)

Time: 1315   Sunglasses and red dark-adaptation goggles
(hour)   were applied.

1700
Fourth Exposure:

> Subject was enclosed in a dark hood, having
> been wearing the red goggles and dark glasses
> for more than 2 hours. After 10 minutes of
> adaptation, his right eye was positioned in
> the beam (Fig. 2B), and a 3-sec exposure was
> given (Position B). Subject was not informed
> when the beam was turned on, and there were
> no audible cues to the best of our knowledge.
> The first thing the subject noted was a

pin-like lights which he described as stars,
white-blue in color, coming at him. There
appeared to be approximately 50 in a total
field, with most of them in the lower left,
relative to the right eye. There were 5 to
10 in the upper right. The field seemed to
be diffusely covered. There was nothing particularly noted in the center of the right
visual field other than, perhaps, a paucity
of these "sparks." The subject expected to
see electrical phosphene-like phenomena with
diffuse streaks or crescents, but these well-
known phenomena were not observed. The subject noted two waves as if the beam had been
modulated. The attached diagram shows what
the subject saw (Fig. 3B).

Subject TB queries whether there was a slow
rise time for the beam, and that the initial
point that he saw, approximately 1 sec before
he exclaimed, was indeed due to a much lower
intensity, by even an order of magnitude.

Summary

Both experiments saw a number of pin-point flashes
while the neutron beam was on. Their descriptions were
very similar. Each experienced light flashes intimately
correlated with exposure to the beam. There appears to
be some lag (less than 1 sec) in recognizing the flashes
after the beam is switched on. Cessation of the flashes
appears to be easier to detect.

POSITIVE PION BEAM EXPOSURE

To explore the possibility of Cerenkov radiation as
the basic light-producing phenomenon from recoil protons
in the above neutron experiment or from heavy charged
primaries, a preliminary experiment was done with positive pions. Assuming the same interaction cross section
for pions as for the previous neutron exposure, approximately one even per sec should be seen during a pion

TABLE 1. Pion Exposures

Intensity	Configuration	Result
< 1 pion cm^{-2} sec^{-1}	Whole body off beam axis	No visual phenomenon
2 pions cm^{-2} sec^{-1}	Head in beam line, beam plug in	No visual phenomenon
200 pions cm^{-2} sec^{-1}	Head in beam	No visual phenomenon

exposure with an incident flux of 200 particles cm^{-2} sec^{-1}. Exposures were done at the Berkeley Bevatron with 1.5-BeV/c momentum π mesons. The dose and intensity measurements were based on total counts from the scintillator beam monitors. The maximum exposure was for 6 sec at 200 pions cm^{-2} sec^{-1}, with a total dose to the head of 0.2 mrem. The beam was free of protons and other particles. The series of three exposures is shown in Table 1. The subject, TB, was dark-adapted for more than 1 hour.

Summary of Pion Exposure:

The dark-adapted subject noted no visual phenomena during or after exposures. As the whole head was bathed in a pion beam of 200 particles cm^{-2} sec^{-1}, each eye received 800 to 1000 particles for a total exposure of about 5000 particles through each retina. Any interactions or Cerenkov light which occurred in the eye were not detected by the subject.

VISUAL OBSERVATIONS AT HIGH ALTITUDE

The same subjects flew repeatedly in commercial airplanes at 10,000 meters (33,000)feet) altitude and in one flight over the Atlantic at geomagnetic latitude 60°N. The cosmic ray particles are more numerous than at ground level by an approximate factor of 60. Subjects dark adapted for periods of 30 min, and, observing for

20 to 30 additional minutes, have not seen any of the
star-like phenomena similar to those observed in the
neutron beam.

X-RAY PHOSPHENE INDUCTION EXPERIMENTS

A Phillips 250-kV therapeutic X-ray machine was used.
The experimental arrangement shown in Fig. 4 was similar
to that used with neutrons. A horizontal X-ray beam of
about 5 cm diam was produced at the dark-adapted subject's
eye level. Dark-adaptation procedures were similar to
those described above. The subjects were otherwise protected by a plywood and lead body shield. The X-ray machine was operated at the lowest rated current (3 mA at
250 kV). A lead pinhole collimator and several absorbers
were used to get the dose rate sufficiently low. The

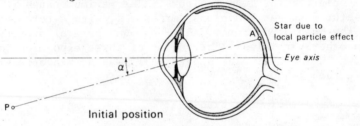

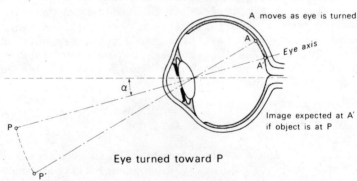

Fig. 4.   An explanation of comma shaped flashes shown in
          Fig. 3.   (See text for details.)

TABLE 2. X-ray Exposures

Dose rate (mR/sec)	Time[a] (sec)	Filters out (see text)	Subject and results
0.05	10		TB, negative
0.40	10	Pb 1.5	TB, negative for stars
0.60	20	Pb 1.5, Al 1.0	TB, negative for stars
0.40	15	Pb 1.5	CT, negative for stars
1.25	10	Pb 1.5, Al 1.0 Cu 20	CT, negative for stars

[a]Note that shutter time of a few seconds keeps the dose rate for the first 2-3 sec lower than given in column 1.

dose rate and total dose were measured by the same Landsverk electrometers as used in the neutron experiments. To reach the lowest dose rate, 0.05 mR/sec, we used a stack of absorbers as follows: Sn (0.06 mm), Cu (3.25 mm), Al (1.0 mm), Pb (1.5 mm), Fe (2.75 mm). The beam, as it emerged, had a half-value layer of 4 mm Cu. Table 2 summarizes all exposures and observations.

Summary of Low-Dose-Rate X-Ray Exposure

The subjects observed no events at all, during any of the exposures, that were similar to the copious starlike scintillations seen in the neutron exposures. Therefore, we conclude that X-rays at a dose rate less than 1.25 mR/sec do not produce phosphenes.

To compare the characteristic of the X-ray phosphene to the neutron beam phosphenes, two subjects were

exposed for 1/30 and 1/60 sec at dose rates of 144 mR/sec
and 72 mR/sec respectively. The X-rays produced by a
Picker clinical X-ray machine set at 80 kVp and 100 mA
produced visual sensations at less than 2 mrad absorbed
dose but at an intensity much hihger than that possible
in the neutron exposure. The light sensation is a soft
bluish-gray-white diffuse light across the visual field
of both eyes, if both are exposed, that does not resemble
the star-like scintillations seen in the neutron beam.

X-ray phosphene characterization studies are being
conducted by one of us (TB) and thus far indicate the
threshold for absorbed dose is below 0.3 mrad at a dose
rate of 24 mrad/sec. This is comparable to the reported
threshold of 0.5 mrad dose at a comparable dose rate [10].
This is still 240 times the dose rate at which neutron
effects were observed.

ELECTRICALLY INDUCED VISUAL SENSATIONS

Subjective sensations of light flashes can be generated in humans by means of 0.3 mA across the head with
a rise time of about 100 msec [11]. Subjects CT and TB
observed electrical phosphenes to note any similarities
to X-ray or neutron-beam phosphenes. The electrical
phosphene is a diffuse bluish-dull-white splash of light
usually in the temporal field if one electrode is placed
over the right forehead and the other behind the neck.
This sensation is one of diffuse light filling more than
10% of the visual field (depending on degree of dark
adaptation and electrical parameters), and differs from
the discrete star-like flashes of the neutron exposure.

DISCUSSION

There are clearly two kinds of phenomena observed
in the course of this research. The star-like flashes,
produced in neutron beams of low fluence, differed markedly from the phosphenes seen from a short burst of X-
rays delivered at higher dose rate. These latter were
rather similar to electrical phosphenes. We shall

examine several alternative explanations in an effort to
understand the processes that have led to the phenomenon,
and to obtain guidance for future experiments. In the
following we shall assume that the relevant interactions
must occur in the eye, that is, in the retina or vitreous fluid. The validity of this assumption will be examined later.

   Assumption 1: The neutron-induced flashes were due
to recoils or spallation products:

   These would come from nonelastic collisions with
carbon, nitrogen, oxygen, phosphorus, sulfur, calcium, or
other nuclei in tissue. The ranges of elastic recoils
are very short for all these nuclei except hydrogen,
whose recoils have considerable range for energies involved. The number of events, E, expected per second in one
eye are:

$$E = \phi \cdot t \cdot a \sum_j N_j \sigma_j.$$

According to our measurements, ϕ, the neutron flux density, was 1.4×10^4 cm^{-2} sec^{-1}. The number, N_j, of
nitrogen, oxygen, and carbon atoms per cm^3 was assumed to
be that characteristic of tissue shown in Table 3. The
effective area of the retina was assumed to be a = 4 cm^2;
t is the effective range of the recoils, that is, the
effective distance away from the retina within which the
non-elastic collis on must occur if the recoiling particle is to reach the retina. We assume for this critical
distance, t = 500 μ or 0.05 cm. This assumption is
equivalent to assuming that in the collisions at least
one heavy recoil has several MeV/nucleon kinetic energy,
otherwise it might not reach the retina. Since spallation occurs, this recoil is probably lighter than the
nucleus hit. These assumptions yield the number of
events, E, as about 43 per second per eye.

   There were 25 to 50 events observed, or about the
same as the actual heavy recoils expected. However, our
calculation could be in error by a factor of 100. Also,
it is possible that a heavy recoil can cross the retina
without causing a visible event.

TABLE 3.

	Percent in tissue[a]	No. of atoms per cm^3 tissue, N_j	Nonelastic scattering cross section,[b] σ_t
C	7.2	1.0×10^{22}	$0.28 \times 10^{-24} cm^2$
N	1.2	1.4×10^{21}	$0.39 \times 10^{-24} cm^2$
O	27.1	2.8×10^{22}	$0.44 \times 10^{-24} cm^2$
H	64	6.6×10^{22}	$0.05 \times 10^{-24} cm^2$[c]

a. Heavier tissue constituents such as P, S, and Ca were neglected due to their low abundance.

b. Taken for this beam. The cross section is largest at about 20 MeV and declines with increasing energy.

c. Total cross section.

The assumption that high-LET, heavy nuclear fragments cause the events is in agreement with the fact that no flashes were observed with π^+ mesons or with low-intensity X-rays.

Assumption 2: Ionization excitations from proton recoils produced in the vicinity of the retina by the primary neutrons cause the majority of flashes:

Protons are produced in elastic collisions, by charge exchange, or in nonelastic collisions with nuclei. Thus, a considerable thickness of the tissue around the retina may serve to generate these. If we assumed this thickness to be $t_p = 2$ cm, the number of "proton events" is

$$E_p = \phi \cdot t_p \cdot a \cdot \sigma_p \cdot N_p.$$

The fluence of proton recoils for each eye, 370 sec^{-1}, is about 10 times the neutron-flash observations estimated by both observers. It seems plausible that some of the protons would miss the rods or that some of the faster protons would not register a flash due to their low LET and low yield of Cerenkov quanta [12].

Slow protons might be more effective than fast protons in producing scintillations. The idea that slow protons with their higher LET could cause light flashes, whereas fast protons could not, is in agreement with the fact that the fast π^+ did not produce flashes; these particles ionize like fast protons, moving with the same velocity.

Assumption 3: The light flashes observed originated from Cerenkov light:

Fazio *et al.* made a suggestion that light flashes observed by astronauts in space flight are Cerenkov radiations from cosmic ray particles [7], and previously, D'Arcy and Porter [5] claimed to have seen light flashes in coincidence with fast μ mesons, possibly due to this effect. In a medium of refractive index 1.34 (the vitreous fluid), only protons with greater than 470 MeV kinetic energy could produce this effect; these would be a relatively small fraction of the 370 protons per second produced in the vitreous fluid by the neutron beam.

In view of the fact that 1.5-GeV π^+ mesons did not produce light flashes in the retina, we doubt Cerenkov effect from protons as the cause of scintillation in this experiment. Contrary to the statistical conclusions of D'Arcy and Porter, we have not been able to see any flashes at ground level or in a plane at 10,000 meters that could be attributable to cosmic ray mesons. We are also informed that a number of astronauts, who have flown orbital missions below the Van Allen radiation belt in near equitorial orbits, failed to observe such flashes.

We conclude that Cerenkov effect from fast particles of charge Z = 1 did not cause the observations in the neutron beam at ground level. It is quite possible, however, that Cerenkov light could contribute to phosphenes produced by very fast heavy nuclei, since the intensity of the light varies with Z^2.

Assumption 4: Production of a visible light flash requires deposition of a minimal ionization energy within a critical time interval and spatial domain:

There have been indications from earlier work by
Lipetz [13] that a single electron passing through a
retinal rod in isolated frog retina can produce measurable
alterations in electrical responses of single fibers in
the frog optic nerve. If single electrons or ionization events could produce light sensation, we would see
frequent scintillation-like flashes (when dark adapted)
due to cosmic ray ionizations in the retina.

The experiments reported in this paper with X-rays
clearly demonstrate that X-rays at low dose rate, below
1.25 mR per second, do not produce visible flashes in a
period of several seconds. On the other hand, at a considerably higher dose rate of 24 mR sec^{-1}, a dose of
0.3 mR was sufficient to produce a generalized white
flash over the entire visual domain. This phenomenon is
dependent on the dose rate of X-ray quanta, whereas all
observations point to the expected proportionality between the number of flashes observed and the total number of neutrons.

The retinal architecture and neurophysiology are
not known in sufficient detail to explain all phenomena
with certainty. We offer the following as a starting
point for more elaborate experimental approaches. We
know that neural integration has a time constant: Events
in sensory elements must be nearly simultaneous to contribute to an image. The time constant is related to
the flicker-fusion frequency, which for light sensation,
is about 20 to 60 per second.

It is well known that the threshold for light re-
ception in the dark-adapted eye is about five photons
distributed over a small area [14]. Thus several rods
must receive one photon each in less than about 50 msec
in order for the subject to perceive light. These individual rods are synapsed to neutrons (bipolar and
horizontal cells) in the region between photoreceptors
(rods and cones) and ganglion cells in a highly complex
manner. The output of the ganglion cell to the brain
thus represents the spatial summation of inputs from a

variable number of rods depending on the cluster of pho-
ton-rod interactions and some as yet unknown bipolar or
horizontal cell modulation (or both).

We believe that the discrete star-like events that
we have seen result from discharge of 20 to 100 rods in
a very small area of the retina. High-LET particles have
associated dense ionization, and we believe that they can
cause energy absorption leading to electrical signals in
a number of neighboring rods they cross. It is possible
that in a 10-μ-diam region of the eye as many as 20 rods
(1.3 μ diam) are activated, giving the sensation of a
pinpoint bright light.

Diffuse light perception such as experienced by
electrical or X-ray phosphenes probably results from the
integrated response of perhaps one in 10,000 rods. The
ionization created by X-rays is relatively evenly distributed across the retina. Local energy density is
nowhere high, and the mechanisms for creating contrast
are absent. Thus, it is reasonable to expect a "gray"
or "white" flash over the whole visual field; and this
is what was observed. There is a low probability of
many ionizing events in a local area, as is the case for
high-LET particles. Hence, one does not expect to see
luminous "stars" from diffuse X-radiation.

There is a contrast mechanism that favors visibility
of high-LET particles. At the low intensity used in our
experiments, the energy is concentrated in the densely
ionizing tracks; there is considerable distance between
particles. In the intervening space there is practically
no ionization at all, providing a light-to-dark contrast
between track core and surrounding region.

*Location of the Primary Interaction Between Radiation and
Tissue to Produce Flashes*

The studies described here suggest that exposure of
regions at or near the eye is responsible for appearance
of visual flashes. It has been known for sometime that
photosensitive receptors or muscle fibers in various
species can be stimulated to produce action potential or

contraction (or both) with a much smaller radiation dose,
by several orders of magnitude, than nerves, receptors,
or muscle fibers that are not sensitive to light stimulation [15]. However, in principle, any part of the
nervous system that participates in handling of visual
information, including the optic nerve and the cerebral
cortex, could be a site of interaction for a visual
signal. For example, the occipital lobe has been suggested as a possible stimulation site [16]. However,
it has been shown that X-ray phosphenes are not produced
by irradiation of the optic tract and visual cortex [17].
It is, of course, possible to direct small doses of fast
particles or neutron irradiation to a preselected site,
and definitive experiments using neutrons or heavy-part-
icle-induced phosphenes are planned to explore the role
played by the optic track or visual cortex.

Within the eye, the retina is prime candidate for
the locus of interaction with radiation. The vitreous
humor and iris, though they strongly fluoresce, appear
to play only a minor role as a site of action for production of X-ray phosphenes [18]. Lipetz [13] has shown
that visual purple can be bleached *in vitro* by a very
high dose of X-rays. On the other hand, a few secondary electrons in an X-ray beam, impinging on the retina,
can alter neural responses in the frog optic nerve.

In man, it is more likely that rods are affected,
rather than cones, as evidenced by the lack of specific
color of the flashes. If the action of particles is
due to ionization or excitation, then it seems likely
that the particles must pass through the light-sensitive
cells (e.g., rods) that they affect.

The Possibility of Aftereffect

We already know that a small dose of X-rays administered to the retina effects retinal threshold for
an appreciable period afterwards [19], and this is also
true for electrical effects on frog retina [13]. Most
of such effects are believed to be reversible. An important aspect of future studies should be evaluation of
such aftereffects following heavy-particle exposure.

Geometric Considerations

Exposure to a lateral beam of neutrons that passed through both eyes caused sensation of small luminous stars with tails (Fig. 3A), quite similar to the appearance of short electron tracks in the continuously expanding cloud chamber. When the beam passed head-on into one eye only, the stars appeared to be better localized and had no tails (Fig. 3B). Subjectively, it was impossible to tell whether the observations were made with one eye or both eyes.

The appearance of tracks in lateral view might signify the existence of "streaks" or tracks within the retina, with the older part of the track appearing fainter as it becomes extinct. However, it is also possible that the tails are optical illusions and are the result of an unsuccessful effort to focus the eyes on the origin of the light. This is ilustrated in Fig. 4. Initially, when the subject's eyes are pointing forward, a flash at A on the retina may cause the illusion that there is a luminous source at point P external to the subject. The subject instinctively turns his eyes toward P; during these eye movements the location of the source appears to recede to P' as light sensation fades. The subject thus has the subjective sensation of seeing a luminous star and a track between P and P'.

Two different stars produced simultaneously by two independent particles, one in each eye, may create the illusion that both images originate from one point in space.

Biological Effects of Heavy Ions in Relation to Light Flashes

Evidence is accumulating to show that light flashes and streaks observed in spaceflight are indications of heavy primary cosmic rays crossing the eye and retina. The flux of nuclei in the iron group is about 160 cm^{-2} day in a 4π solid angle, whereas that of the C, N, O group is more than 10 times as great [20]. We know that X-rays at 2000 R dose can cause irreversible degeneration of the light-sensing cells of the retina and

of the electroretinogram;[21] however, the damage might
be reversible at 1000 R [22]. The minute ionizing core
of heavy nuclei represents an energy exchange that corresponds to more than 10 [8] rads in dose terms within
a few angstroms of the core. If passage of such particles causes irreversible deterioration of retinal cells
and of neurons, then in spaceflights of long duration
(several months or more) outside the earth's magneto-
sphere a significant degree of random cellular damage
may result.

SUMMARY AND CONCLUSIONS

1. When a high-energy neutron beam from the Berkeley 184-
inch cyclotron was passed through the region of one or
both eyes in two human subjects, both subjects observed
many small, star-like light flashes.

2. The energy of the neutrons was greater than 20 MeV
and less than 640 MeV, with maximum fluence around 300
MeV. At 1.4×10^4 neutrons sec^{-1} cm^{-2}, about 25 to 50
star flashes were seen at any given time in the visual
field, seemingly more at the periphery and fewer at the
center. The dose rate was about 0.1 mR/sec, or about
1.25 mrem/sec. The beam was on for several seconds.

3. The same dark-adapted subjects observed no similar
star-like flashes, over a period of 1 hour, when the
beam was off. The subjects saw no such light flashes
over 30- to 60-min periods in dark adaptation while fly-
ing in a plane at 10,000 meters at geomagnetic latitudes
of 60°N and 40°N.

4. A beam of π^+ mesons at the Berkeley Bevatron (momentum 1.5 GeV/c, fluence 200 mesons cm^{-2} sec^{-1}) failed to
produce any kind of visual effect in one of the subjects,
exposed for a total of 6 sec.

5. A 250-kV X-ray beam failed to produce any kind of
light sensations at dose rate up to 1.25 mR/sec. This
dose rate is 12.5 times the neutron dose rate that produced the star-like light flashes.

6. Light flashes (phosphenes) due to X-ray exposure are seen only when the dose rates are twenty or more times as high as in the above cited neutron exposures. At a dose rate of 24 mR/sec, a dose of 0.3 mR can produce a flash. Such X-ray phosphenes are not localized; rather they flash across the whole visual field; they are of whitish-blue color.

7. Electrical phosphenes that can be produced by passing an electrical current though the retina are similar in timing and appearance to the X-ray phosphenes. Electrical stimulation of the visual apparatus does not result in star-like or pinpoint flashes.

8. It appears likely from the above observations that star-like flashes in high energy neutron fields are due to high-LET nuclear recoils (from spallation) when the neutrons interact with the nuclei of tissue. Since most recoil nuclei travel too slowly to produce Cerenkov effect, the visual phenomena are more likely due to ionization or excitation.

9. The lack of observations of light in a π^+ -meson beam would indicate that Cerenkov light from singly charged particles might be too weak to produce frequent light flashes. It is possible that Cerenkov light from multiply charged, fast nuclei, such as the particles of heavy primary cosmic rays, could produce an effect.

10. Since visual effects can be produced by exceedingly low doses of fast neutrons and of other radiations, well below the recognized permissible exposure limits, it appears feasible and safe to further explore the visual effects produced by fast, accelerated particles and to compare such effects observed at ground level with light flashes and streaks that have been observed by a number of astronauts in lunar flights. Of immediate interest are (a) the location of regions in the eye and brain that respond to particles by producing light sensation, (b) the LET (linear energy transfer) charge and velocity of particles that cause these effects, (c) the effects of small radiation doses on the responses of the eye to light stimuli, and (d) reversible and irreversible

sequelae of particle exposure and high energy proton irradiation on man's vision.

11. Since the star-like light flashes observed in space
and at accelerators appear to be caused by high-LET
particles, these findings call attention to the necessity of studying the biological effects of such particles,
particularly in tissues with nondividing cells, such as
brain and retina. The biological effects of such particles should be carefully evaluated before long-term,
manned spaceflight in interplanetary space or to the
planets.

ACKNOWLEDGMENT

The authors benefited from discussions of the flash
effect with Astronaut Edwin Aldrin, Dr. Charles Berry,
and Dr. Charles Barnes at a Committee Meeting of the
Radiobiological Advisory Panel of the Space Science
Board (Wright Langham, Chairman); with the staff of
Ames Research Center-NASA (Hans Mark, Director); and
with Dr. Richard Benson, Dr. Philip Chapman, Dr. G. Fazio,
Dr. Donald Hagge, and Dr. Larry Pinsky at the Manned
Spacecraft Center, Houston. We are indebted to Mr. Wade
Patterson and Dr. Ralph Thomas of the Health Physics
Department and Mr. Jimmy Vale and the operating crew of
the 184-inch cyclotron for their indispensable assist-
ance.

Since the International Congress of Radiation Research in June 1970, it has been learned that astronauts
on lunar flights Apollo 13, 14 and 15 regularly observed
light flashes and streaks. The authors have conducted
further experiments on the light flash phenomena at three
different accelerators.

Weak flashes of light have been observed by six subjects at the University of Washington's 60" cyclotron,

from neutrons of 25 MeV maximum energy*. Using accelerated helium ions of about 250 MeV kinetic energy it was shown that individual helium ions in the last cm of their path can produce light flashes and short streaks if they cross the retina of one eye (National Conference on Natural and Manmade Radiation in Space, Las Vegas, Nevada, March 1-4, 1971). Finally, three dark adapted subjects have been exposed to accelerated 4 GeV nitrogen (7+) particles at the Berkeley Bevatron and have reported observations of relatively intense streaks and stars due to individual particles (report in preparation). All these observations add to the evidence that individual heavy ionizing particles crossing the retina at nonrelativistic velocities often produce light sensation in human subjects.

REFERENCES

1.   From debriefing records and conversations with Appollo astronauts, Manned Spacecraft Center, Houston, Texas, 1970.

2.   LIPETZ, L.E., X-Ray and Radium Phosphenes, *Brit. J. Opthamol.*, *39*, 577-598, 1955.

3.   TOBIAS, C.A., Radiation Hazards in High Altitude Aviation, *J. Aviation Med.*, *23*, 345-372, 1952.

4.   TOBIAS, C.A., *Radiation Hazards in Space Flight*, UCRL-8115, Jan. 1958 (unpublished).

5.   D'ARCY, F.J. and PORTER, N.A., Detection of Cosmic Ray μ Mesons by the Human Eye, *Nature*, *196*, 1013, 1962.

6.   FREMLIN, J.H., Cosmic Ray Flashes, *New Scientist*, Letter to the Editor, July 2, 1970.

---

*T.F. Budinger, Hans Bichsel, and Cornelius Tobias, Visual Phenomena Noted by Human Subjects on Exposure to Neutrons of Energies Less Than 25 Million Electron Volts, *Science*, 172, 868-870, May 21, 1971.

7. FAZIO, G.G., JELLEY, J.V. and CHARMAN, W.N., Light Flashes Generated by Primary Cosmic Ray Nuclei Within the Eyes of Apollo Astronauts, 6th Inter-american Cosmic Ray Seminar, La Paz, Bolivia, July 19, 1970.

8. Presented by TOBIAS, C.A., BUDINGER, T.F. and LYMAN, J.T. at the Symposium on Space Radiobiology of the Fourth International Congress of Radiation Research, Evian, France, June 29, 1970.

9. McCASLIN, J.P., A High Energy Neutron Flux Detector, *Health Phys.*, 2, 399-407, 1960.

10. PAPE, R. and ZAKOVSKY, J., Die Röntgen-Strahlensensi-bilität der Retina, *Fortschr. Gebiete Röntgenstrahlen*, 80, 65-71, 1954.

11. BUDINGER, T.F., *Indirect Electrical Stimulation of Visual Apparatus*, UCRL-18347, 1968 (unpublished).

12. JELLEY, J.V., *Cherenkov Radiation and Its Applications* (Pergamon Press, London, 1958).

13. LIPETZ, L.E., *An Electrophysiological Study of Some Properties of the Vertebrate Retina* (Ph.D. thesis), UCRL-2056, Jan. 1953 (unpublished).

14. HECHT, S., SHLAER, S. and PIRENNE, M., Energy, Quanta, and Vision, *J. Gen. Physiol.*, 25, 819-840, 1942.

15. GANGLOFF, H. and HUG, O., The Effects of Ionizing Radiation on the Nervous System, In: *Advances in Biological and Medical Physics*, Academic Press, N.Y., pp. 1-90, 1965.

16. HAYMAKER, W. (Ames Research Center, NASA), private communication.

17. GURTOVOI, G.K. and BURDIANSKAIA, Y.O., Exact Dose of
     X-Irradiation of Various Regions of the Head and
     Visual Sensations, *Biofizika, 5,* 354-361, 1960,
     translated.

18. NEWELL, R.R. and BORLEY, W.E., Roentgen Measure-
     ment of Visual Acuity in Cataractous Eyes, *Radio-
     logy, 37,* 54-61, 1941.

19. MOTOKAWA, K., KOHATA, T., KOMATSU, M., CHICHIBU, S.,
     KOGA, Y. and KASAI, T., A Sensitive Method for De-
     tecting the Effect of Radiation Upon the Human Body,
     Tohoku J. Exptl. Med., 66, 389-404, 1957.

20. FOWLER, P.H., ADAMS, R.A., COWEN, V.G. and KIDD,
     J.M., The Charge Spectrum of Very Heavy Cosmic Ray
     Nuclei, *Proc. Roy. Soc. (London) A., 301,* 39-45,
     1967.

21. GAFFEY, C., Bioelectric Sensitivity to Radiation of
     the Retina and Visual Pathways, In: *International
     Symposium on the Response of the Nervous System to
     Ionizing Radiation,* 2d, Los Angeles, 1963, Ed.
     Thomas J. Haley and Roy S. Smith, (Little-Brown,
     Boston, 1964, pp. 243-270).

22. MARMUR, R.K. and MANTURO, N.A., On the Vulnerability
     of the Retinal Membrane of the Eye to X-Rays,
     Radiobiologica, 6 [3], 431-433, 1966.

ON THE ROLE OF RADIO-PREVENTIVE SUBSTANCES IN THE CREATION OF BIOCHEMICAL RADIORESISTENCE BACKGROUND

Yu.B. KUDRYASHOV and E. GONCHARENKO

Moscow State University, U.S.S.R.

According to vast material in radio-biological literature the radio-protective substances provoke numerous disturbances of biochemical processes. The irradiation of an object takes place against the background of these numerous changes. It won't be correct to assume that all the changes in organisms and cells caused by the injection of radio-protective drugs increase the radioresistance of the organism. Of all the changes we must distinguish those, which cause radioresistance of the organism. If we take into consideration only one process or one group of substances there is some danger that we can lay obstacles for the further investigation of the mechanisms of radio-protective effect.

We have in view the study of those substances in organisms which could provoke the radio-protective effect themselves. That's why in this paper we study the andogenic drugs, serotonin and hystamin as well as andogenic radiosensitizer - e.g.; Lipid Toxic Substances (LTS).

We assumed that even slight changes of the quantity of biogenic radiosensitizers and the increase of andogenic substances with the potential radio-protective effect can't be indifferent in the mechanism of radioresistance.

Some part of the injected radio-protector penetrates

into the cell; that's why the additional increase of
the substance in the cell, having the radio-protective
effect is able to strengthen it.

MATERIALS AND METHODS

The male laboratory rats were the material under
investigation: the body weigh 120-150 grams. The water solution of radio-protector was injected to animals.
After various periods of time the serotonin content [2]
in various organs and tissues was measured together
with the activity and the content of the oxidized products of high unsaturated fatty acids (The polarography
method [1]) and phospholipids (The thin-layer chromo-
tography). The conditions for hypoxia were arranged in
a special camera by means of lowering the air pressure
to 200 mm of mercury column. The radiation exposure,
whole-body and single on the cobalt installation (the
power is 50 rads per minute). The criterion of the protective effect of the drugs was the magnitude-the factor
of decrease of the dose (FDD by LD 50/30).

1. *Decrease of Radiosensibility Effect is one of the*
   Factors Provoking the Background of High Radio-
   resistance

In our previous papers [1] it was shown that Lipid
Toxic Substances (LTS) present a damageable complex,
which consists of hydroperoxides, apoxides, aldehydes
and ketones of high unsaturated fatty acids. The LTS
drugs, obtained from the tissues of irradiated animals
have the radiomimetic effect on different biological
systems and objects, e.g., rats, mice erythrocytes,
yeast cells, ascid carcinomas, cells and intercellular
structures.

One of the most convenient methods of determining
the LTS activity is the eritrogram, used in this paper.

It was previously shown that the radiosensitive
activity of LTS depends not only on the content of

oxidized products in cells, but also on the fraction
of loose-tied phospholipids, e.g., inhibitors LTS.
Therefore, in this paper, besides the quantitative
determination of LTS, we studied the content of
tissue phospholipids.

Having discovered the direct dependence between
the radiosensibility and the LTS activity in various
biological objects [1], we assumed that one of the
factors increasing the radioresistance, is the reduction of LTS activity in the tissues of animals.

The results of the experiments are shown in Table 1.

The table shows that the hypoxia and the injection
to rats of the highly effective radio-protective substances (AET, MAA-β-mercapto-atil-amin, 5HT - five hy-
droxytryptamin), belonging to different classes of chemical drugs reduce the LTS activity in a number of tissues. This decrease depends on the reduction of the
quantity of the oxidized products of high unsaturated
fatty acids and (or) on the increase of the phospholipids content. For example, the injection of 5HT pro-
vokes the decrease in the quantity of peroxides and the
LTS activity in the small intestine, without changing the
content of phospholipids, while in the testes and liver the level of phospholipids increases reliably. But
the LTS activity and the quantity of peroxide remains
unchanged.

The injection of control drugs (serin or physiological solution) into rats (the drugs have no radioprotective activity) significantly influences neither the
LTS activity nor the content of the oxidized products,
nor of their inhibitors, e.g. phospholipids.

The tables reflect the changes in tissues of
animals during maximum radioresistance period, that is
15 minutes after the injection of radio-protectors and
5 minutes after the creation of the maximum hypoxia condition. The changes in LTS activity of oxidized products and in the quantity of phospholipids in the entire
process of high radioresistance are presented in Table 1.

TABLE 1 . LTS and PhL in the Tissues of Rats after the

Dose of substance (mg /kg)	Time after injection	Factor of dose decrease by LD 50/30	LTS Small Intestine
Hypoxia 215 mm of mercury column	at once	1.6	1.02±0.09 / 89±6
	past 3 minutes		1.08±0.10 / 102±6
5 - HT (60)	15 minutes	1.4	0.68±0.02** / 81±3**
	4 hours		0.90±0.07 / 97±3
	6 hours		1.09±0.08 / 101 ± 2
6 MOT	15 minutes	1.0	0.98±0.07 / 100±2
AET (250)	15 minutes	1.4	0.81±0.04** / 73±7**
	4 hours		0.84±0.06 / 93±3
	6 hours		1.04±0.07 / 120±12
MET (400)	15 minutes	1.5	0.84±0.03*** / 84±4
	1 hour		0.86±0.05*** / 98±6
	3 hours		1.05±0.08 / 98±3
Serin (1200)	15 minutes	1.0	0.96±0.08 / 96±5
Norm			1.0 / 100±3

Above line: Coefficient of LTS activity = Time of 50% hemolys:
(control/experimen

Below line: LTS content in %
*p<0.001, **p<0.01, ***p<0.02

Injection of Radio-protectors and Hypoxia Condition

LTS		Phospholipids (%)		
Testes	Liver	Small Intestine	Testes	Liver
0.09±06** / 70±3*	1.00±0.08 / 84±4**	113±8	102±5	146±2**
1.04±0.07 / 106±5	1.00±0.09 / 104±5	102 ±5	102±5	87±8*
0.96±0.08 / 103±3	0.97±0.06 / 100±3	113 ±6	131±5**	146±3*
1.04±0.08 / 109±10	1.10±0.09 / 121 ±21	85±4*	102±2	102±1*
1.01±0.07 / 100±3	1.00±0.07 / 102±2	78±1*	85±4*	100±2
1.04±0.09 / 100±3	0.98±0.08 / 105±7	100±1	101±2	98±2
0.78±0.02** / 73±8**	0.96±0.10 / 82±2**	108±7	100±4	94±2***
0.89±0.08 / 100±6	1.15±0.10 / 125±12	90±4	102±1	100±1
0.98±0.07 / 98± 4	1.00±0.09 / 98±14	122±6**	100±1	81±1*
0.91±0.02** / 92±10	0.96±0.01 / 97 ±6	92±3	97±5	114±3*
0.99±0.05 / 98±5	1.00±0.06 / 100±4	80±2*	100±1	106±1*
1.00±0.06 / 100±3	1.05±0.07 / 100±2	95±3	100±1	109±1
1.13±0.11 / 97±5	0.97±0.10 / 105±6	102±2	100±1	102±2
1.0 / 100±3	1.0 / 100±2	100±2	100±3	100±2

The table shows that the maximum changes of the investigated products are observed in the maximum radioresistance period of animals (15 minutes after the injection of drugs). Then it decreases and disappears
completely in 4 - 6 hours after the injection or at
the beginning of the hypoxia condition, namely, during
the extinction period of the high background of radioresistance.

2. *The Content in Tissues of Animals of Andogenic*
    Serotonin and Histamine during the Period of
    High Radioresistance

The content changes in tissues of serotonin and
histamine can't be indifferent to the organism, when
we have a radio-protective effect because, the biogenic
amines themselves have the antiradiation capacity. The
serotonin and histamine content in tissues was studied
after the injection of drugs, having various activity.
Thus, from Table 2, it is clear that the active radio-
protector substances, e.g., aminothiols, provoke a considerable increase of the serotonin content in the small
intestine, stomach and spleen.

In the liver and brain the increase of the serotonin quantity occurs only in case of some active radio-
protective drugs, and these changes are not essential.
The substances of the average radio-protective activity (that is histamine and adrenalin) bring about only
a slight increase of serotonin in tissues. The control drugs of alamine and serin, as well as the physiological solution don't cause any definite changes of
serotonin in tissues.

The hypoxia causing a high radio-protective effect
doesn't change the level of serotonin in any of the
exploratory tissues. Probably this factor is to be
investigated once again, and once more discussed.

What is the mechanism of the serotonin in the tissues under the influence of aminothiols. To answer this

TABLE 2. Serotonin Content in Tissues of Rats 10 minutes after the Injection of Radio-protective Substances (mg/g)
loose-tied form
whole form

Substance	Small intestine	Stomach	Liver	Brain	Spleen
AET	3.07+0.30	2.56+0.23	0.35+0.04	0.36+0.03	-
	4.16+0.47	4.30+0.39	0.64+0.06	0.51+0.05	-
Cystaphos	1.51+0.51	2.29+0.16	0.38+0.04	0.34+0.04	-
	3.95+0.40	3.41+0.17	0.64+0.05	0.84+0.04	-
MEA	1.95+0.18	2.01+0.20	0.39+0.04	0.42+0.04	1.50+0.12
	3.87+0.31	3.83+0.19	0.54+0.04	0.73+0.06	5.26+0.31
Cystamine	2.14+0.23	2.31+0.14	0.46+0.05	0.38+0.04	2.70+0.15
	5.05+0.37	3.96+0.04	1.03+0.08	0.79+0.08	5.45+0.33
Cysteine	0.66+0.05	1.83+0.14	0.45+0.05	0.40+0.03	-
	3.46+0.31	4.15+0.26	0.61+0.06	0.81+0.05	-
Alanine	0.66+0.07	1.79+0.16	0.35+0.03	0.35+0.03	-
	2.90+0.25	3.08+0.28	0.56+0.06	0.69+0.07	-
Serin	0.60+0.03	1.62+0.08	0.35+0.02	0.37+0.02	-
	2.04+0.17	2.80+0.19	0.65+0.04	0.68+0.07	-
Hystamine	0.87+0.07	1.92+0.12	0.44+0.03	0.37+0.03	1.87+0.11
	2.96+0.13	3.42+0.21	0.73+0.06	0.62+0.05	3.51+0.27
Adrenalin	0.60+0.06	1.73+0.15	0.37+0.04	0.38+0.04	1.86+0.09
	3.40+0.03	2.82+0.23	0.79+0.08	0.65+0.07	5.04+0.18
Hypoxia	0.71+0.07	1.80+0.10	0.39+0.03	0.46+0.04	1.69+0.14
	2.25+0.23	2.46+0.31	0.57+0.04	0.73+0.06	3.27+0.31
Control	0.71+0.07	1.75+0.14	0.35+0.02	0.36+0.02	1.87+0.07
	2.55+0.20	2.97+0.22	0.61+0.05	0.66+0.05	3.45+0.25

question we studied the activity of the enzymes responsible for the new formation and disturbance of this biogenic amine, e.g., -5-oxytryptophandecarboxilase (OTDC)
and monoaminoxidase (MO).

As it is clear from the Table 3 the 5-OTDC activity increases considerably after the injection of the
effective amine-alkyl-thiols whereas the activity of MO
doesn't change as a rule. A slight decrease of MO activity in the small intestine was observed only after
the injection of AET. If we compare these results with
those of serotonin both whole and loose-tied, we may ar-
rive at a conclusion that the injection of aminothiols
strengthenthe process of new formation of serotonin in
tissues due to the activation of 5-OTDC.

The increase of loose-tied forms is the sign of
its release: the change of another biogenic amine, e.g.,
histamine in tissues under the influence of radio-protectors differ from that of serotonin. Table 4
shows that not only active drugs of aminothiols but
also indolyl-alkyl-amines as well as hypoxia provoke a
considerable increase of hystamine level in tissues.

The control drug serin doesn't bring about the increase of either loose or whole hystamine in any of the
investigated tissues. Particularly considerable changes
occur in the content of the whole histamine. The increase of the whole and loose-tied histamine in tissues is the sign of the release of andogenic histamine
under the influence of radio-protectors as well as of
their new formation.

With respect to the given factual material about
the change of biogenic amines, we can draw the following conclusion: during the maximum radioresistance of
rats, created in the first minute after the injection
of radio-protectors of hypoxia condition there occurs
the new formation and loosening of histamine. Aminothiols give rise to another new formation and loosening of serotonin. To make the question about the association of the investigated change with the disturbances in radioresistance under the influence of radio-

TABLE 3. Enzyme Activity after the Radio-protector Injection to Rats

	Substances	Dose mg/kg	Small intestine	Stomach	Liver	Brain
MO (µm NH₃/hr)	AET	310	10.9±1.1 p<0.05	8.3±0.41 —	8.45±0.45 —	—
	Cystamine	200	16.0±1.22	7.44±0.42	7.8±0.59	—
	Norm		14.7±0.9	8.3±0.5	8.7±0.14	—
5OTDK (µmg/mg 5HT/hr)	Cystamine	200	36.1±3.4 p<0.01	0.51±0.05	31.5±2.8 p<0.03	5.22±0.6 —
	Cystaphos	461	39.4±1.9 p<0.01	0.54±0.06	34.8±2.1 p<0.01	4.7±0.5 —
	MEA	180	44.8±2.4 p<0.001	0.56±0.06	39.4±3.7 p<0.001	7.0±0.5
	AET	310	32.7±0.96 p<0.001	0.38±0.04	35.2±2.7 p<0.02	5.48±0.6
	Norm		19.6±0.97	0.54±0.03	22.8±0.72	4.8±0.4

TABLE 4. Histamine Content in Tissues of Rats 10 minutes after the Injection of Radio-protective Drugs (mg/g) loose form whole form

Substance	Skin	Stomach	Liver	Kidney
AET	15.3±0.8 / 53.0±1.1	10.8±0.6 / 26.7±0.9	7.2±0.4 / 12.4±1.1	5.0±0.3 / 10.1±0.7
MEA	12.2±0.7 / 59.5±1.9	11.5±0.5 / 27.5±1.1	6.9±0.5 / 9.9±0.8	5.7±0.3 / 12.1±1.1
Cystamine	14.6±0.9 / 50.4±1.2	10.9±0.9 / 27.0±1.3	9.7±0.7 / 15.1±1.2	5.4±0.4 / 15.0±1.2
Serin	13.7±0.5 / 31.3±1.0	11.0±0.6 / 20.4±1.0	6.5±0.4 / 10.8±1.0	3.7±0.3 / 8.6±0.7
Serotonin	18.6±0.8 / 56.8±1.1	15.7±0.9 / 55.0±1.5	8.05±0.7 / 13.5±0.9	5.8±0.4 / 15.0±1.2
Control	12.7±0.5 / 37.2±2.9	11.5±0.4 / 20.3±1.7	6.3±0.2 / 9.3±0.7	4.4±0.1 / 9.7±0.8

protective means clear, we studied the amine content in various periods after the injection of the substances.

The maximum accumulation of amines occurs in the period cf high radioresistance, namely, 15 minutes after the drug injection. After 4 to 7 hours the content of amines becomes fully normal.

The given data show that after the drug injection the increase of biogenic amines is only during the period of high radioresistance.

Special emphasis is placed on the fact that not only andogenic serotonin and histamine are able to raise the biochemical background of radioresistance. First and foremost it concerns the substances, including SH-groups, as well as a number of biologically active substances which are not mentioned in this paper (Bacq and Concly).

Considering the question about the reasons of the

radioresistance background increase on the whole, we must once again emphasize that one of these reasons is the complex of changes, including the increase of the andogenic substances having radio-protective effect and decrease of biogenic radiosensibilizers in cells. The injection to organism of different from the point of view of their chemical structure radio-protectors may, in various ways influence separate links of the entire complex of changes which provoke the short-time increase of radioresistance of organisms.

CONCLUSION

One of the reasons of the increase of radioresistance caused by the injection of radio-protectors is the complex of changes: the decrease of the activity of biogenic radiosensibilizers (LTS) and the increase of the content of the andogenics of serotonin and histamine

REFERENCES

1.   KUDRYASHOV, YU., and GONCHARENKO, E.N., On the role of biologically active substances (radiotoxins) in radiation damage, *Radiobiology*, *10*, 2, 212, 1970.

2.   YUDENFRIEND, S., Fluorescence assay in biology and medicine N.Y., L., 1962.

HEAVY GALACTIC PARTICLES

P.H. FOWLER

*H.H. Wills Physics Laboratory, Tyndall Avenue,
Bristol B58, ITL, England*

The cosmic ray primaries were shown to be nuclei of various elements over 20 years ago, when photographic emulsion was flown by balloon at a sufficient altitude to sample the primary radiation. In these early experiments primaries with Z = 2, and the CNO group and nuclei up to and including Fe, Z = 26, were found to be prominent.

A remarkable feature of the cosmic radiation is the high energy possessed by many of the primaries - the median energy is $\sim$ 1. Ge V/nucleon - a figure much higher for complex nuclei than any radiation available for study in the laboratory.

Fig. 1 shows examples of tracks of relativistic nuclei in photographic emulsion from the early work. The track density in photographic emulsion is not proportional to the rate of energy loss - at high values of charge and velocity the track center is saturated and the overall response is closely proportional to the energy deposited by δ-rays having an initial energy $\gtrsim$ 20 keV. The energy deposited per unit volume is given for emulsion by the relation:

$$\rho = 2.4 \frac{Z^2}{\beta^2 \Gamma_\mu{}^2} \left| 1 + 0.012 \ln \frac{\beta^2}{1-\beta^2} \right| \text{ eV } (\mu m)^{-3},$$

$$\text{for } \beta > 0.25 \left[\Gamma_\mu\right]^{0.30}$$

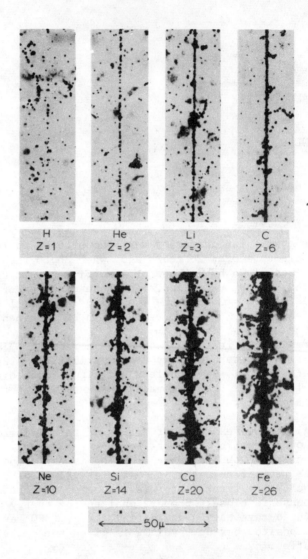

Fig. 1. Photomicrographs of segments of tracks produced by relativistic
heavy nuclei of the Cosmic Radiation. The kinetic energy was
determined to be excess of 1 GeV/nucleon from measurement of the
small degree of multiple coulomb scattering on the track length
available, which exceeded 1 cm for each track.

Γ_μ is the perpendicular distance from the track, measured
in microns. The restriction on the values for β follows
because of the need for $r \ll R_{max}$, the range of a δ-ray
with an energy at the kinematic limit. At lower values
of high energy δ-rays. See Fig. 2.

In the early work using photographic emulsion as the
detector, the two ways in which these heavy primaries are
attenuated was vividly demonstrated. They are:
   (a) being brought to rest through ionisation loss,
and
   (b) undergoing nuclear interactions.

Fig. 2 shows an example of the track of a cosmic ray
primary coming to rest in emulsion - the track shows a
characteristic taper towards the end of its range - as explained above.

Fig. 3 shows a nuclear interaction of an Fe primary
of relatively low energy, $\sim$ 100 MeV/n. This illustration
emphasizes an important feature of these interactions,
the incoming nucleus is not necessarily destroyed,
usually a substantial fragment remains which emerges from
the collision with very nearly the same speed and direction as that of the incident nucleus. Other fragments,
principally α-particles, proton and neutrons often may
emerge with similar speeds and direction to that of the
incident nucleus.

Recent work has given us much improved resolution of
charge and estimation of energy. At lower energies the
best measurements for discussion here have been made on
satellites, and at higher energies the heavier payloads
needed, still required balloon exposures. In each case
the charge resolution is $\sim$ 0.3 charges over the whole
spectrum. The principal results of these beautiful experiments may be summarised:
   (a) The charge spectrum seems to be well established
up to Z = 26, and to be almost independent of the energy/
nucleon (or speed) of the particles. The small differences in energy spectra for various charges are of course
very interesting and informative concerning the source
and propagation of the cosmic rays but perhaps need not

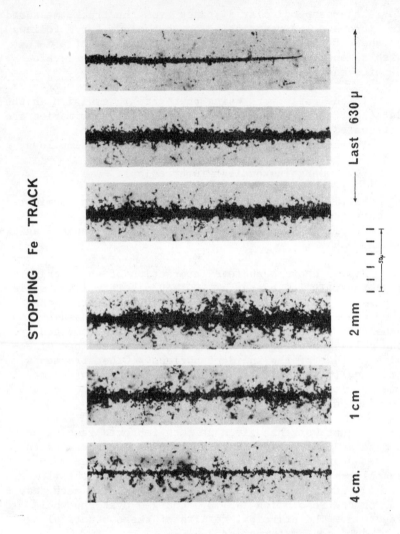

Fig. 2. Photomicrographs of segments of a track of an Fe nucleus of long
         range that come to rest in a stack of emulsion pellicles of total
         volume ∿ 5 litres. The characteristic taper is clearly visible
         in the last few hundred microns of track. The maximum energy
         loss occurs at a residual range ∿ 20μ, whereas the maximum num-
         ber of Ag grains occurs at a residual range ∿ 1mm when the en-
         ergy is ∿ 50 MeV/n.

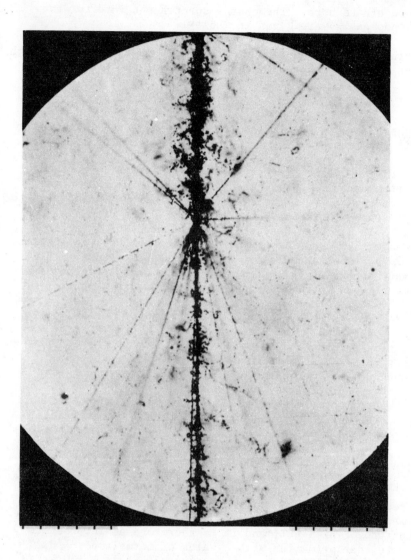

Fig. 3. Photomicrograph of an interaction of an Fe nucleus of energy ∿ 100 MeV/n with a nucleus of Ag or Br of the photographic emulsion. A substantial fragment of the incoming nucleus survives the encounter and emerges with only a small deflection. Twelve other fragements from both collisions partners can be discerned, many pass out of focus within a short distance.

concern us here. The charge spectra obtained for two
bands energy are given in Table 1.

(b) The energy spectrum has a peak at a value of
kinetic energy/nucleon of 0.3 Ge V/n and falls off at higher energies according to the empirical relation

$$dN \propto \left(\frac{E}{A}\right)^{-2.5} dE$$

where $E = T + Mc^2$ is the total energy, and A is the atomic mass number.

The energy spectra, obtained principally from satellite work, are illustrated in Fig. 4. The graphs are
from the review article of P. Meyer, 1969. In addition to
the recent work for $Z \leq 26$, a low fluence of nuclei with
$Z \gg 26$ has been detected from the study of large area
photographic emulsion detectors flown by balloon (Fowler
1967). Some examples of these tracks are shown in Fig. 5
and, as one might expect, the tracks are prodigious in
comparison to the far more abundant tracks of nuclei of
more modest charge. Their abundance is $\sim 10^{-4}$ of Fe nuclei or $\sim 3 \times 10^{-8}$ of all cosmic rays! Nevertheless we
have obtained ~ 200 tracks and there promises to be ex-
citing information about the cosmic ray source and propagation of the cosmic rays from this rare component. The
spectrum of energy/nucleon for this component appears
from our preliminary measurements to be the same as that
of the lighter elements. The relative abundance of various charge groups is shown in Table 1. The available
data pertain mainly to high energy particles as indicated.

From the known Z and energy spectrum of the cosmic
ray primary radiation we can determine the spectrum of
dE/dx expected - as shown in Fig. 6. Also indicated
separately are the contributions from significant elements or groups of elements. We are concerned with radiations of high LET, and it is therefore of interest to
note that primaries with a value of normalised $dE/dx \sim$
676, (relativistic Fe) or a value of $LET_{(\infty)} \sim 130$ keV/μ
have a fluence of ~ 1.3 m^{-2} ster^{-1} sec^{-1}, and are contributed almost exclusively by the Fe group. One does not
have to be so concerned about the more abundant primaries with lower charge. The ultra heavy nuclei appear to

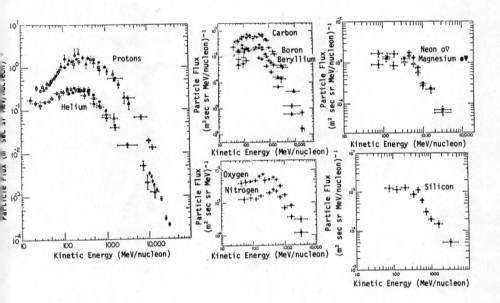

Fig. 4. Energy spectra for various elements in the Cosmic Rays, reprinted from the review article by P. Meyer.

TEXAS   1966

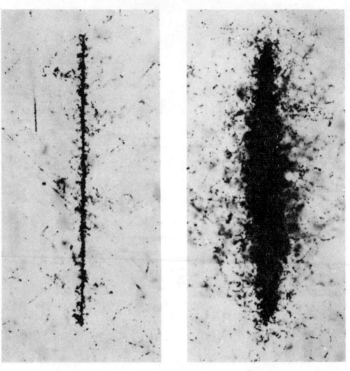

Fe Z = 26   Z = ~ 90

Comparison of tracks of Fe nucleus and that
of a very heavy primary.

Fig. 5.   Photomicrograph of the first track of an ultra-heavy primary.
          The particle was known to be fast as it penetrated $\sim$ 4g/cm^2
          of detector with no discernable change in track density.

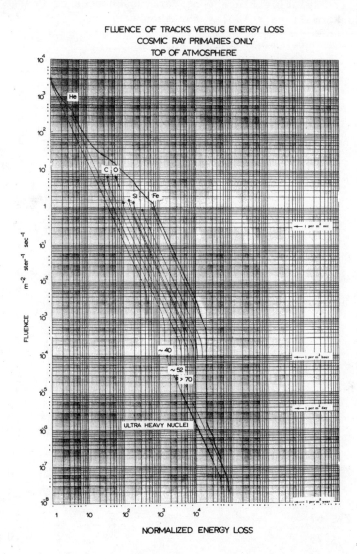

FLUENCE OF TRACKS VERSUS ENERGY LOSS
COSMIC RAY PRIMARIES ONLY
TOP OF ATMOSPHERE

NORMALIZED ENERGY LOSS

Fig. 6.   Fluence of tracks having values of normalised energy loss in
          excess of the figure quoted. Unit energy loss is that for a
          proton of minimum ionisation, i.e. ~ 2 MeV cm^2 g^{-1} in H$_2$O.
          Contributions from individual elements or groups of elements
          are indicated. The dominance of the Fe group in the interval
          $6 \times 10^2 - 2 \times 10^4$ for the normalised energy loss is apparent.

Table 1. Relative Fluence of Various Charges or Charge
Groups Normalised to Unity for the Fe Group.

Element	50-200 MeV/n	> 1.5 GeV/n
H	1600	3300
He	300	330
Li	1.3	2.0
Be	0.6	1.1
B	2.2	2.6
C	6.7	7.5
N	1.6	2.2
O	6.7	6.7
F	0.03	0.1
Ne	1.2	1.4
Na	0.3	0.3
Mg	1.9	1.6
Al	0.2	0.4
Si	1.3	1.4
P - V	0.8	0.9
Cr-Ni (Fe Group)	1.0	1.0
$29 \leq Z \leq 35$	unknown	uncertain
$36 \leq Z \leq 43$	"	2×10^{-5}
$44 \leq Z \leq 51$	"	2×10^{-5}
$52 \leq Z \leq 59$	"	1.2×10^{-5}
$60 \leq Z \leq 67$	"	4×10^{-6}
$68 \leq Z \leq 75$	"	8×10^{-6}
$76 \leq Z \leq 83$	"	5×10^{-6}
$84 \leq Z$	"	6×10^{-6}

be so rare that unless one is concerned with values of
LET$_\infty$ > 4000 keV/μ, their contribution is overshadowed by
the slowing members of the Fe group. The fluence tracks
with LET$_\infty$ $\gtrsim$ 10 MeV/μ is only $\sim$ 10/m^2 year.

We must also be concerned with the propagation of the
cosmic rays through tissue or shielding. Nuclear interactions mentioned earlier certainly reduce the ionising
power of the primary as its secondaries produce less ionisation. More significant is the reduction of fluence as
a result of primaries being brought to rest. The range
spectrum of primaries can be calculated from Z $\propto$ E spectrum and is shown in Fig. 7. It is empirically well
filled by:

$$\left[\frac{dN}{N}\right]_Z \simeq \frac{0.267}{(X + R) + 33.3 \dfrac{A}{Z^2}} \, ,$$

for
$$(X + R) \frac{Z^2}{A} \gtrsim 400 \text{ g/cm}^2$$

where $\frac{dN}{N}$ is the proportion stopping per g/cm^2 of any component with charge Z and atomic mass number A, possessing
a residual range R under X g/cm^2 of shielding. Also
shown in Fig. 6 are the range spectra under various quantities of overlying material X. It is seen that the number of short range and hence heavily ionising primaries is
rapidly reduced by quite small quantities of matter.
This process is much more effective than that of nuclear
interaction at reducing the fluence. Table 2 gives some
representative figures. Using the empirical formula we
see that passage through an amount of material equal to

$$y = \frac{33.3A}{Z^2} \quad \text{g/cm}^2$$

results in an attenuation of the number of very low range
particles by a factor of y + 1. At high values of LET
where the Fe group dominates the value of

$$\frac{33.3A}{Z^2} \simeq 2.7 \text{ g/cm}^2$$

so that the space capsule and the human body provide appreciable shielding.

Table 2. Mean Free Paths for Nuclear Interaction and
Attenuation by Ionisation for Cosmic Ray Primaries in H_2O.

Primary	Nuclear λ_I	Ionisation $\div 2$	$\div 10$
^1H	80 g/cm^2	33 g/cm^2	300 g/cm^2 H_2O
^4He	46	33	300
^{12}C	27	11	100
^{16}O	23	8	75
^{28}Si	17	5	43
^{56}Fe	12	2.7	25
^{90}Zr	8.8	1.9	17
^{126}Te	7.2	1.6	14
^{190}Pt	5.6	1.0	9.4
^{238}U	4.9	0.8	7.3

The estimates provided above used data collected 4
or 5 years ago. More recent data refers to a phase of
the Solar sunspot cycle when the magnetic shielding provided by the enhanced solar activity provides a considerable measure of shielding for low energy primaries in
the vicinity of the earth. Even when the lowest values
of solar activity prevail - as in 1966 there seems likely to be appreciable shielding in the vicinity of the
earth. It is possible that in the region of the orbit
of Jupiter and at greater distances from the sun the
fluence of that low energy heavy primaries may be as high
as 2 or 3 times that given for 1966, and used as the
basis of calculation for Figs. 6 and 7.

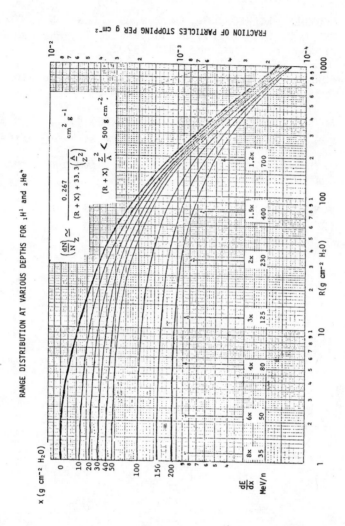

Fig. 7. The differential range distribution for primary Cosmic Ray H
and He nuclei is plotted under various amounts of shielding,
X. Also indicated is the energy scale and the value of $\frac{dE}{dx}$
normalised to the minimum value for the appropriate charge.
An empirical formula is also given which applies to all values
of Z for the range of R + X indicated.

REFERENCES

CORYDEN PETERSON, O., DAYTON, B., LUND, N., MELGAARD, K., OMO, K., PETERS, B. and RISBO, T., *Nuclear Instruments and Methods, 81,* 1970.

2.   FOWLER, P.H., ADAMS, R.A., COWEN, V.G. and KIDD, J.M., *Proc. Roy. Soc., A301,* 1967.

3.   FOWLER, P.H., CLAPHAM, V.M., COWEN, V.G., KIDD, J.M. and MOSES, R.T., *Proc. Roy. Soc.,* 1970, in press.

4.   MEYER, P., *Annual Review of Astronomy and Astrophysics, 7,* 1969.

5.   VON ROSENVINGE, T.T. and WEBBER, W.R., *Nuclear Instruments and Methods, 66,*

TRADESCANTIA EXPERIMENT IN BIOSATELLITE II*

A.H. SPARROW, L.A. SCHAIRER and K.M. MARIMUTHU

*Biology Department, Brookhaven National Laboratory,
Upton, L.I., N.Y., 11973, U.S.A.*

The *Tradescantia* experiment on board Biosatellite II
was designed to determine the effects of low-gravity
(weightlessness) and other spacecraft environmental conditions on spontaneous and radiation-induced mutation
rates and on various cytological changes in a special
clone of the higher plant, *Tradescantia*, commonly called
spiderwort. This hybrid clone of *Tradescantia* has a
chromosome number of 12; it is heterozygous for flower
color; and it has high radiation-induced mutation rates.
Since numerous experiments have been done with this plant,
its normal response to ionizing radiation is well documented. During the two-day Biosatellite flight, 32 young
plants were arranged in a plastic housing so that the
flower buds were exposed to about 220 R of gamma rays
while the roots, immersed in nutrient, were exposed to
known radiation levels from about 125 to 285 R. Thirty-
two flight control plants were flown in the spacecraft
behind a tungsten radiation shield and similar unflown
control packages (with and without irradiation) were
maintained at the Cape Kennedy launch site.

The spacecraft environment was rigorously controlled
and conditions monitored throughout the flight with tem-
peratures held between 65 and 70°F in the *Tradescantia*

---

*Research supported in part by the U.S. Atomic Energy
Commission and in part by the National Aeronautics and
Space Administration (Purchase Order R104-7 and W-12,792).

packages and the vehicle atmospheres at about 55% relative humidity. Similar conditions were maintained in the
unflown vehicle held at the launch site. The gravitation-
al force was maintained at about 10^{-5} g during the 42-hour
irradiation phase of the 5-hour orbital flight. Tele-
metered and on-board records were made of levels of vibration, shock, acceleration, etc. for use in subsequent
Earth-based tests.

Immediately after retrieval of the spacecraft near
Hawaii, samples of root-tip, ovary and stamen tissues were
fixed. These and the intact plants were flown to Brookhaven for observations on several end points. In the
fixed material, chromosome aberrations and abnormal cell
division were scored in the root tips; micronuclei, disturbed spindle function, and cell death were analyzed in
early and late binucleate pollen. In the intact plants,
stamen hairs were scored daily for 28 postflight days for
somatic mutations (blue to pink or colorless cells), cell
size (giant or dwarf), loss of reproductive integrity
(stunted hair growth); petals were observed daily for the
occurrence of pink mutations. Also, effects on embryo sac
development and pollen viability were followed using tissues fixed from mature flowers as they opened daily postflight.

After preliminary analysis of the engineering and
biological data from Biosatellite II, several postflight
Earth-based experiments were performed under conditions
as close as possible to those of the flight. These tests,
run in the same packages and spacecraft (capsules) as used
in the flight experiment, were designed to establish or
recheck base-line data on the effects of irradiation, vibration, biocompatibility of the spacecraft, etc. (see
Table I). These data were to be used to help interpret
the results of the actual flight. Many of the end points
studied have been described in detail elsewhere [3, 4, 5,
6, 7] and therefore will be discussed only briefly below.

RESULTS

Following retrieval of the packages from the flight

Table I. Summary of environmental factors in Biosatellite
          II and various postflight experiments

Experiment	Vehicle	Gravity	Dynamic Factors*	Environment[†]
Biosatellite II				
Flight	301	10^{-5} g	Yes	Closed
Nonflight	201	1 g	No	Open
Phase B				
Nonflight	301	1 g	No	Closed
Nonflight	201	1 g	No	Open
Phase C				
Nonflight	301	1 g	Yes[‡]	Closed
Nonflight	201	1 g	No	Open
Vibration				
Nonflight	None	1 g	Vibration	Open
Clinostat				
Nonflight	None	Gravity compensated	No	Open

*Includes vibration, shock, centrifugation, etc.

[†]In the 301 vehicle the same capsule air was re-
cycled (3.5 centimeters per minute) for humidity and temperature control. In the 201 vehicle conditioned room
air was circulated at the same rate of flow as that in
the 301 vehicle.

[‡]Simulated

and postflight experiments daily records of the flower
production were made. The plants used in each experiment
were randomly assigned to the four packages prior to
treatment so that flower production should be comparable
between packages within each experiment (Biosatellite II,
Simulated Flight and Component Tests). Despite the fact
that more buds blasted in both the flown and unflown 301
samples during the first eight days after each treatment
(Table 2 C), there was a significant increase in the
total number of flowers produced in both flight samples

over their respective nonflight controls (Table 2B).
In the postflight Phase C test no such increase in
flower production in the 301 samples was observed.

The numbers of pink mutant sectors in the petals
from flight material are given in Fig. 1 and Table 2A.
Computed peak values given in Table 2 are based on a
theoretical curve fitted through the actual data points.
The curves for the pink-celled mutation data from the irradiated flight and nonflight control petals are nearly
superimposed. Similar results were obtained from irradiated samples for all the other ground-based postflight tests (Phase B, Phase C, Clinostat). Where differences did occur around day 16 to 18 post treatment,
either the standard errors are too large or the day-to-
day variability is too great to conclude that this difference is real. All nonirradiated control samples had
consistently low mutation rates and showed no difference
between flight and nonflight samples.

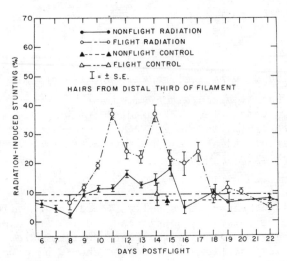

Fig. 1. The frequencies of pink mutations in *Tradescantia* petals for all
4 treatments vs. time in days postflight.

Table 2. Summary of computed peak aberration rates ± S.E. for various Tradescantia end points from Biosatellite II and nonflight tests showing effects indicated

End points	Biosatellite II Flight (301) Irrad.	Flight (301) Nonirrad.	Nonflight (201) Irrad.	Nonflight (201) Nonirrad.	Simulated flight (Phase C) 301 vehicle Irrad.	301 vehicle Nonirrad.	201 vehicle Irrad.	201 vehicle Nonirrad.	Component test Clinostat Irrad.	Erect Irrad.
A. No significant effect										
Pink/petal	16.9 ± .85	1.37 ± .17[*]	13.3 ± .63	1.10 ± .20[*]	18.7 ± .66	1.47 ± .48[*]	18.7 ± 0.7	2.22 ± .28[*]	23.1 ± .80	20.8 ± 0.7
Colorless/100 stamen hairs	10.7 ± .83	.132 ± 0.1[*]	11.1 ± 1.8	0.32 ± .26[*]	5.88 ± 1.1	0.09 ± .09[*]	5.11 ± .59	0.26 ± .16[*]	6.21 ± .37	5.5 ± 0.8
Dwarf cells/100 hairs	11.2 ± .65	3.05 ± .83[*]	13.1 ± 1.1	3.44 ± 1.2[*]	3.84 ± .39	0.53 ± .27[*]	2.47 ± .97[+]	0.72 ± .26[*]	4.29 ± .30	4.1 ± 0.3
Giant cells/100 hairs	5.69 ± .46	--	4.96 ± .19	--	1.83 ± .42	0.59 ± .50[*]	1.95 ± .38	0.65 ± .34[*]	1.4 ± 0.1	1.4 ± 0.1
Chromosome aber./cell in roots (194 R)[+]	0.53 ± .09	0.04 ± .02	0.48 ± .10	0.02 ± .01	--	--	--	--	--	--
B. Enhanced flight effects										
Loss of reprod. integrity (stunting)/100 hairs	26.9 ± 1.3	9.60 ± 3.8[*]	11.6 ± .73	7.26 ± .70[*]	14.8 ± 1.5[*]	13.2 ± 1.5[*]	18.9 ± 1.8[‡]	10.7 ± 1.4[*]	11.1 ± 1.6	--
Pollen abortion (%)	69.5 ± 2.4	36.5 ± 2.2[*]	49.6 ± 2.5	41.0 ± 2.5[*]	69.2 ± 2.5	47.0 ± 2.1	58.8 ± 3.0	47.1 ± 1.9	90.0 ± 2.7	83.8 ± 3.1
Micronuclei/100 pollen	15.4 ± 3.2[*]	3.59 ± 0.7	6.5 ± 0.8	3.0 ± 0.3	33.3 ± 15.6	--	22.9 ± 10.0	--	--	--
Flower production (26-day total)	227	244	162	191	221	229	243	261	333	328
Disturbed spindles (%cells) Roots[+]	0.55 ± .08	0.25 ± .05	0.06 ± .03	0	0.08 ± .03	0	0	0	0	0
Microspores[+]	All aborted	27.5 ± .92	0.3 ± .09	0.18 ± .07	0.93 ± .21	0.50 ± .11	0.15 ± .06	0.12 ± .05	--	--
Megaspores[*]	6.2 ± 1.3	4.48 ± 0.9	1.2 ± .68	1.94 ± .86	1.39 ± .79	0.50 ± .50	1.54 ± .88	--	--	--
C. Enhanced effects attributed to internal vehicle environment										
Pink/100 stamen hairs	4.89 ± .27	0.31 ± .24[*]	8.21 ± .39	0.20 ± .10[*]	6.13 ± .19[§]	0.11 ± .08[*]	9.95 ± .54[§]	0.13 ± .09[*]	10.7 ± .33	9.3 ± 0.3
Microspore developmental abnormalities (% cells)	--	3.28 ± .28	--	0.43 ± .10	--	4.73 ± .34	--	0.33 ± .09	--	--
Microspore death(% buds)[+]	100	100	16.7	33.3	100	100	25	12.5	--	--
Bud blasting/plant[*]	5.75 ± .39	5.31 ± .27	4.16 ± .29	4.94 ± .33	8.19 ± .39	9.16 ± .39	6.94 ± .75	5.47 ± .44	--	--
Embryo sac abortion (%)[*]	52.1 ± 5.0	17.6 ± 2.8	35.0 ± 6.1	19.0 ± 6.0	50.1 ± 5.1	13.3 ± 3.6	35.9 ± 5.9	14.3 ± 4.4	--	--

[*] Average of daily observations over extended posttreatment scoring period.

[+] Observations of single postflight tissue collection.

[‡] Average of daily observations over extended posttreatment scoring period of Phase B nonflight test.

[§] Computed peak values from Phase B nonflight test.

The radiation-induced frequencies of pink mutations per 100 stamen hairs increase with time from 8 day to about day 16 postflight in a response curve similar in shape to that of Fig. 2 by 28 days drop to frequencies

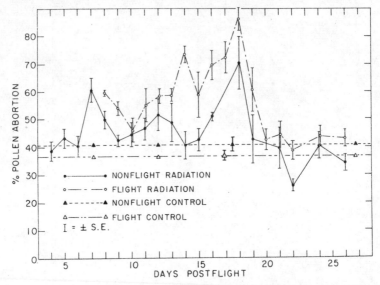

Fig. 2. The percentage of stunted *Tradescantia* stamen hairs for irradiated flight and nonflight sample vs. time in days postflight.

approaching the control values. Although the data are quite variable from day to day, a statistical analysis showed the computed peak for the nonflight radiation mutation rate to be significantly higher than that of the flight radiation rate (Table 2C). A simultaneous rise of mutation rates of irradiated nonflight and flight material from 8 to 12 days postflight indicates no alteration in the rates of bud development after the flight. In a ground-based postflight experiment (Table 2C, Simulated Flight) utilizing the flight (301) and nonflight (201) capsules a similar reduction in mutation rate was observed in the plants irradiated in the flight capsule when compared with data from plants in the nonflight control capsule. This significant difference may therefore be attributable to some environmental factor inherent in the 301 vehicle itself and not necessarily dependent upon flight factors. The mutation rates in all nonirradiated plants (flight and postflight tests) were generally low throughout the experiments with no statistically significant differences between the flight and nonflight samples.

The computed peak rates of radiation-induced colorless-cell mutations in the stamen hairs are given in Table 2A. Although a slightly lower mutation frequency is evident in data from the irradiated flight sample, compared with the irradiated nonflight sample, this difference is not significant in view of the relatively large standard errors and day-to-day variability of the data. Unflown postflight tests in the 201 and 301 capsules also showed little or no difference in mutation rate. At the control level, again, the data showed no statistically significant difference between the flight and nonflight samples.

The loss or partial loss of reproductive integrity of terminal or subterminal stamen hair cells results in a short or stunted hair. Hair lengths normally vary somewhat, but the occurrence of stunted hairs increases with postirradiation time up to about day 14. Fig. 2 shows that in the period between 9 and 17 days after retrieval the percentage of stunted hairs was consistently higher in the flight-irradiated than in nonflight-irradiated samples. Many more very short hairs (5 cells or less) were observed in the flight sample than in comparable nonflight sample, indicating that the same exposure produced a greater deleterious effect on cell division in the biosatellite than in the Earth-based plants.

Mature pollen was collected daily, and, after staining with cotton blue, the percentages of aborted pollen were determined for all four treatments. Although it should be stated that this clone of *Tradescantia* is characterized by an abnormally high rate of spontaneous pollen abortion, the data indicate that there is generally a higher abortion rate in the flight-radiation sample than in the nonflight-radiation sample with some points being significantly different at about the one percent level (Fig. 3 and Table 2B). Peak abortion rates occurred about 8, 14 and 19 days after irradiation reflec-

ting treatment during the more sensitive stages of mitosis and meiosis. Comparable postflight tests showed
considerable variability, but, in general, data from the
301 and 201 samples showed no consistent differences.

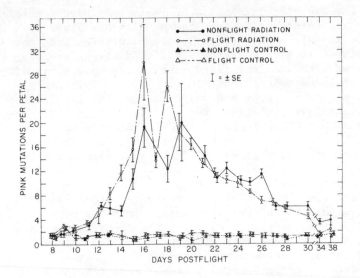

Fig. 3. The percentage of pollen abortion in flight and nonflight buds.
Unirradiated control lines are averages of combined daily observations.

Other mature pollen samples were Feulgen-stained and
scored for the presence of micronuclei. In general, the
same pattern of response as that for pollen abortion was
found, again reflecting greater radiosensitivity of cells
in mitosis and meiosis. During the period from 13 to 19
days after irradiation the average frequency in the flight
sample was significantly higher than the nonflight sample
(15.4 vs 6.5 micronuclei per 100 cells, respectively).
Nonirradiated control levels for the flight (3.59) and
nonflight (3.0) samples, however, were not significantly
different (Table 2B).

Collections of young microspores made immediately

after the flight showed an unexpectedly high death rate
in both flight samples (Table 2C). In the flight material, microspores in 11 out of 14 buds treated during
microspore mitosis had an abortion rate of more than 95%
while the remaining 3 buds (treated only during late mitotic stages) were only slightly above normal in percentage of aborted microspores. Subsequent Earth-based tests
in the flight vehicle (301) produced similar microspore
death to that of the orbited material. This effect may
therefore be due to some environmental variable in the
301 vehicle rather than to flight conditions. Data on
abnormal cell division in the surviving fraction (<5%) of
the microspores are given in Table 2B. Abnormalities reflecting disturbances in the spindle mechanism (cell division in an atypical plane of orientation) were observed
at a much higher frequency in the flight control (27.5%)
than in the nonflight control (0.18%) (Table 2B).

Evidence of a disturbance in the spindle mechanism
was also seen in root tips of flight material in the form
of multinucleate cells and in peculiarly-shaped nuclei.
Table 2B gives the percentage of such cells in flight and
nonflight root tips. The percentages are small when expressed as a percent of all cells scored including those
which presumably had not undergone division during flight,
but would be much larger if only cells which had just
completed division were scored. However, it was apparent
that not all cells in division showed evidence of a
spindle inhibition or malfunction.

Chromosome aberrations were scored at metaphase in
root-tip cells fixed shortly after treatment. No significant differences were found between data from the respective control and irradiated flight and nonflight samples
(Table 2A).

Embryo sac development was studied in serial sections
of ovaries collected daily as the flowers bloomed. When
the normal megaspore development was interrupted, presumably by spindle malfunction, the nuclei became either
clumped or scattered within the embryo sac and the data
are given in Table 2B. The frequency of embryo sacs
showing such spindle effects was significantly higher in

both the irradiated and nonirradiated flight samples (6.2 and 4.5%) than in their respective nonflight controls (1.2 and 1.9%). Other postflight tests had consistently low frequencies (1.4, 0.5 and 1.5%) of these embryo sac abnormalities whether irradiated or nonirradiated.

The postflight tests included studies of the effects of vibration and clinostat on the various end points used. Work with the clinostat (2 revolutions per minute) with and without irradiation can be quickly summarized as having had no effect on any of the end points scored as compared with its control (Table 2). Flight-simulated vibration tests, along the longitudinal axis only, on either the entire capsule or individual packages also failed to show any significant effect on the *Tradescantia* plants.

DISCUSSION AND SUMMARY

The *Tradescantia* Biosatellite experiment was designed to study the effects and possible interactions of weight-lessness and other spaceflight factors on both irradiated and nonirradiated samples. Data from nonirradiated flight and nonflight samples were used to study the effects or interaction of spaceflight factors on spontaneous aber-ration and mutation rates while the irradiated samples provided a means to determine if there is any interaction with a predetermined amount of gamma radiation. The end points used in these determinations are listed in Table 2 along with a summary of the effects noted.

Nonirradiated Material

Comparisons of data from nonirradiated flight and nonflight samples showed that significant differences at-tributed to flight factors were found only in the end points reflecting meiotic or mitotic spindle disturbance and flower production. Increased occurrence of cells with disturbed spindle function was observed in three different parts of the orbited plants. This spindle malfunction re-sulted in misoriented nuclei following microspore division, scattered or clumped nuclei in underdeveloped embryo sacs

and irregularly shaped or fragmented nuclei in the roots.
These effects have been attributed primarily to the
weightlessness factor of the space environment because
1) the effects occurred only in the orbited plants, 2) no
such abnormalities were observed in postflight experiments
incorporating simulated dynamic factors such as vibration
(along the longitudinal axis only), shock, acoustic noise
and centrifugation, and 3) there are supportive data of
Delone *et al.* from their Vostok 5 and 6 experiments which
show a rate of spindle disturbance in *Tradescantia palu-
dosa* microspores increasing with time in orbit [1]. At
present no logical mechanism can be suggested for the increased flower production in the orbited samples.

Irradiated Material

        Irradiated samples showed a higher degree of vari-
ability within and between flight and nonflight samples
than in nonirradiated material. However, there was no
significant flight effect on chromosome aberration rate
in roots and, with one exception (an apparently lower
pink-celled mutation rate in the irradiated stamen
hairs), there was no effect on mutation rate in the petal
or stamen hair tissues. This one exception was discredi-
ted when a similar response was observed in a postflight
test using the flight (301) vehicle. Therefore, our interpretation of these data is that there was, in general,
no significant effect of spaceflight factors on chromosome aberration in root tips or on mutation rates in the
flowers.

        Radiation-induced loss of reproductive integrity (as
represented by stunted hairs), pollen abortion, and micronuclei frequency in pollen, were all significantly higher
in the flight samples. These differences were not noted
in Earth-based postflight experiments although data for
these end points were quite variable from day to day after
treatment. Exposing plants to simulated flight dynamic
factors and to clinostat stresses had no apparent effect
on stamen hair stunting, pollen abortion or micronuclei
frequency. It is improbable that the relatively low
levels of vibration measured on board Biosatellite II [2]
would contribute to effects observed in flight material,

but it is difficult to exclude it completely from consideration as a possible factor.

Spindle effects observed in the irradiated flight samples were similar in type but higher in frequency than those in nonirradiated flight samples (Table 2B). The spindle effects were not observed in postflight tests, including vibration and clinostat stresses, and therefore appear to be attributable to weightlessness.

Table 2C lists several effects observed in irradiated and nonirradiated material which were considered to be due to some internal vehicle environmental factor and not flight factors. The exact cause (or causes) of this vehicle effect is unknown but may be related to the closed gas management system employed in the 301 vehicle as opposed to the open air circulation of the 201 vehicle (see Table 1).

The mechanisms responsible for the above effects or interactions and their possible long-term effect on growth and development remain a problem for future research in deep space probes or orbiting laboratories.

CONCLUSIONS

A modified frequency of several spontaneously occurring or radiation-induced effects in *Tradescantia* plants was attributed to orbital flight environments. These effects are rather small but significant and appear to be related to effects on normal cell division and cell survival. High rates of pollen abortion, micronuclei, and stamen hair stunting are unique to the irradiated, orbited sample and reflect an enhanced interaction between radiation and weightlessness. Nuclear misorientation and flower production were increased significantly in both irradiated and nonirradiated flight samples. Although these effects have been attributed to weightlessness alone, they may conceivably be due to weightlessness preceded and/or followed by vibration or other dynamic factors associated with orbital flight. Several of the effects studied either showed no modification attributable to the flight environment or showed a modification not thought to be caused by weightlessness.

ACKNOWLEDGEMENTS

The authors wish to acknowledge with thanks the
dedicated efforts and personal sacrifices in connection
with various phases of the Biosatellite experiment by
Priscilla M. Baetcke, Brenda M. Floyd, F.K. German, Julie
Klee, Leanne Puglielli, E.E. Klug, C.H. Nauman, Marta M.
Nawrocky, Anne F. Nauman, R. Sautkulis, Marie U. Schairer,
Susan S. Schwemmer, Rhoda C. Sparrow and R.G. Woodley.
Thanks are also expressed to K.H. Thompson for statistical
analyses and consultation. Last, but not least, thanks
go to the NASA and General Electric personnel for their
support and cooperation in carrying out the experiment.

REFERENCES

1.   DELONE, N., BYKOVSKIY, V., ANTIPOV, V., PARFENOV, G.,
      VYSOTSKIY, V. and RUDNEVA, N., *Kosmicheskiye Issledo-
      vaniya*, 2, 320, 1964.

2.   LOOK, B., *BioScience*, *18*, 560, 1968.

3.   MARIMUTHU, K., SCHAIRER, L. and SPARROW, A., *Radi-
      ation Botany*, *10*, 249, 1970.

4.   MARIMUTHU, K., SCHAIRER, L., SPARROW, A. and NAW-
      ROCKY, M.M., *Am. J. Botany* (submitted).

5.   MARIMUTHU, K., SPARROW, A. and SCHAIRER, L., *Radi-
      ation Res.*, *42*, 105, 1970.

6.   SCHAIRER, L., SPARROW, A. and MARIMUTHU, K., In:
      W. Vishniac and F.G. Favorite (eds.), *Life Sciences
      and Space Research*, VIII North-Holland Publ. Co.,
      Amsterdam, p. 19-24, 1970.

7.   SPARROW, A., SCHAIRER, L. and MARIMUTHU, K., *Bio-
      Science*, *18*, 582, 1968.

EFFETS DE PARTICULES ACCELEREES SUR
LE VIEILLISSEMENT DE DROSOPHILES

H. ATLAN*,**

*N.A.S.A. Ames Research Center, Moffett Field,
Calif. 94035, U.S.A.*

G. WELCH

*Donner Laboratory of Biophysics and Medical Physics,
University of California, Berkeley, Calif. 94035, U.S.A.*

J. MIQUEL

*Experimental Pathology Branch, Ames Research Center,
N.A.S.A., Moffett Field, Calif., 94035, U.S.A.*

Bien que les doses utilisées chez la Drosophile
soient beaucoup plus élevées que chez les mammifères on
sait que l'utilisation de ces insectes présente certains
avantages pratiques et théoriques: populations homogènes
permettant d'obtenir de bons résultats statistiques; durée de vie normale ne dépassant pas 120 jours; petite
taille qui permet de les irradier facilement en grands
nombres dans des faisceaux d'accélérateurs de particules;
de plus, les cellules somatiques des drosophiles adultes

---

*U.S. National Research Council Sen. Post. doct.
Research Associate.

**Adresse actuelle: Laboratoire de Biophysique,
Polymer Dept., Weizmann Institute, Rehovot, Israel.

ne se renouvelant pas, ces animaux peuvent être considé-
rés dans une certaine mesure comme des modèles de tissus
à cellules non reproductives (nerveux et musculaire) chez
les mammifères.

ETUDES PRELIMINAIRES A L'AIDE DES RAYONS γ DU ^{60}Co

La nature des effets des radiations ionisantes sur
la durée de vie des drosophiles est encore très contro-
versée. Les partisans de la théorie du "vieillissement
accéléré" [5, 6] se sont opposés à ceux du "vieillissement anticipé" [2, 3]. Deux d'entre nous [1] avons pu-
blié dans un précédent article des résultats qui nous ont
conduit à adopter une troisième position: le raccourcissement de la durée de vie serait provoqué par un syndrome
spécifique retardé des radiations plutôt que par un effet
sur les processus du vieillissement (Figs. 1 et 2).
Cette façon de voir a été confirmée par des études his-
tologiques comparatives sur des mouches irradiées et des

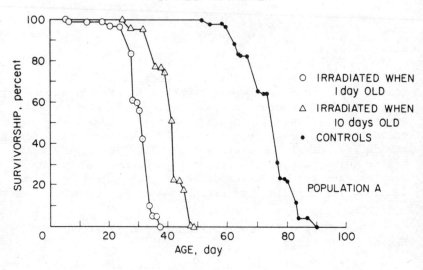

Fig. 1. Courbes de mortalité de *D. melanogaster* mâles adultes (groupes
d'environ 150 individus).

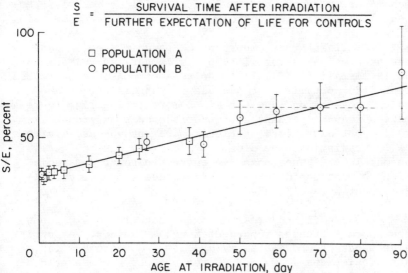

Fig. 2.   Raccourcissement de la durée de vie après 50 kR de rayons γ du ⁶⁰Co délivrés à des âges différents, chez *D. melanogaster* mâle adulte. (S/E = tèmps de survie après irradiation/Espérance de vie pour des groupes témoins du même âge non irradiés). L'accroissement de S/E avec l'âge de l'irradiation est statistiquement indubitable pendant la première partie de la durée de vie, et correspond à une valeur de S qui reste constante tant que la mort survient dans le plateau des courbes de mortalité des groupes témoins (voir Fig. 1).

mouches sénescentes: les lésions présentent des différences évidentes [7].

En cherchant les raisons de ces désaccords nous avons été amenés à préciser un certain nombre de points sur les conditions d'expérience.

1) Une précision statistique suffisante est indispensable pour pouvoir servir de base à telle ou telle théorie. C'est ainsi que faute d'y atteindre, les résultats de Baxter et Blair sont utilisés aussi bien par ces auteurs eux-mêmes pour un modèle de vieillissement anti-

cipé que par Lamb et Maynard-Smith pour un modèle de
vieillissement accéléré. Les résultats de M. Lamb [5]
échappent en grande partie à cette critique mais ils res-
tent insatisfaisants en ce qui concerne le deuxième point.

2) Il est très important de pouvoir séparer dans
une population la mortalité produite par les radiations
de la mortalité naturelle. Cela n'est possible que si la
courbe de mortalité est presque rectangulaire, ou au
moins présente un long plateau à mortalité nulle: toute
mort survenant pendant cette période dans un groupe ir-
radié peut alors être attribuée sûrement aux seuls effets
de l'irradiation. De plus, ce n'est que dans ce cas
qu'une interférence possible entre syndromes des radiations à mort rapide et à mort retardée (aigu et chronique) peut être éliminée.

Les *conditions expérimentales* dans lesquelles nous
nous sommes trouvés répondent à ces exigences. A partir
d'un stock de *Drosophila melanogaster* "Oregon R wild",
des populations de mâles adultes ont été élevées et conservées à 22°C dans des bouteilles contenant un milieu
nutritif à la farine de maïs enrichi par des levures.
Après éclosion et séparation des femelles, les populations étaient conservées par flacons de 10 individus dont
la nourriture était changée (par transfert dans de nou-
veaux flacons) 2 fois par semaine. Dans ces conditions,
les courbes de mortalité présentaient un long plateau
ainsi qu'on peut le voir sur la Fig. 1. Ce n'était pas
le cas dans les expériences de M. Lamb et on peut com-
prendre par là pourquoi ses résultats sont différents des
nôtres. Après avoir traité nos résultats à l'aide d'un
modèle mathématique [4] basé sur l'addition de 2 taux de
mortalité indépendants, l'un dû à l'irradiation, l'autre
au vieillissement, nous sommes arrivés aux conclusions
suivantes - que ne contradisent pas, d'ailleurs, les résultats exéérimentáux de M. Lamb (voir "discussion" dans
réf. [1]).

1) La survie après irradiation est totalement indé-
pendante de l'âge de l'irradiation tant que la mort par
vieillissement naturel ne vient pas s'ajouter à celle due
au syndrome spécifique des radiations (Fig. 1 et 2).

2) Quand la mortalité naturelle ne laisse pas au syndrome post-irradiation le temps d'arriver à son terme, il semble bien qu'un certain synergisme soit observé entre les deux causes de mortalité: le rapport S/E tend à devenir constant (Fig. 2, droite en pointillés), en accord avec les résultats de M. Lamb, ou au moins à augmenter avec une ponte beaucoup plus faible. Mais compte tenu du 1), (que cet auteur n'a pas pu observer à cause de l'absence de long plateau sur ses courbes de mortalité), ce synergisme doit être interprété comme *une augmentation de l'efficacité de l'irradiation due au vieillissement, plutôt qu'un vieillissement accéléré sous l'effet des radiations*; en particulier, une augmentation de la radiosensibilité pour un syndrome aigu des radiations pourrait fort bien rendre compte des résultats durant cette partie de la vie où il est difficile sinon impossible de séparer sur une population de mouches les morts par syndrome aigu de celles par syndrome chronique et de celles par vieillissement naturel. Une telle augmentation avec l'âge, de la radiosensibilité pour un syndrome aigu, avait d'ailleurs été observée par Baxter et Blair.

EFFETS D'IONS He^{++} ACCELERES

Les conditions d'élevage et de survie des populations étaient les mêmes que celles précédemment décrites pour les irradiations gamma. Les ions He^{++} étaient produits et accélérés par le Cyclotron de 88" du Lawrence Radiation Laboratory de Berkeley. Des énergies de 103 et 118 MeV ont été utilisées, ce qui représente des TEL de 8,5 et 7,7 KeV/μ respectivement. Ces valeurs caractérisent ce que nous appelons les particules α à faibles TEL. Les particules α à TEL élevés étaient obtenues en plaçant entre l'échantillon et la sortie du faisceau des plaques absorbantes d'aluminium, d'épaisseur convenable, de telle sorte que le parcours résiduel dans l'eau, des particules, soit de 0,9 mm épaisseur moyenne des mouches. De cette façon, les mouches, disposées au niveau du pic de la courbe de Bragg, étaient irradiées par des particules qui couvraient un large spectre d'énergies au-dessous de 36 MeV, pour lesquelles le TEL varie de 22 à 60 KeV/μ. Au contraire, au cours des irradiations par particules α à

faibles TEL les mouches étaient disposées au niveau de la
partie plate de la courbe de Bragg. Cela était réalisé
dans tous les cas à l'aide d'un dispositif ad hoc où, par
groupes de 100, les mouches étaient maintenues en une
seule couche perpendiculaire au faisceau, par une mince
feuille de mylar. Elles gardaient cependant la possibi-
lité de se mouvoir, de sorte que leur orientation dans
cette couche était laissée au hasard.

Pour chaque expérience, des groupes pris d'une même
population étaient irradiés le 2e ou le 3e jour après
éclosion, dans exactement les mêmes conditions par des
faisceaux de particules α à faibles TEL, et par des faisceaux à TEL élevés, et dans des conditions aussi voisines
que possible par des rayons γ d'une cellule à irradiation
au ^{60}Co, tandis que des groupes témoins étaient placés
dans les mêmes conditions à l'exception de l'irradiation.
Pour chaque dose, 2 groupes de 100 mouches étaient utilisés; ils mouraient ensuite en moyenne en même temps avec
des taux de mortalité très similaires, ce qui constituait
une démonstration a posteriori de l'homogénéité de la population. C'est pourquoi presque toujours les résultats
ont été réunis et la longévité moyenne calculée sur des
groupes d'environ 200 individus

*Effets comparés des particules α à faibles TEL et a
à TEL élevés et des rayons γ du ^{60}Co (Fig. 3 et 4)*

a) Les courbes de longévité moyenne en fonction de
la dose sont de type exponentiel, en accord avec la plu-
part des auteurs. Une EBR a donc pu être mesurée facilement pour les 3 types de radiations étudiées.

b) L'efficacité des particules α à faibles TEL (7 à
8 KeV/μ) est identique à celle des rayons γ du ^{60}Co.

c) Les particules α à TEL élevés ("pic de Bragg",
22 à 60 KeV/μ) ont une efficacité plus grande que celle
des deux autres types de radiations, avec un coefficient
d'EBR ∿ 1,3..

d) Pour des populations dont les longévités moyen-
nes sont différentes, les pentes des courbes survie-dose
en coordonnées semi-logarithmiques pour un même type de
radiations sont différentes. Une comparaison des Figs.

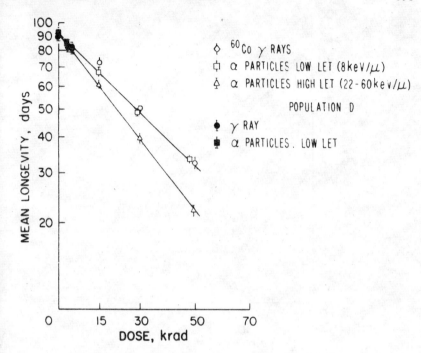

Fig. 3.   Effets de rayons γ du ^{60}Co et de particules α à faibles TEL et à
          TEL élevés sur la longévité moyenne de *D. melanogaster* mâles, ir-
          radiés par dose unique le 2e ou 3e jour après éclosion (population
          à grande longévité).

3 et 4 qui concernent deux populations à longévités différentes montre comment les temps de survie des groupes
ayant reçu 50 krad de rayons γ ou d'α à faibles TEL sont
très voisins dans les 2 populations, alors que ceux des
groupes témoins sont très différents, ce qui se traduit
évidemment par des pentes différentes. En ce qui concerne les particules α à TEL élevés, le même résultat peut
être observé pour une dose sensiblement inférieure à 50
krad (∿ 40 krad). Nous reviendrons sur ce phénomène dans
la discussion de ces résultats.

Effets des faibles doses

        Certains auteurs avaient observé que des doses consi-
dérées comme faibles pour des Drosophiles (3 et 5 krad),

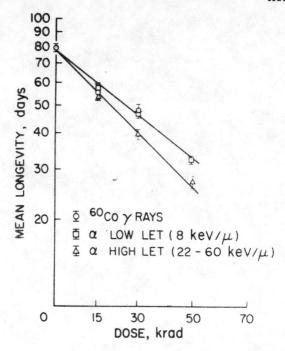

Fig. 4.   Effets de rayons γ du ^{60}Co et de particules α à faibles TEL et à
          TEL élevés sur la longévité moyenne de *D. melanogaster* mâles, ir-
          radiés par dose unique le 2e ou 3e jour après éclosion (population
          à longévité moyenne).

délivrées en une fois dans les premiers jours après
l'éclosion, provoquaient un allongement de la durée de
vie, tandis que d'autres n'observaient aucun effet, et
décrivaient ainsi le raccourcissement de la durée de vie
comme un effet à seuil. Nous avons observé dans tous les
cas une diminution significative de la durée de vie après
irradiations par 3 ou 5 krad de rayons γ du ^{60}Co ou de
particules α de 120 MeV. En fait, les temps de survie
que nous avons mesurés, s'inscrivent parfaitement (Fig. 3,
population D) sur les courbes survie-dose de type exponentiel et témoignent ainsi d'un effet sans seuil. Les
différences observées entre les différents auteurs nous
semblent devoir encore être attribuées à la force des
courbes de mortalité. Les allongements de durée de vie

moyenne n'ont été observés que sur des populations à mau-
vaises courbes de mortalité, et, comme le notait déjà
Sacher [8] l'allongement de la moyenne était toujours ac-
compagné d'un raccourcissement de la durée de vie maximum.
Autrement dit, ces faibles doses n'auraient un effet pro-
tecteur que contre des facteurs de mortalité précoce.

Effets du débit de dose

Les irradiations γ étaient réalisées avec un débit
de 4350 R/min. Comme il est facile de faire varier con-
sidérablement le débit de dose des particules accélérées,
un effet possible de celui-ci a été recherché. En le
faisant varier dans un intervalle de 4 à 256 1rad/min
nous n'avons pas observé de différences significatives
dans les temps de survie de groupes qui avaient reçu 50
krad de particules α à faibles TEL le 2e jour après éclosion. Toutefois une très faible diminution d'efficacité
semble se manifester avec le débit très élevé de 256
krad/min.

DISCUSSION

Le fait que des populations à longévités différentes
présentent des temps de survie identiques après une certaine dose d'un même type de radiations est en accord
avec nos résultats précédents en faveur d'un syndrome
spécifique des radiations indépendant du vieillissement.
Les doses moins élevées entraînent une survie moyenne
suffisamment longue pour que la mortalité naturelle se
superpose à celle due à l'irradiation. Mais la forme
exponentielle simple des courbes est plus difficile à
expliquer que dans l'hypothèse du vieillissement accéléré
de Lamb et Maynard-Smith, car elle laisse supposer un
seul mécanisme à l'origine des effets observés dans l'intervalle des doses utilisées. Ces auteurs en rendent
compte très simplement par la théorie de la cible en sup-
posant une analogie entre les "cibles" (organes ou organelles) des lésions des radiations et celles du vieillissement. Mais cette simplicité est peut être trompeuse
car ils appliquent, directement et sans intermédiaire, la
théorie de la cible à un phénomène où le paramètre biolo-
gique mesuré est un *temps*, alors que la théorie concerne

un nombre de cibles distribuées dans *l'espace*. Le passage de l'un à l'autre est simplement effectué en appli-
quant le formalisme de la théorie à des temps de survie.
(Ils écrivent que la diminution dS du temps de survie,
provoquée par une dose dD est proportionnelle à l'espérance de vie S en l'absence d'irradiation, ou dS =
- k S dD, ce qui donne par intégration la relation exponentielle $S = S_0 e^{-kD}$). Mais il n'est pas sûr que ce
passage doive s'effecteur de cette façon et que cette
application de la théorie de la cible soit légitime. Une
étape logique intermédiaire nous semble nécessaire entre
le nombre de cibles éventuelles et le temps de survie;
c'est en suivant cette ligne que nous proposons l'inter-
prétation - négative - suivante. Le nombre N de cibles
restantes après une dose D est $N = N_0 e^{-kD}$ où N_0 est le
nombre total en l'absence d'irradiation et k la radiosensibilité. Il s'agit là de la théorie de la cible sous
sa forme la plus simple. La mesure des temps de survie
nous conduit à admettre que ceux-ci sont proportionnels à
N. De plus k (mesurée par la pente des exponentielles en
coordonnées semilogarithmiques) et N_0 varient avec la
longévité des populations en dehors de toute irradiation.
Cela ne veut pas dire pour autant que les "cibles" des
radiations soient nécessairement les mêmes que celles du
vieillissement. Tout ce qu'on peut affirmer est qu'elles
sont moins nombreuses chez des mouches à espérance de vie
plus faible mais *cette variation n'est pas forcément uni-
forme pendant toute la durée de vie*; en particulier, les
expériences d'irradiations à des âges différents montrent
qu'elle doit être très lente (au point d'être négligeable)
pendant la première partie de la durée de vie. De plus,
cette variation, chaque fois qu'elle est décelable, s'ac-
compagne d'une variation dans le même sens de la radiosensibilité k, ce qui est normal si on interprète celle-
ci comme une probabilité d'atteinte: celle-ci doit augmenter si le nombre de cibles augmente alors que le volume moyen des mouches reste le même. Autrement dit le
fait que leur nombre varie avec la longévité, ne nous
force pas à identifier ces cibles avec des organes ou
organelles qui joueraient un rôle central dans les méca-
nismes du vieillissement. La difficulté vient de ce
qu'on applique la théorie de la cible à un phénomène où

la grandeur mesurée se trouve être un temps. Ceci impli-
que une transformation espace → temps entre un nombre de
cibles distribuées dans l'espace et un nombre de jours.
Cette transformation n'obéit pas à des lois qui sont im-
médiatement évidentes. L'hypothèse la plus simple était
évidemment de supposer une relation étroite entre les lésions produites par les radiations et celles dues au
vieillissement, considéré comme le simple passage du
temps. Mais il est clair que le temps lui-même ne peut
pas être destructeur et que les lésions du vieillissement
proviennent d'un ensemble de facteurs exogènes et endo-
gènes accumulés dans le temps. Par conséquent la relation supposée entre les lésions des radiations et celles
du vieillissement peut être considérée comme plus appa-
rente que réelle, comme un espèce d'artefact provoqué par
la transformation espace-temps qu'on observe dans la manifestation des effets retardés des radiations. Tout
facteur d'agression, qui présenterait une telle propriété,
poserait la même sorte de problèmes.

RESUME

    Des courbes de longévité moyenne en fonction de la
dose de type exponentiel ont été obtenues après irradiations de *Drosophila melanogaster* par dose unique de rayons
γ ou de particules α à faibles TEL et à TEL élevés. L'EBR
de ces dernières par rapport aux rayons γ du ^{60}Co et aux
particules α à faibles TEL était de 1,3. Les faibles
doses (3 et 5 krad) ont provoqué un raccourcissement si-
gnificatif de la durée de vie. Aucun effet de débit de
dose n'a été observé dans un intervalle de 4 à 256
krad/min. Ces résultats sont discutés et interprétés
dans le cadre de conclusions antérieures qui avaient
conduit à la théorie d'un syndrome spécifique tardif des
radiations indépendant des processus du vieillissement
naturel.

REMERCIEMENTS

    Nous voulons exprimer combien l'aide de Mrs. R.M.
Binnard a été appréciée pour les manipulations et la

surveillance des populations de Drosophiles, ainsi que
celle du personnel du Cyclotron de 88" de Berkeley pour
le contrôle du faisceau de particules.

REFERENCES

1.   ATLAN, H., MIQUEL, J. et BINNARD, R.M., *J. Geron-
      tology*, *24*, 1. 1969.

2.   BAXTER, R.C. et BLAIR, H.A., *Radiation Res.*, *30*,
      48, 1967.

3.   BAXTER, R.C. et BLAIR, H.A., *Radiation Res.*, *31*,
      287, 1967.

4.   DOLKAS, C., ATLAN, H. et MIQUEL, J., en préparation.

5.   LAMB, M.J., *Radiation and Ageing* (P.J. Lindop & G.A.
      Sacher eds).   Taylor & Francis, London, 163, 1966.

6.   LAMB, M.J. et MAYNARD-SMITH, J., *Radiation Res.*, *40*,
      450, 1969.

7.   MIQUEL, J., ATLAN, H. et BINNARD, R.M., *The Geron-
      tologist*, 20th Ann. Meet. Gerontol. Soc., *7*, n.3,
      1967.

8.   SACHER, G.A., *Physiological Zoology*, *36*, 295, 1963.

HABROBRACON IN THE BIOSATELLITE EXPERIMENT*

R.C. VON BORSTELL**, ROGER H. SMITH and ANNA R. WHITING

*Biology Division, Oak Ridge National Laboratory,
Oak Ridge, Tennessee 37830, U.S.A.*

DANIEL S. GROSCH

*Department of Genetics, North Carolina State University,
Raleigh, North Carolina 27607, U.S.A.*

Biosatellite II was launched into space from Cape
Kennedy on September 7, 1967, and the spacecraft was
brought down in the vicinity of Hawaii on September 9
after 28 orbits. A radiation source on the spacecraft
was activated for 42 hours, so that enhancing or antagonistic effects of radiation in conjunction with effects caused by the space flight itself might be detected and studied. Males and females of the small
parasitic wasp *Habrobracon juglandis* Ashmead were
contained separately in five different packages within
the spacecraft affording data from animals that were
irradiated before the flight or during the flight with
different exposures, as well as some that were shielded
from the strontium-85 source.

Numerous genetic and physiological parameters were
assayed in Habrobracon after the spacecraft was

*Research jointly sponsored by the National Aero-
nautics and Space Administration (through NASA Research
Grant No. NsG678) and the U.S. Atomic Energy Commission
under contract with the Union Carbide Corporation.

**Present address: Department of Genetica, University
of Alberta, Edmonton, Canada.

recovered. Many of these are listed in Tables 1 and 2
along with the effects of flight relative to effects
obtained in animals held in the ground-based control set-
up where geometric, temperature, and radiation conditions
were maintained that closely approximated those in the
spacecraft itself. Detailed discussions of Habrobracon
data obtained from the flight are presented elsewhere
[1, 2]. Suffice it to say that the largest effects were
on fecundity and hatchability of transitional and primitive oogonia [3]. Here the damaging effects of radiation, easily recognizable at exposures below five
hundred roentgens, were eliminated by the journey in
space at all exposures including one of over 2500 R.
Even animals irradiated with exposures of 2000 R before
the flight had very little damage done to oogonia in
these stages of development. Other effects, such as
increased recessive lethal mutation frequency in the
sperm of males, the disoriented mating behavior of the
males after the flight, and the increased life-span
of the females, were observed, but none of these was as
dramatic or as great as the antagonistic effect of space
flight to radiation of the oogonia.

The observed effects of the space flight on Habrobracon probably derived from one or both of two principal conditions of the flight that are difficult, if
not impossible, to reproduce in the laboratory. These
are weightlessness, as defined as a freely orbiting
state, and the three-dimensional vibration profile exhibited by a space vehicle during its launch and recovery phases.

The enhancement of spontaneous recessive lethal
frequencies in sperm of Habrobracon seen from analysis
of the flight animals was reproduced during one of the
post flight tests in which the flight vehicle was vi-
brated and centrifuged; thus this effect seems clearly
to have been induced by something other than weightlessness. The enhancement of embryonic, larval, and pupal
deaths in the nonirradiated flight females was dependent upon their placement at different positions within
a package during the flight; thus these too may be
attributed to vibration. We have deduced by genetic

TABLE 1. Genetic Effects Obtained in the Habrobracon
         Experiment in Biosatellite II Relative to Those
         Obtained on Earth

	Effect of flight dynamics	
End points	Flight alone	Flight + radiation
Sperm		
Dominant lethal mutations	null	null
Recessive lethal mutations	increased	null
Translocations	null	null
Oocytes		
Hatchability		
Metaphase I	reduced	reduced
Late prophase I	null	null
Early prophase I	null-reduced	reduced
Recombination		
Late prophase I	null	null
Transitional oogonia		
Hatchability	null	increased
Primitive oogonia		
Hatchability	null	increased

TABLE 2. Physiological Effects Obtained in the Habrobracon Experiment in Biosatellite II Relative to Those Obtained on Earth

End points	Effect of flight dynamics	
	Flight alone	Flight + radiation
Survival		
Males	null	null
Females	null	null
Fecundity		
Transitional oogonia	null	increased
Primitive oogonia	null	increased
Behavior		
Mating of males	disoriented	disoriented
Oviposition of females	null	null
Other effects		
Fertilizing capacity of sperm	null	enhanced
Xanthine dehydrogenase activity in males	reduced	reduced
Life-span of females	increased	increased

reconstruction experiments that these effects were chromosomal aberrations and recessive lethal mutations which were induced in the eggs.

At this time, the best candidates for an effect of weightlessness from the flight appear to be the following: (a) enhancement of fecundity and hatchability of primitive and transitional oogonia, (b) disorientation of male mating behavior, (c) life-span of females, and (d) decreased xanthine dehydrogenase activity. Two remaining effects found in the flight, enhanced fertilizing capacity of sperm and the reduced hatchability of eggs from females irradiated as metaphase I and early prophase I oocytes, could be either from weightlessness or from other factors of spaceflight.

SUMMARY

Numerous genetic and physiological parameters were assayed in Habrobracon after they had been carried for two days in orbital flight. Most effects from the flight were small or nonexistent. Some large effects (e.g. recessive lethal mutations) could be attributed to vibrations associated with launch; two large effects (enhancement of fecundity and hatchability in oogonia) could be attributed to weightlessness.

REFERENCES

1. VON BORSTEL, R.C., SMITH, R.H., GROSCH, D.S., WHITING, A.R., AMY, R.L., BAIRD, M.B., BUCHANAN, P.D., CAIN, K.T., CARPENTER, R.A., CLARK, A.M., HOFFMAN, A.C., JONES, M.S., KONDO, S., LANE, M.J., MIZIANTY, T.J., PARDUE, M.L., REEL, J.W., SMITH, D.B., STEEN, J.A., TINDALL, J.T. and VALCOVIC, L.R., *Bioscience, 18*, 598, 1968.

2. VON BORSTEL, R.C., SMITH, R.H., WHITING, A.R. and GROSCH, D.S., In: *Biosatellite Project* (J.F. Saunders, ed.) in press.

3. GROSCH, D.S., *Mutat. Res., 9*, 91, 1970.

CHAPTER 2

THE SIGNIFICANCE OF "RESTING" CELL POPULATIONS FOR HEMATOPOIETIC REGENERATION AFTER IONIZING RADIATION OR APPLICATION OF RADIOMIMETIC SUBSTANCES*

T.M. FLIEDNER, R.J. HAAS and H. BLATTMANN

*Abteilung für Klinische Physiologie,
Zentrum für Klinische Grundlagenforschung,
Universität Ulm, Parkstrasse 11, Ulm/Donau, Germany*

INTRODUCTION

There is accumulating evidence, that most of those cells, that are capable of restoring hematopoietic cell production in a radiation or chemically induced bone marrow aplasia, are "resting" as far as their proliferative activity is concerned [1-6]. Further, these cells appear to be able to restore cell production in the erythrocytic, granulocytic and megakaryocytic series as well as of the lymphocytic organs [7, 8]. Whether there is actually *one* type of "uncommitted" stem cells capable of restoring all types of blood cell formation by becoming "committed" or produce specific cell types after being stimulated by humoral, nerval or cell ecological factors, or whether there are more than one type of such stem cells remains to be determined. However, it appears clear that "uncommitted" stem cells can be found among blood leukocytes [9, 10] as well as in bone marrow cell suspensions in dogs, rats, mice and other species [5, 11-15] and in certain species (e.g. mouse) in the spleen. However, hema-

*Research supported by EURATOM Contract Nrs. 072-68-1 BIOD, 079-69-1 BIAC and the Bundesministerium für Bildung und Wissenschaft.

topoietic stem cells have not been found in the thoracic
duct lymph nor in cell suspensions from lymphnodes [16,
17, 18].

Despite numerous attempts, it has not been possible
until now to identify morphologically the - presumably -
uncommitted, cytokinetically resting stem cells in an
unequivocal manner. All tests used until now to characterize such cells have been function oriented. Therefore,
it has been the purpose of our studies to develop a
method that would allow the radioactive labelling of
cells by means of tritiated thymidine (^{3}H-TdR) throughout
all hematopoietic organs - such as bone marrow, spleen
lymphnodes and thymus - that are at rest cytokinetically,
to identify them morphologically and to investigate their
generative response after treatment with whole and
partial body irradiation as well as the administration
of radiomimetic agents.

2.   METHODS USED TO LABEL "RESTING" CELLS
   THROUGHOUT THE HEMATOPOIETIC ORGANS

In principle, the method used to label "resting"
cells of the hematopoietic tissues consists of the repeated or continuous administration of tritiated thymidine
from the onset of organogenesis of an organism at least
until its birth or until any desired time thereafter.
The hematopoietic organs are studied autoradiographically
for the kinetics of resting cells after a suitable time
interval after discontinuation of ^{3}H-TdR administration
in order to allow the disappearance of label from the
rapidly renewing cell types.

A useful approach to establish the presence of
"resting cells" already at birth of an animal has been to
infuse pregnant rats with tritiated thymidine continuously from day 9 of pregnancy until term and to study the
hematopoietic tissues of the offspring serially [19-21].
At birth for example, all cell nuclei of bone marrow,
spleen, lymphnodes, thymus and peripheral blood are
^{3}H-TdR-labeled. Within 10-14 days the label disappears
from the bulk of cells and only a few cells in these

organs retain label, indicating their slow turnover rate.
About 2 weeks after birth, in the bone marrow there were
still about 100% of the endothelial cells, about 90% of
all reticular cells, and 5% of small lymphocytes labelled.
Other cell types, such as myelocytic, erythrocytic and
megakaryocytic cells, had diluted their label to such an
extent that it was not distinguishable from background.
In the spleen, there is a marked hematopoiesis early
after birth but little lymphocytopoiesis. 10-14 days
after birth, most labelled cells had disappeared. However, endothelial cells and reticular cells continue to
be labelled as well as a small fraction of small and medium sized lymphocytes. In lymphnodes a small fraction
of lymphocytes were found labelled 2 weeks after birth
when the administration of ^{3}H-TdR was discontinued at
birth. The thymus shows a rapid decline of the labelling
over all cells except a small fraction of small lymphocytes. In the peripheral blood, the only cell type that
remains labelled 10-14 days after birth were medium sized
and small lymphocytes (about 8%). From the growth curve
of the completely labelled newborn rats it was obvious
that the decline of labelling activity over "slowly turning over" hematopoietic cells corresponded to the growth
of the various organs and that the respective cell types
or systems had obviously not come to a state of complete
cytokinetic rest [21].

Therefore, if experiments are designed to study the
response of resting cells of the hematopoietic organs to
different stimuli, the prenatal administration of ^{3}H-TdR
has to be complemented by a series of repeated postnatal
injections of ^{3}H.TdR. When ^{3}H.TdR (2 mCi/mM) was continuously administered before birth (1.6 µCi/g/day to the
mother) and for 4 weeks thereafter (0.5 µCi/day/g, divided in 2 doses 12 hours apart) followed by serial tissue
sampling, the following labelling pattern was observed
10-14 days after the last ^{3}H-TdR administration. In the
marrow, the reticular and endothelial cells were 100%
labelled. Of the bone marrow lymphocyte population,
about 15% of the small type were labelled. The label had
disappeared from all other hematopoietic cell elements.
In the *thymus* little if any label was seem anymore at
this time in large and medium sized lymphocytes. However,

a small fraction of about 3% of small lymphocytes retained
the label. In *spleen* and *lymphnodes* some medium sized
and (in lymphnodes) about 40% of small lymphocytes retain
their label. Thus, the fact that about 17% of all small
and about 10% of all medium sized lymphocytes were still
found to be labelled in the peripheral blood some 2 - 3
weeks after the last ^{3}H-TdR injection is taken to indicate that it is mainly the small round cell type, called
lymphocyte, for which cellular traffic exists between the
various sites of blood cell formation. The differences
in the fraction of cells that continue to be labelled in
the various organs may be strong evidence, however, that
the mixing of the "lymphocyte"-populations throughout the
body is not uniform. In any event, it cannot yet been
determined accurately, what the contribution of the various organs is as far as the delivery of "resting" lymphocytes to the blood is concerned.

When the cytotoxic action of various agents on the
resting cell populations of hemopoietic organs was studied, ^{3}H-TdR was administered continuously before birth
and every 8 hours (0.33 µCi/g) for 6 weeks after birth.
Thereafter, a period of 6 weeks elapsed without ^{3}H-TdR
administration to allow the label to clear from all rapidly turning over cell types. At this time it was found,
that the *bone marrow* contained a fraction of 10% labelled
small marrow lymphocytes while 100% of endothelial and of
reticular cells were still labelled. In the *thymus*,
about 1% of medium and small lymphocytes were labelled.
In the *lymphnodes*, 23% of lymphocytes were labelled and a
similar fraction in the *peripheral blood*.

From the data it was obvious that there is a clear-
cut distinction in the bone marrow between "resting cells"
such as endothelial and reticular cells and a fraction of
small marrow lymphocytes and the majority or rapidly turning over differentiated hematopoietic cells. In the lymphatic organs there is evidence of a continuing labelling
also of larger lymphocytes, in addition to the resting
cell types, such as endothelial and reticular cells,
which may indicate that such larger cells originate from
labelled smaller lymphocytes by transformation.

CYTOKINETIC PROPERTIES OF "RESTING CELLS"
IN HEMATOPOIETIC ORGANS

After having established the identity and presence
of at least 2 cell categories of different cytokinetic
properties - the slowly and the rapidly turning over cell
types - in bone marrow, spleen, lymphnodes and thymus, it
appeared to be of interest to establish renewal rates of
the slowly turning over cells.

The study of slowly turning over bone marrow cells
in rats that received ^{3}H-TdR before birth and for 3 weeks
thereafter indicates (Fig. 1), that the labelling intensity of about 25 grains per endothelial and per reticular
cell decreased to about 15 per cell within 30 weeks.
Thus, the time for *all* of these cells to undergo at least
one division must be in excess of 30 weeks (= > 7 months).
The fact that about 20% of these slowly turning over
cells lost their label altogether during this time indicates that there may be a wide distribution of cellular
turnover: while some of the cells must have undergone
several divisions in order to loose all detectable label
and thus reduce the labeling index to 80%, others may not
have undergone any division during this time. This is
supported by the fact that highly labelled cells (= 20
grains per cell) were present with equal frequency 10,
20 and 30 weeks after the last ^{3}H-TdR administration.
This behaviour is reasonable since the labelling pattern
is determined in smears of the marrow, while the study of
sections indicates that the more intense dilution of
label occurs in the growth zones of the bones.

Among the marrow lymphocytes, only about 5% retain
their ^{3}H-TdR label for at least 30 weeks without significant dilution. A similar fraction of small blood lymphocytes retained their label during this time (Fig. 2). In
lymphnodes at the same time about 20% of small lymphocytes were found to be labelled.

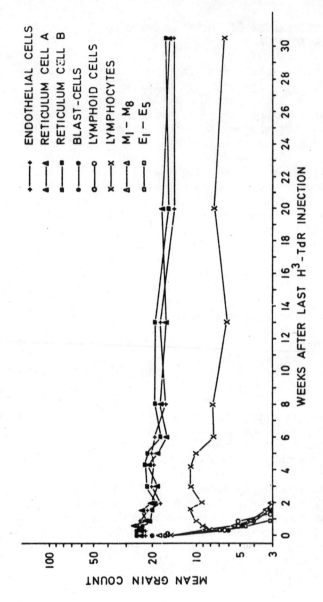

Fig. 1. Labeling intensity as a function of time of various bone marrow cell categories in animals, which obtained ³H-TdR before birth and during 3 weeks afterwards. (Blood 34, 794, 1969).

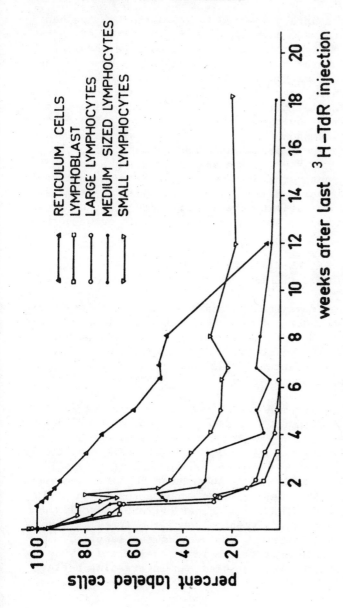

Fig. 2. Labeling index of various cell categories of lymphnodes in animals which obtained ³H-TdR before birth and during 3 weeks afterwards.

Thus, the data presented indicate that in the bone marrow of rats, the physiological regeneration of endothelial and of reticular cells is based on a turnover measured in months rather than in days or hours. Among the majority of marrow lymphocytes appears to be a small fraction turning over at a similar slow rate than reticular or endothelial cells, whereas in lymphnodes a larger fraction exists having a slow turnover time. Since there are labelled lymphocytes in the blood at all time intervals studied, their origin and destiny may be in bone marrow, lymphnodes or spleen and indicates the possibility of a continuing exchange of such a cytokinetically resting cell pool. However, it is not possible at the present time to estimate the relative contribution of the different organs to such a cellular traffic between them.

THE RESPONSE OF "RESTING CELLS" TO SEVERAL CYTOTOXIC AGENTS

The model described to characterize morphologically cell types that are "at rest" cytokinetically was used to investigate, which of these resting cell types respond with a proliferative activity during hematopoietic regeneration and, more recently [22] during an immune response after antigenic stimulation.

Suitable prepared rats (^{3}H-TdR given before and 4 weeks after birth, no ^{3}H-TdR during 4 weeks prior to experiment) were given 750 R 250 kV x-rays to the entire body with the right hind-limb shielded. This resulted in a severe bone marrow depletion within 2.5 to 3 days in the irradiated femur with a subsequent cellular recovery, while the shielded femur did not show a change in cellularity (Fig. 3). The total number of labelled cells did not change significantly in neither, the irradiated nor the unirradiated marrow. However, if the labelled populations of endothelial and reticular cells and of the marrow lymphocytes were studied, an interesting pattern

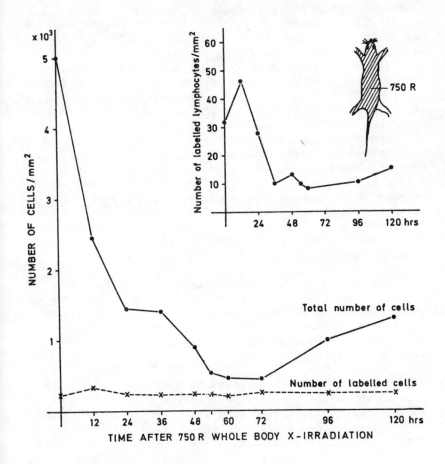

Fig. 3.   Number of labeled and unlabeled nucleated bone marrow cells per
          mm² as a function of time after x-irradiation in group A (750 R
          with the right hind leg shielded). *(Cell and Tissue Kinetics,*
          4, 31, 1971).

evolved. In the irradiated tibia there is no change in
the labelling intensity of endothelial nor of the reticular cells during the first 5 days after ionizing irradiation. However, the labelling intensity of the small
fraction of labelled bone marrow lymphocytes decreases
from the original value prior to radiation of 16 grains
per cell to about 4 to 5 grains per cell within 2 to 3
days after irradiation. When the total number of lymphocytes was counted during this time (Fig. 3), it was seen
that the number of labelled lymphocytes per mm^2 bone marrow section increased during the first 12 hours and
thereafter declined to about 1/3 of the initial level
within 2 to 3 days. This level was maintained thereafter
throughout the period of observation. In the shielded
tibia a similar pattern of decrease of labelling intensity over the small bone marrow lymphocytes was observed
while endothelial cells and reticular cells did not show
a change in the labelling intensity.

These findings have been interpreted to indicate
that the endothelial and reticular cells of the marrow do
not respond with a proliferative activity after this dose
of ionizing radiation and hence may not be involved in
the process of hematopoietic cell regeneration in the
sight of irradiation.

However, it is of interest to note that during the
time in which the bone marrow prepared itself for the
cellular recovery, i.e. during the first 12 hours resting
marrow lymphocytes appears to proliferate indicated by
the decrease in the labelling intensity while the number
of labelled cells increases transiently. That the increase in the number of labelled lymphocytes does not
continue beyond 12 hours, may indicate that the cells
transform into cell types of different morphological
identity and are hence not any more counted within the
labelled lymphocyte population. The first sign of hematopoietic cellular regeneration was observed between 2
and 3 days as evidenced by the appearance of young blast
cells with a deep blue cytoplasm and nucleoli. That the
study did not provide evidence for a significant degree
of labelling of these cells was explained on the basis of
the rather low labelling intensity of the lymphocytes

from which such a label could have originated. The labelling pattern in the shielded marrow was taken to indicate
the possibility that the destruction of hemopoiesis in
the irradiated part of the body was so severe, that it
caused a proliferative activity in the shielded labelled
lymphocyte population. The lymphocytes have either migrated out stimulating the remainder to divide or they
divided and some of the divided cells migrated out to
other sites of the body.

In order to investigate the migration possibility,
another radiation experiment has been performed. Rats, in
which the resting cells of the bone marrow were selectively
labelled were given 1500 R irradiation only to the right
limb. During the first 5 days after this local irradiation, the bone marrow was studied autoradiographically
in the irradiated and in the non-irradiated collateral
tibia. In the irradiated tibia, the labelling intensity
of reticular and endothelial cells did not change. However, in the population of small lymphocytes, the labelling intensity decreased within 48 hours in a similar
fashion seen after irradiation with 750 R with only one
hind limb shielded. However, it is of great interest to
observe that there is a re-appearance of labelled lymphocytes between 48 and 120 hours after irradiation. This
finding is substantiated when the histogram of the
labelled cells is being studied. In the shielded tibia,
the labelling intensity does not decrease over endothelial cells and over reticular cells, but the labelled
lymphocyte population did show a small decrease in the
labelling intensity which however was not very dramatic.
These findings can be interpreted to mean that there is a
migration of labelled lymphocytes from non-irradiated
parts of the body into the irradiated field. Although it
cannot be proven that the labelled lymphocyte population
functions as a stem cell population, it is highly suggestive that the pattern observed is associated with the
bone marrow recovery in the irradiated site [23].

For the nitrogen mustard experiment, rats were used
in which the labelled cell populations of the bone marrow
were obtained by prenatal and postnatal ^{3}H-TdR labelling
in the fashion described above. Animals in which the

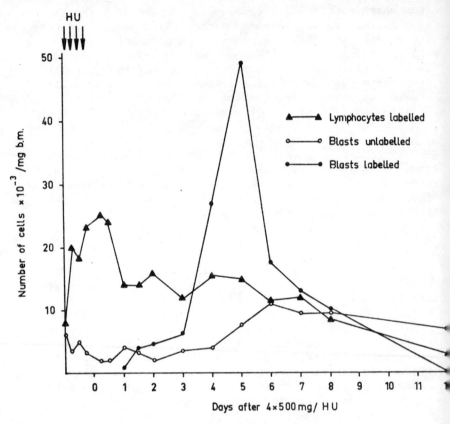

Fig. 4.   Number of labeled lymphocytes, labeled and unlabeled blast cells
          per mg bone marrow as a function of the time after HU-treatment
          (4 × 500 mg Hu/kg body weight). *(Brit. J. Haemat., 19, 533, 1970).*

resting cells were labelled were given 0.9 mg/kg body
weight of nitrogen mustard, a dose which is known to produce a severe pancytopenia of the peripheral blood and a
marked bone marrow aplasia with, however, a rapid recovery followed.

The endothelial cells and the reticular cells did not
loose any of the labelling intensity, while the small

fraction of labelled bone marrow lymphocytes decreased
the labelling intensity to very low levels within 36 to
48 hours. The disappearance of highly labelled bone marrow lymphocytes coincided with the beginning of bone marrow regeneration. Although there was suggested evidence
that some of the very early regenerating hematopoietic
cells did show label over the nuclei, the labelling intensity of these cells was not high enough to prove the
theory that these cells were derived from the population
of labelled small bone marrow lymphocytes [24].

This was the reason why, in another experiment,
hydroxyurea was used as a cytotoxic drug to investigate
the regenerating pattern of the labelled lymphocyte population. There is strong evidence, that hydroxyurea acts
only on cells in DNA synthesis [25].

The next figure indicates the cellular response of
the bone marrow to 4 doses of hydroxyures given 6 hours
apart (4 × 500 mg/kg body weight). Within 1 and 2 days,
this dose results in a very severe bone marrow aplasia
which is followed by a rather rapid recovery during the
next 10 to 14 days. The investigation of the labelled
cell population in the bone marrow indicates that the reticular cells and the endothelial cells did not change
the labelling intensity. However, the small fraction of
labelled bone marrow lymphocytes decreased the labelling
intensity within 2 days to almost background levels. It
is of interest now that there was a population of early
blast cells between 2 and 6 days after 4 doses of hydroxyurea that showed a definite labelling intensity.

In Fig. 4 the absolute number of labelled lymphocytes, of labelled and unlabelled blast cells is plotted
at different times after 4 doses of 500 mg.kg body weight
of hydroxyurea. This shows that there is an increase in
the number of labelled blast cells between day 1 and day
3 after hydroxyurea (no labelled cells of this type were
observed earlier), and a rapid increase in the number of
labelled blast cells between 3 and 6 days, the time in
which the bone marrow recovery proceeds at a most rapid
rate. It is of interest also to see that the number of
labelled small lymphocytes increases during the first day

after the last administration of hydroxyurea. In a similar pattern as was observed in the shielded leg when the
rest of the body was irradiated with 750 R. During this
time the labelling intensity over these small bone marrow
lymphocytes decreased, so that an intervening cell division without cell transformation was feasible. There was
no doubt that on day 2 and during the phase between day 2
and day 6 there was evidence of the appearance of labelled
early myelocytic and erythropoietic precursors. Although
a final proof cannot be given, it is suggestive that the
label over these regenerating early hemopoietic cells
originated in the labelled lymphocyte population.
Although it cannot be excluded as yet that the label seen
resulted from reutilisation of decaying labelled lymphocytes, it is suggestive that the observed pattern indicates the potentiality of bone marrow lymphocytes to divide and to transform into hematopoietic precursors [26].

     It was of interest in this context to investigate
the behaviour of the labelling pattern of labelled lymphocytes in the lymphatic organs. Radiation, nitrogen
mustard and hydroxyurea had no effect on the labelling
intensity of thymus lymphocytes. The same was true for
the labelling intensity of labelled lymphocytes in the
submandibular lymphnodes after radiation, nitrogen mustard or hydroxyurea.

     These findings indicate that the small labelled bone
marrow population of lymphocytes behaves entirely different than similar populations of lymphocytes in the lymphatic organs. This fact is taken to indicate that small
round cells in the bone marrow and in the lymphatic organs that are cytokinetically resting are not identical
as far as their function is concerned, and are not necessarily in an exchange with each other. It remains to be
determined whether among the labelled cells of the blood
are some that are in exchange between the various sites
of the bone marrow, and some that are in exchange with
the various lymphatic organs.

CONCLUSIONS AND SUMMARY

1) ^{3}H-thymidine (^{3}H-TdR) has been successfully employed to identify morphologically cytokinetically "resting" cells of hematopoietic tissues of the rat. ^{3}H-TdR
was administered before and for several weeks after birth
to obtain 100% labelled animals. 2 weeks after the last
^{3}H-TdR injection in hematopoietic tissues reticular cells
and a small fraction of lymphocytes were found to have a
very slow turnover time.

2) In bone marrow there was no evidence that any of
the differentiated cells remain labelled, so that there
appeared to be no feed in of "resting cells" into differentiated cells under normal steady state conditions.

3) In the lymphatic tissues morphologically similar
cell types were detected to be labelled 2 weeks after the
last ^{3}H-TdR injection. However, in lymphnodes there were
in addition to those cell types large and medium sized
lymphocytes found to be labelled even month afterwards
indicating a continuous influx from "resting cells" of
this organ.

4) The data presented suggest that a possible cellular traffic of cells which are cytokinetically "resting"
is apparently restricted to cells morphologically identified as small lymphocytes.

5) Administration of x-irradiation or radiomimetic
agents allows the identification of those resting cells
that respond with proliferative activity after perturbation of hematopoietic cell renewal systems. The findings suggest that only the small fraction of resting bone
marrow lymphocytes respond with proliferative activity
indicated by the reduction of the labelling intensity and
a parallel increase of their number.

6) If hydroxyurea was used as an agent to eliminate
a large fraction of rapidly turning over cells in addition to the former findings, labelled early hematopoietic precursor cells in the bone marrow were found at
the early phase of regeneration of this organ.

Our tentative conclusion is that these cells are derived by transformation of labelled small bone marrow
lymphocytes whereas other resting cells, namely reticular
and endothelial cells of the bone marrow do not contribute to this process.

REFERENCES

1. LAJTHA, L.G., OLIVER, R. and CURNEY, C.W., *Brit. J. Hem*
    8, 442, 1962.

2. BECKER, A.J., McCULLOCH, E.A., SIMINOVITCH, L. and
    TILL, J.E., *Blood*, *26*, 296, 1965.

3. BRUCE, W.R. and MEEKER, B.E., *J. Nat. Cancer Inst.*, *34*,
    849, 1965.

4. BRUCE, W.R., MEEKER, B.E. and VALERIOTE, F.A.,
    J. Nat. Cancer Inst., *37*, 233, 1966.

5. FLIEDNER, T.M., THOMAS, E.D., MEYER, L.M. and
    CRONKITE, E.P., *Ann., N.Y. Acad. Sci. 114*,
    510, 1964.

6. STOHLMAN, F. Jr., EBBE, S., MORSE, B., HOWARD, D.
    and DONOVAN, J., *Ann. N.Y. Acad. Sci.*, *149*,
    156, 1968.

7. FORD, C.E., HAMERTON, I.L., BARNES, D.W.H. and
    LOUTIT, B.F., *Nature*, *177*, 452, 1956.

8. BECKER, A.J., McCULLOCH, E.A., TILL, J.E., *Nature*,
    197, 452, 1963.

9. GOODMAN, J.W. and HODGSON, G.S., *Blood*, *19*, 702,
    1962.

10. BARNES, D.W.H. and LOUTIT, J.F., *Lancet*, *75*, 26,
    1138, 1967.

11. TILL, J.E. and McCULLOCH, E.A., *Rad. Res. 14*, 213, 1961.

12. HODGSON, G.S., *Blood, 19*, 460, 1962.

13. CUDKOWICZ, G., BENNET, M. and SHEARER, G.M., *Science, 144*, 866, 1964.

14. SMITH, L.H., *Am. J. Physiol., 206*, 1244, 1964.

15. BLACKETT, N.M., *Brit. J. Haemat., 13*, 915, 1967.

16. MICKLEM, H.S. and FORD, C.E., *Transpl. Bull., 26*, 436, 1960.

17. GOODMAN, J.W., In: *La Greffe des Cellules Hémato-poiétiques Allogéniques*, p. 31, Paris, Editions du CNRS, 1965.

18. STORB, R., EPSTEIN, R.B. and THOMAS, E.D., *Blood, 32*, 662, 1968.

19. LITTLE, J.R., BRECHER, G., BRADLEY, T.R. and ROSE, S., *Blood, 19*, 236, 1962.

20. FLIEDNER, T.M., HAAS, R.J., STEHLE, H. and ADAMS, A.C., *Lab. Invest., 18*, 249, 1968.

21. HAAS, R.J., BOHNE, F. and FLIEDNER, T.M., *Blood, 34*, 791, 1969.

22. HAAS, R.J., MEYER-HAMME, K.D., TREPEL, F. and FLIEDNER, T.M., Held at the *XIII International Congress of Hematology*, Munich, August 2 - 8, 1970.

23. HAAS, R.J., BOHNE, F., HARRIS, E.B. and FLIEDNER, T.M., *Cell and Tissue Kinetics, 4*, 31, 1971.

24. HAAS, R.J., FLIEDNER, T.M. and STEHLE, H., In: *Effects of Radiation on Cellular Proliferation and Differentiation*, IAEA Vienna, p. 205, 1968.

25. PHILIPS, F.S., STERNBERG, S.S., SCHWARTZ, H.S.,
     CRONIN, A.P., SODERGREN, J.E. and VIDAL, P.M.,
     Cancer Research, 27, 61, 1967.

26. BOHNE, F., HAAS, R.J., FLIEDNER, T.M. and FACHE, I.,
     Brit. J. Haemat., 19, 533, 1970.

REGENERATION OF CELL RENEWAL SYSTEMS WITH PARTICULAR REFERENCE TO STEM CELL TRAFFIC*

HARVEY M. PATT

Laboratory of Radiobiology, University of California, San Francisco, California 94122, U.S.A.

The rate at which a cell renewal system will run down and recover when its stem cells are depressed can depend upon a multiplicity of variables [17, 20]. However, irrespective of these variables, recovery clearly requires a certain nidus of cells with a potential for stemness. Such cells may represent the characteristic stem cells of the system or, conceivably, other undifferentiated cells that can be appropriately programmed. In this paper, I shall consider in a general way the origin and traffic of cells responsible for initiation of regeneration under different conditions of damage. Since most of the work in this area has been concerned with hematopoiesis, our attention will be focused on bone marrow.

REQUIREMENTS FOR REGENERATION

Little is known about the precise mechanism involved in the initiation of regeneration after irradiation or other insults. The basic stimulus is presumed to be local in origin, but the recovery process may be influenced by various homeostatic factors when a sizeable part of a system is damaged. This applies to a fairly simple renewal tissue such as the intestinal mucosa or to a more complex system such as bone marrow.

---

*Work performed under the auspices of the U.S. Atomic Energy Commission.

Unlike wounding, radiation-induced injury is somewhat discriminate. With moderate irradiation, the reactions of cell renewal systems are referable mainly to the characteristic renewing population rather than to the supporting matrix. This is in contrast to the picture after heavy irradiation or after mechanical injury or removal of a part of the system. Here, regeneration depends upon the interplay of a number of reparative processes involving the stroma and vasculature as well as the characteristic population. The healing of a bone fracture or the reconstitution of bone marrow in a depleted medullary cavity are examples of this type of regenerative program.

In theory, the characteristic population of a cell renewal system could recover if only a single viable progenitor or stem-type cell remained in its proper environment. This is improbable, however, particularly in those instances where cell traffic is limited or where a critical level of mature cells is necessary for the system's integrity. In most cases, a certain number of stem cells is required for successful regeneration, the number depending upon various attributes of the system. One such attribute is the potential for stem cell turnover or recruitment relative to the steady state condition [17]. Another is the possibility of stem cell migration. When only a part of the system is damaged, for example, after partial body irradiation, the requirements for regeneration may be quite different because of cell traffic. In this respect, there appear to be two types of cell renewal systems: 1) local traffic and 2) distant traffic. In the former, migration of progenitor cells is generally restricted to contiguous areas, while in the latter migration can occur from one region to another via the blood and lymph. Thus, stem cell requirements can differ widely depending upon the system and the conditions of damage. A single spermatogonium may restore a seminiferous tubule, while in the intestine the critical mass needed to reconstruct a functional cover on the surface seems to be one to a few cells per crypt in a few crypts per villus [20]. On the other hand, because of the possibility of seeding, very few cells may suffice to repopulate an entire bone marrow.

As in the repair of a wound, some physiological interplay is evident between irradiated and adjacent unirradiated areas. A protective effect of unirradiated tissue is apparent in corneal epithelium when areas of different size are exposed to X-rays [21]. A comparable
sparing action may occur in the lens and in the intestinal mucosa as well. Although the mechanism of these apparently local effects is imcompletely understood, cell
migration from the margins of neighboring areas is probably a contributing factor.

The most dramatic effects of cell migration are, of
course, seen in recovery of irradiated tissues and organs
such as bone marrow, thymus, lymph nodes and spleen after
appropriate shielding or transplantation. This has led
to the belief that there is a significant traffic of hematopoietic stem cells even in the normal steady state [9]
and to the concept that such stem cells may be principally circulating cells which become fixed in an *inductive
microenvironment* [13]. Stem cell traffic could provide a
unifying mechanism for control of the widely disseminated
hematopoietic tissues. Unfortunately, this does not seem
to be so.

SIGNIFICANCE OF CIRCULATING STEM CELLS

The presence of hematopoietic stem cells in the circulating blood has been established in numerous studies.
Colony-forming units (CFU's) can be recovered from peripheral blood and their release from marrow to blood and
transfer from blood to hematopoietic tissues have been
demonstrated in a variety of radiation experiments with
mice [8]. Stem cell migration has also been noted in phenyl-
hydrazine-induced hemolytic anemia [9] and after grafting
of semisyngenic heterotopic bone marrow under the renal
capsule [6]. Despite the vast array of evidence, the
physiologic significance of circulating stem cells in
the normal animal remains a moot point.

It has been estimated that such cells represent perhaps 0.1 percent or less of CFU's in the mouse [8]. The
average transit time in blood is reported to be only a

matter of about 10 minutes, based on the disappearance rate of intravenously injected cells [9]. Although the latter technique may not provide a valid measure of the transit time, taken at face value, this time would signify a daily turnover from blood of some 5 to 10 percent of the total CFU's in a mouse. After several injections of phenylhydrazine, the turnover apparently increases several-fold [9]. As an alternative to the circulation of all CFU between marrow and blood, it has been proposed that only a very small fraction (less than 1 percent) of marrow CFU's can be exchanged rapidly with blood [8]. There is, however, no definitive proof that a rapid interchange between such cells in peripheral blood and a small subpopulation in marrow is a normal occurrence. The initial rapid release of colony-forming cells from a shielded part could simply refect a non-specific response to irradiation as in the case of the early transient mobilization of granulocytes. Conceivably, a mere change in marrow blood flow could be an important contributing factor. Whatever the mechanism, it seems from the experience with phenylhydrazine [9] that a rather substantial increase in CFU emigration from marrow can occur when hematopoiesis is stimulated.

The most convincing evidence against a meaningful bone marrow to blood to bone marrow stem cell traffic in the steady state comes from experiments with chromosome-marked bone marrow [5, 16]. In these studies, there was no suggestion of any equilibration of donor cells (CBA-T6T6) between irradiated (femur) and unirradiated (humerus) bone marrow. A majority of donor cells persisted in the femur for up to two years and, significantly, the number in the humerus was unchanged from the low level seen soon after transplantation (Fig. 1). It has been inferred from the same studies with chromosome markers that there is normally a continuous stem cell traffic between marrow and thymus [5]. The data obtained for the thymus were quite variable, however, unlike the marrow data. Moreover, even if the proportion of donor cells in the thymus increased to a stable level over a several week period, as has been claimed [5] this need not signify a continuing influx of stem cells. It could simply reflect the time required for the proliferating progeny of originally implanted cells to achieve a steady state in thymus.

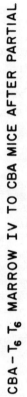
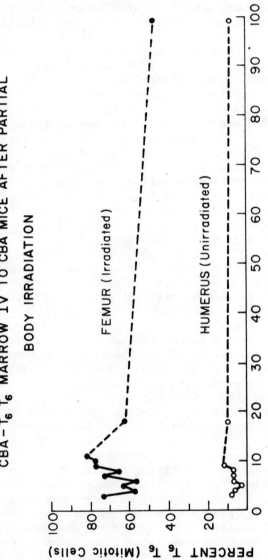

Fig. 1. Distribution of chromosome-marked cells in irradiated and unirradiated marrow. (Data of Ford et al. [5].)

More recently, we have observed that the regeneration of bone marrow in a mechanically depleted medullary cavity is independent of circulating stem cells [18]. There is no delay in repopulation of a shielded evacuated femur shaft when the remainder of the body is X-irradiated. However, irradiation of only the femur leads to a definite impairment of marrow regeneration (Fig. 2). A similar situation obtains with fracture repair; an unirradiated bone transplanted to an irradiated site and subsequently fractured heals normally, whereas an irradiated bone placed in an unirradiated area fails to heal [3]. Further evidence for the local, in contrast to the hematogenous, origin of the regenerative cells has been provided in our experiments with marrow transplants [18]. It was found that the evacuated femur shaft was repopulated by host cells even though many donor cells were evident in hematopoietic tissue elsewhere including the epiphyseal marrow adjacent to the evacuated area.

The several lines of evidence concerning the significance of circulating hematopoietic stem cells could be reconciled in the following manner. It seems reasonable to assume that there is a random loss of stem cells from marrow and blood. Emigration from marrow to blood would be a function of (1) the number of stem cells in close proximity to blood vessels and (2) the rate of marrow perfusion. It is expected that ordinarily only a minor fraction of the stem cell population would be adjacent to marrow sinuses, which agrees with the suggestion of a small rapidly mobilizable pool [8]. Apropos of the finding of a few CFU's in the peripheral blood, it is noteworthy that a small number of immature hemic cells are also present in blood normally. Like the circulating CFU, these may be thought of as a biological artifact without particular hematopoietic significance under normal conditions. Since there is no sensitive functional assay for such cell types, they are usually not detected unless a large sample is counted. The uptake and eventual proliferation of circulating stem cells in marrow must depend on marrow cellularity and environment as well as on the number in blood and the rate of blood flow. It follows that the probability of successful seeding would be low, for example, in a normal relative to an aplastic marrow.

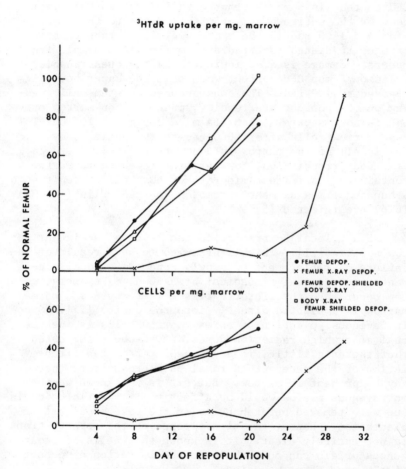

Fig. 2.   Effect of local and body X-irradiation on initiation of marrow
           restoration in a mechanically depleted femur shaft.   (Reprinted
           with permission from Science *165*, 71, 1969, M.A. Maloney and
           H.M. Patt.   Copyright 1969 by the American Association for the
           Advancement of Science.)

It is expected that the significance of hematopoietic stem cell traffic in perturbed states would be determined by the nature and magnitude of the perturbation.
There seems to be little difference in the depression of
CFU content in a mouse femur with 100 rad to the lower
body or the entire body, or with 100 rad to the lower
body and 1000 rad to the upper body [2]. That traffic
from unirradiated to irradiated marrow is minimal with
moderate damage is also indicated by the questionable effects on femur CFU content when only the upper body is
exposed to 100 rad. The consequences of stem cell seeding on CFU content are readily apparent when marrow damage is more severe. When CBA mice are given 10^5 CBA-T6T6
bone marrow cells after 1000 rad to the entire body, virtually all of the marrow is donor-type [16]. With partial body irradiation, however, the regenerated marrow
contains a significant minority of host cells even though
a hundred times as many chromosome-marked cells (10^7 CBA-
T6T6) are injected [5].

Heavy local X-irradiation can lead to persistant marrow aplasia [11]. This is presumed to be a result of the
failure of replacement of slowly renewing stromal elements and eventual sinusoidal breakdown. Regeneration
can occur when the fibrotic tissue is removed and normal
marrow is implanted directly into the cavity [12]. Since
intravenous injection of normal marrow cells is ineffec-
tual after high radiation doses, it has been suggested
that there is little, if any, seeding from the circulation of the necessary stromal cell progenitors that
may be present in marrow. But, it is not known whether
intravenous marrow would be effective if the fibrotic tissue were removed beforehand as in the case of direct implantation. Hence, the significance of this observation
is not entirely clear. It is known that cells of hematogenous origin can contribute to the formation of connec-
tive tissue after wounding.

It is significant that marrow can be reconstituted
in an evacuated femur shaft without the apparent inter-
vention of circulating stem cells [18]. In this instance
reconstruction of the marrow reticulum and vasculature
are a prelude to hemic cell repopulation. The picture is,

therefore, quite different from that seen after moderate
irradiation, where regeneration depends mainly upon the
survival or seeding of a certain number of hematopoietic
stem cells within an existing matrix. Although it might
be argued that the emptied medullary cavity is not accessible to circulating stem cells, this is not a likely explanation for their neglibible role since blood flow is
restored rather rapidly [18]. Moreover, it is important
to note that regeneration of the diaphyseal marrow does
not even depend upon cell migration from neighboring intact epiphyseal marrow. There is reason to think that
activation of a local source of hematopoietic progenitors
in the adjacent bone, possibly from the perivascular con-
nective tissue cells in the Haversian canals, accounts
for the repopulation of a mechanically depleted medullary
cavity [18].

We have observed that many of the mesenchymal cells
in the Haversian canals are labeled with tritiated thymidine (^{3}HTdR) during the first few days after femur evacu-
ation; only an occasional flash-labeled cell is seen in
the canals of the contralateral femur. Labeled undifferentiated cells are also evident at this time in the developing granulation tissue within the medullary cavity.
Fig. 3 depicts the changes in labeling indices of such
cells with time after ^{3}HTdR injection and after marrow
removal. The data suggest an influx of labeled cells,
presumably from the Haversian system. It will be noted
that this is closely correlated with the rise and fall of
undifferentiated cells as seen in imprints of the medullary tissue. In this regenerative system, the reappearance of CFU as assayed in spleen or in soft agar cultures
is a relatively late event and occurs *pari passu* with the
reappearance of obvious hemic cells (Fig. 4) [15].

THE CASE FOR A HEMATOPOIETIC STEM CELL HIERARCHY

By definition, stem cells must have a capacity for
self-renewal as well as for differentiation. In respect
to the latter, it is clear that stem cells may be uni-
potent or pluripotent. Bone marrow apparently contains
both committed and uncommitted types of stem cells.

It is usually assumed that stem cells, at least of the uncommitted variety, have infinite reproductive integrity.
However, marrow repopulating capacity is known to decline
with successive transplantation [14]. Does this mean that
the repopulating cell, presumably the CFU, has a limited proliferative capacity, or perhaps that maintenance of
the stem cell pool is compromised by the repeated pressure for differentiation? The latter is unlikely since
a subnormal repopulating capacity has been shown to persist for as long as 150 days. The former would agree
with the inference from tissue culture studies of a limited proliferative potential for all normal mammalian
cells [7]. Indeed, the possibility of eventual stem cell
exhaustion even under normal lifetime requirements has
led to a concept of clonal succession in which exhausted
clones of stem cells are replaced by ancestral clones
[10]. Because of the exponential nature of clonal succession, many fewer generations would satisfy the requirements for differentiation normally and in response to
stress. It might be expected that impairment of the repopulating ability of a recolonized marrow would be a
function of the number of transplanted cells in addition
to the number and timing of repeated transplantations.
That this may be so [4] is consistent with the hypothesis
of clonal succession; however, the data are incomplete
and other interpretations are possible.

In view of the foregoing considerations, we may in-
quire whether cells ancestral to the conventional CFU and
with a potential for hematopoiesis exist outside of the
marrow proper in an adult animal. It seems reasonable
to think that such ancestral (pre-stem) cells could be
present among the mesenchymal elements in bone. There is
some support for this from studies of bone and bone matrix
implantation [22] and of marrow regeneration in a depleted medullary cavity [18]. Still, the fact that donor
marrow cells can more or less permanently recolonize an
irradiated recipient's bone marrow [16] tends to suggest
that an influx of any pre-stem cells from bone is ordinarily very small or limited to certain conditions. As
noted above, recolonization does not necessarily signify
complete recovery; a latent residual injury may remain
even in spontaneously regenerated marrow [1]. The mes-

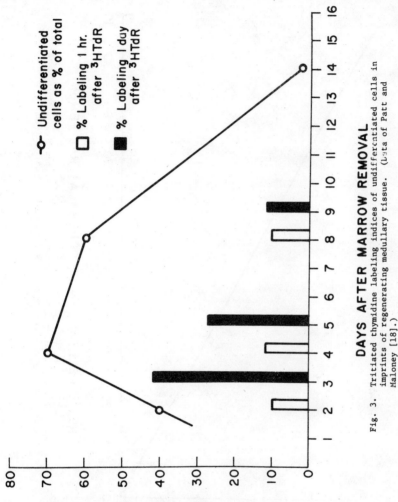

Fig. 3. Tritiated thymidine labeling indices of undifferentiated cells in imprints of regenerating medullary tissue. (Data of Patt and Maloney [18].)

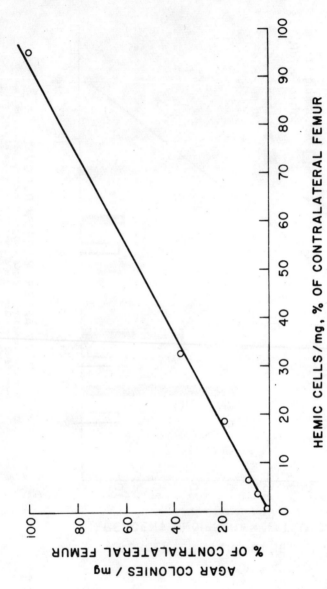

Fig. 4. Relationship between agar colony-forming cells and hemic cells in
regenerating medullary tissue. (M.A. Maloney, unpublished data).

enchymal elements in bone, which ordinarily manifest
little or no turnover, can be quite radiosensitive and by
analogy with hepatic cells may reveal damage only upon
activation [19]. Hence, such irradiated cells may not
contribute perceptibly to a marrow seemingly restored by
transplantation. Conceivably, this could be a factor in
residual injury. Although it is now recognized that stem
cells do not represent a rigidly compartmentalized homogenous population, I suggest that it is also necessary to
recognize that the conventional CFU of marrow may not represent the first echelon in a stem cell hierarchy, even
though it may be the most important operational component
in normal hematopoiesis and in a variety of compensatory
responses.

SUMMARY

    In most cell renewal systems there is a restricted
traffic of stem cells and regeneration of a damaged part
requires cells of local or proximate origin. A notable
exception is the lympho-myeloid complex. Yet, even here,
circulating stem cells are of questionable physiologic
significance in the steady state. Although distant metas-
tases can have an important function in the restoration
of hematopoiesis, this is not always the case. Depending
upon the circumstances of damage, marrow restitution can
involve a hierarchy of stem-type cells. In respect to
hematopoiesis *per se*, it seems necessary to consider the
possible role of a pre-stem cell ancestral to the marrow
CFU and resident in osseous tissue.

REFERENCES

1.   BAUM, S.J., *Radiation Res.*, *32*, 651, 1967.

2.   CARSTEN, A.L. and BOND, V.P., In: *Normal and Malig-
      nant Cell Growth*, R.J.M. Fry, M.L. Griem and W.H.
      Kirsten, Eds., Springer-Verlag, p. 21, New York,
      1969.

3.   COOLEY, L.M. and GOSS, R.J., *Am. J. Anat.*, *102*, 167, 1958.

4.   CUDKOWICZ, G., UPTON, A.C., SHEARER, G.M. and HUGHES, W.L., *Nature*, *201*, 165, 1964.

5.   FORD, C.E., MICKLEM, H.S., EVANS, E.P., GRAY, J.G. and OGDEN, D.A., *Ann. N.Y. Acad. Sci.*, *129*, 283, 1966.

6.   FRIEDENSTEIN, A.J., PETRAKOVA, K.V., KUROLESOVA, A.I. and FROLOVA, G.P., *Transplantation*, *6*, 230, 1968.

7.   HAYFLICK, L., *Exptl. Cell Res.*, *37*, 614, 1965.

8.   HELLMAN, S. and GRATE, H.E., In: *Effects of Radiation on Cellular Proliferation and Differentiation*, p. 187, IAEA, Vienna, 1968.

9.   HODGSON, G., GUZMAN, E. and HERRERA, C., In: *Effects of Radiation on Cellular Proliferation and Differentiation*, p. 163, IAEA, Vienna, 1968.

10. KAY, H.E.M., *Lancet II*, *418*, 1965.

11. KNOSPE, W.H., BLOM, J. and CROSBY, W.H., *Blood*, *28*, 398, 1966.

12. KNOSPE, W.H., BLOM, J. and CROSBY, W.H., *Blood*, *31*, 400, 1968.

13. KRETCHMAR, A.L., *Exptl. Haematol.*, *19*, v, 1969.

14. LAJTHA, L.G. and SCHOFIELD, R., In: *Normal and Malignant Cell Growth*, R.J.M. Fry, M.L. Griem and W.H. Kirsten, Eds., Springer-Verlag, p. 10, New York, 1969.

15. MALONEY, M.A., *Proc. Soc. Exptl. Biol. Med.*, *135*,412, 1970.

16. MICKLEM, H.S., FORD, C.E., EVANS, E.P. and GRAY, J., *Proc. Royal Soc.*, London, Series B, *165*, 78, 1966.

17. PATT, H.M., In: *Effects of Radiation on Cellular Pro-liferation and Differentiation*, p. 3, IAEA, Vienna, 1968.

18. PATT, H.M. and MALONEY, M.A., In: *Hemopoietic Cellu-lar Proliferation*, F. Stohlman, Jr., Ed., Grune and Stratton, New York, p.56, New York, 1970.

19. PATT, H.M. and MALONEY, M.A., *Radiation Res., 41*, 500, 1970.

20. PATT, H.M. and QUASTLER, H., *Physiol. Rev., 43*, 357, 1963.

21. STRELIN, G.S., *Nucl. Sci. Abstr., 4*, 953, 1950.

22. URIST, M.R., HAY, P.H., DUBUC, F. and BURING, K., *Clin. Orthopaed., 64*, 194, 1969.

THE RADIATION RESPONSE OF THE INTESTINAL EPITHELIUM*

A.B. CAIRNIE

*Department of Biology,
Queen's University,
Kingston, Canada*

It is unusual to find in a symposium entitled *Self-renewing Systems in Vivo* that there are six papers on the small intestine and only two on the bone marrow. I now find myself in the position of reviewing papers whose authors will follow me on the programme and I am therefore conscious that while I shall have the first word, they will have the last. I shall try to give an overview, to set the stage for them, and perhaps to provoke some discussion.

INTRODUCTION

The basic organization of the small intestine in mammalian species takes the form of crypts and villi which have on their luminal surface a simple columnar epithelium. There are slight differences between different parts of the small intestine, and a simpler architecture is usually found in embryos and neonatal animals. There is some variation between species in the size of the crypt, and rather more in the shape of the villus, which may be either approximately cylindrical or leaf-like. The work which I shall refer has been

---

*The work reported was supported by the Department of University Affairs, Toronto and the National Research Council, Ottawa.

done on mice and rats, which are qualitatively similar
as regards intestinal cell kinetics and response to radiation, although differing quantitatively in some respects.

While the most abundant cell in the small intestine
is the columnar cell, there are also goblet, Paneth and
argentaffin cells (Fig. 1). The columnar cell prolifer-
ates in the crypt and presumably undergoes self-renewal,
but the goblet and Paneth cells do not [6]. Little is
known about the origin of the argentaffin cells. Goblet cells are post-mitotic cells which are believed to
be derived in the crypts from the proliferating columnar cells and to migrate with them to the villi. Paneth
cells, found only in the base of the crypts, are also
post-mitotic and may arise from progenitor cells situated
outside the crypts, although it is more usually suggested
that they come from columnar cells in the base of the
crypts [7]. Radiation interfers primarily with the proliferating columnar cells and the effect of radiation
on the intestinal epithelium is attributed to this effect rather than to effects on post-mitotic cells.

SCHEMATIC DIAGRAM OF INTESTINAL CRYPT

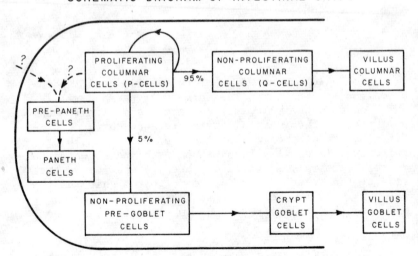

Fig. 1.   The progenitor relationships of the various cell types in the
crypt of the small intestine.

Wimber [17], working in Henry Quastler's laboratory at Brookhaven, pioneered a technique for dissection of single crypts which has recently been taken up by Lesher's group [10], and by myself in turn. This has been used to show that there are about 1.1×10^6 crypts and 2.5×10^5 villi in the mouse small intestine. The mouse crypt contains 300 to 350 cells and the villus an epithelial population of about 1000 cells. The turnover time of the villus cells is 30 to 40 hr.

CONTROL OF PROLIFERATION AND DIFFERENTIATION

One of the reasons for the continued interest in cell renewal systems is the opportuity they afford to study differentiation displayed spatially rather than, as in the embryo, temporally. The crypt is the embryo, in which cell diversification and specialization proceed as the cells approach the villus. The villus represents the adult, the specialized cell lines corresponding to the tissues of the organism. Beyond the villus lies Death, from which no cell returns. One would hope and expect that an understanding of the control of cell renewal would have a profound bearing on our ideas on differentiation in general. It is perhaps too early to say yet whether this optimism is justified, but certainly our knowledge of the regulation of haematopoiesis is rapidly extending to the level of gene regulation [9]. In the intestine our understanding is much less complete, and it would be undully optimistic to anticipate that our understanding of differentiation would come from this tissue. The intestine is often described as the simplest cell-renewal tissue; it is also one of the least accessible. I would however like to return later to this subject of control, especially of proliferation.

In the meantime I would like to draw your attention to the interpretation I published in 1965, along with Steel and Lamerton, of the distribution in the normal crypt of cells in S-phase and M-phase in terms of a "cut-off" of proliferation in a particular zone of the crypt [2,3]. This zone was later stated as being between one-third

and just above one-half of the way up the crypt from the
base.   In the bottom third of the crypt each cell divides
to give two-daughter cells which will in turn divide.
In the cut-off zone there is a gradual changeover to the
production of post-mitotic cells, and above the cut-off
zone only post-mitotic cells are produced.

Dr. Galjaard, who is contributing to this symposium,
together with Dr. Bootsma, has recently correlated this
distribution of proliferating cells with another characteristic of cell specialization in the intestine, namely
the non-specific esterase activity [8].   They have shown
that after 400R of x-rays the expansion of the zone of
proliferating cells which ensues in the crypts is accompanied by an absence of esterase, and the two parameters
return to normal in synchrony.   They state, "From this
negative correlation it might either be concluded that
the non-specific esterases might play a role in the
"critical decision phase" of the crypt cells or that
only a parallelism exists of two effects: as soon as a
crypt cell does not proliferate any more it shows esterase activity as one of its features of maturation".

MANIFESTATIONS OF CONTROL - RESPONSE TO RADIATION

The effect of continuous irradiation on cell-renewal systems has been intensively studied in the group
which developed around Len Lamerton at the Institute of
Cancer Research in Sutton, England.   He has on a number
of occasions [13] written of the advantages of this approach, particularly the slowness and subtlety of the
changes which can be evinced by the application of a
constant physical stress, in contrast to the transients
in the response to acute radiation.

With intestine we have worked mainly at a dose-
rate around 400 rads/day since it was shown in 1959
that the rat intestine could establish a steady state
under these conditions [16].   To summarize the more
recent findings [4,5]; this steady state is associated
with a slight reduction in crypt population, a reduced
villus size (and presumably population) but normal turn-

over time, an extension of cell proliferation to higher
levels in the crypts, a small decrease in cell cycle
time, but a net reduction in cell production rate per
crypt. One unresolved problem is that the percentage
of cells which label with ^{3}H-thymidine is much lower in
the bottom half of the crypt than one would expect
from the cell cycle data if all the cells were in cycle.
It was suggested, rather reluctantly, that there were
cells present which were unable to continue in the cycle
because of radiation damage, but which could persist and
presumably migrate to the villi [4].

There are transient changes observed shortly after
the start and end of a period of continuous irradiation
[4]. During the first 18 hours of irradiation proliferation moves to a minimal level from which it subsequently
partially recovers. Particularly marked are the reduced
percentages of cells which label with ^{3}H-thymidine and
of mitotic cells, and the increase in length of $(G_2+1/2M)$
the time to the 50% point on the upswing of the labelled
mitosis curve. It is not possible to measure other
phases of the cell cycle promtly and therefore they
cannot be followed through a transient response. As I
mentioned, these are minimal levels below those reached
when the steady state is finally established. When irradiation is terminated there is a remarkable increase in
the percentage of cells in the crypt which take up ^{3}H-
thymidine, and these cells are found even at the top of
the crypt. We have no idea what signals the cessation
of radiation. Within two days all parameters of the
intestine, so far as we know, have returned to normal.

What we are observing here, in this complex of
action and reaction, is homeostatic control of:
    crypt population
    villus population
    villus turnover time
    distribution of proliferating cells in the crypt
    cell cycle time
    cell production rate

While many of these are undoubtedly inter-related,
the compexity and precision of control is impressive.

Our understanding of the mechanisms involved is at the
early stage of untested hypotheses.

Lesher has recently studied the response of the
small intestine in terms of cell kinetics to acute doses
between 75R and 1000R [14]. His group has been extremely
productive and I do not have time to review all their
findings. Using Wimber's crypt dissection technique,
they have shown that the number of cells in DNA synthesis and in mitosis drops, recovers, and then overshoots
transiently. This is another manifestation of the homeostatic control of cell proliferation.

RADIOSENSITIVITY OF THE INTESTINE

The ability of the intestinal epithelium to achieve
a proliferative steady state in the face of 400 rads/day,
and the rapidity and degree of the response in the crypt
to acute irradiation betoken in qualitative terms high
radio-resistance in comparison with other tissues. The
importance for survival of an intact epithelial layer,
and the short turnover time of the cells, would lead
one to expect that the small intestine would be always
the critical tissue. As we all know, the bone marrow in
fact fails to maintain its structural integrity at a
lower dose than is the case for the intestine. This
degree of radio-resistance can be attributed to the dose-
survival characteristics of the epithelial cells, shown
by Hornsey and Vatistas [12] to have a D_Q of 400R, much
greater than that found in other mammalian cells. I am
not aware of any studies of the molecular or chemical basis of this, but possibly the approach used by O'Hara
and Terasima [15] in correlating the cyclic changes in
sensitivity to x-rays with cellular sulphydryl content
could be fruitfully applied.

The response of the cells to x-rays has been further analysed in an import series of papers by Withers
and Elkind [18,19] using a nodule assay similar to that
used by Withers for skin. The slope of the dose-survival curve is given by a D_0 of 97.3 rads, which lies in
the normal range for mammalian cells, but the extrapo-

lation number is between 50 and 160, depending on the method of estimation used. Since

$$D_Q = D_o \ln n$$

we have a D_Q of 380 to 490 rads, in good enough agreement with Hornsey and Vatistas' less direct measurement of 400R. Such a dose-survival curve indicates an unusually broad shoulder, a high resistance to continuous irradiation, and a large capacity for repair of sublethal damage; conclusions already reached using other less-direct approach [4,5,12].

With this information it was of course possible for Withers and Elkind to estimate the number of cells which survive in the intestine after various doses. Using Lesher's figure of 130 proliferative cells per crypt, 7 cells in each crypt on average would survive a dose of 660 rads. If one makes the assumption that any proliferative cell is capable of repopulating the crypt, one would not expect to find a measurable number of crypts sterilized by this dose. In this way they were able to account for the absence of detectable residual damage from a first dose of 660 rads when the fractionation interval was 4 days or longer.

TABLE 1. Total Number of Crypts in the Small Intestine at 7 Days After Irradiation

X-Ray Dose (R)	Calculated* Survival Level of Crypts	Measured Number of Crypts (Mean ± S.E.)
0	100%	$1.47\pm0.11 \times10^6$ (100%)
400	100%	$1.41\pm0.10 \times10^6$ (96%)
800	71%	$1.54\pm0.11 \times10^6$ (105%)
1200	<0.5%	$1.03\pm0.05 \times10^6$ (70%)
1600	∿0%	$0.64\pm0.06 \times10^6$ (45%)

*Mean number of surviving cells per crypt was calculated from Withers and Elkind's data [18]. Poisson statistics give percentage of crypts with one or more surviving cells.

However, if there are only 2 surviving cells per
crypt, which one would expect after 840R, some 40 per cent
of the crypts would be sterilized. Table 1 sets out a
series of doses, the anticipated level of reduction in
numbers of crypts, and that actually found after 7 days
in irradiated mice using Hagemann *et al.*'s [10] technique for counting crypts. The mice used were LAF1 males
about 8 weeks old. They were exposed at 21R/min. with
their hind limbs shielded and using the following regime - 225kV, 15m.a., 1/2 mm. Cu + 1 mm. Al filtration,
F.S.D. 108 cm. It can be seen that although there was
some loss of crypts after 1200R and 1600R, the numbers
present were much greater than the calculations would
suggest.

The limitation of this approach can be seen in the
next experiment, where the total numbers of crypts and
villi in the small intestine were followed for 3 weeks
after 1600R (Fig. 2). The number of villi may show a
slight drop, but these results are not conclusive. However, the number of crypts shows a dramatic drop and
then undergoes a gradual recovery which is not complete
even after 3 weeks. At 3 days there are a very few
structures present which look in the dissection microscope like normal crypts. At 5 and 7 days there are
many more crypts and they are much larger. At 14 and
21 days the crypts are almost reduced to normal size.

Using Withers and Elkind's data for the dose-survival
curve, and Lesher's figure of 1.1×10^8 proliferative
cells in the whole intestine, one can calculate that after 1600R there would only be 1800 surviving cells in
the intestine. Of the original 1.1 million crypts only
1800 would contain a surviving cell. If each crypt is
a separate clone, self-sustaining, and with no possibility of re-inforcement or replenishment from a central
reserve, only 1800 crypts can regenerate. Contrast
this with the situation of the bone marrow stem cell
which we know circulates, even through the peripheral
blood stream, and which can give rise to a clone of a
million or more cells.

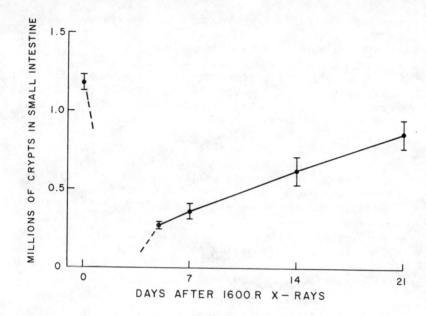

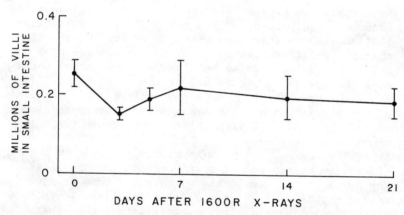

Fig. 2. Numbers of villi and crypts present at various time intervals
after the administration of 1600 R X-rays.

Since the experiment I have described deomonstrates
the regeneration of crypts far in excess of 1800, and
moreover a progressive increase in the number, one must

conclude that the crypt is not a closed system. Either
crypts can divide into more or less equal parts, or new
crypts can be seeded by stem cells.

I have some reservations about Withers and Elkind's
assay system. Their macrocolonies obtained by local
irradiation are much bigger than crypts and at the time
they assay, 14 days, I see only relatively normal crypts
in my mice using a dose in the same range. Since the
number of crypts increases with time, crypts cannot be
regarded as clones and numbers of crypts cannot be used
as an assay for surviving cells. What is the relation
between the macro- and micro-colonies of Withers and
Elkind on the one hand, and crypts on the other? I do
not know. It may be that their colonies are derived
from single cells but at the moment I am sceptical about
this. This is an important point to settle as the assumption is absolutely basic to their interpretation.

The demonstration that the crypt is not a closed
system raises interesting questions concerning stem
cells in the intestine, that is cells which can produce their own kind as distinct from those cells which
produce cells proceeding along the pathway of specialization. Up to this point in this paper I have assumed
that all proliferative cells in the crypts are stem
cells, but as we pointed out in 1965, one cannot determine the degree of "stemness" of the crypt cells [3].
Since we know that in bone marrow only a small fraction
of the population has the ability to function as stem
cells, the number of stem cells in the mouse crypt is
almost certainly much less than 130, the number of proliferative cells. Crypt numbers may increase during regeneration by fission of crypts or as a result of seeding by migrating stem cells which might come from existing crypts or even from a different tissue. In this
connection, I have already suggested that the Paneth
cells may have a progenitor outside the crypt [6]. I am
intrigued by observations such as those of Andrew [1],
who described what he called "lymphocyte transformation"
in intestinal epithelium, and the suggestion by Hard, Martinez and Good [11] of a possible trephocytic role of
the thymus lymphocyte in the small intestine. We may
be on the brink of important discoveries in developmen-

tal biology, which may even link cell renewal in the
small intestine to other cell renewal systems through
the existence of a common multi-potent stem cell.

REFERENCES

1.   ANDREW, W., *J. Nat. Canc. Inst.*, *35*, 113, 1965.

2.   CAIRNIE, A.B., LAMERTON, L.F., and STEEL, G.G.,
     Exp. Cell Res., *39*, 528, 1965.

3.   CAIRNIE, A.B., LAMERTON, L.F. and STEEL, G.G.,
     Exp. Cell Res., *39*, 539, 1965.

4.   CAIRNIE, A.B., *Radiation Res.*, *32*, 240, 1967.

5.   CAIRNIE, A.B., *Radiation Res.*, *38*, 82, 1969.

6.   CAIRNIE, A.B., *Cell Tissue Kinet.*, *3*, 25, 1970.

7.   CHENG, H., MERZEL, J. and LEBLOND, C.P., *Amer. J.
     Anat.*, *126*, 507, 1969.

8.   GALJAARD, H. and BOOTSMA, D., *Exp. Cell Res.*, *58*,
     79, 1969.

9.   GOLDWASSER, E.,   *Current Topics in Developmental
     Biology*, 1, 173, 1966, Academic Press.

10. HAGEMANN, R.F., SIGDESTAD, C.P., and LESHER, S.,
     Cell Tissue Kinet., *3*, 21, 1970.

11. HARD, R.C., MARTINEZ, C., and GOOD, R.A., *Nature*,
     204, 455, 1964.

12. HORNSEY, S., and VATISTAS, S., *Brit. J. Radiol.*,
     36, 795, 1963.

13. LAMERTON, L.F., *Radiation Res.*, *27*, 119, 1966.

14. LESHER, S., and BAUMAN, J., *Nat. Cancer Inst.*,
     Monograph No. 30, 185, 1969.

15. O'HARA, H., and TERASIMA, T., *Exper. Cell Res.*, *58*, 182, 1969.

16. QUASTLER, H., BENSTED, J.P.M., LAMERTON, L.F., and SIMPSON, S.M., *Brit. J. Radiol.*, *32*, 501, 1959.

17. WIMBER, D.E., QUASTLER, H., STEIN, O.L., and WIMBER, D.R., *J. Biophys. Biochem. Cytol.*, *8*, 327, 1960.

18. WITHERS, H.R., and ELKIND, M.M., *Radiation Res.*, *38*, 598, 1969.

19. WITHERS, H.R., and ELKIND, M.M., *Int. J. Radiat. Biol.*, *17*, 261, 1970.

RADIOSENSITIVITY OF INTESTINAL CRYPT CELLS IN RELATION TO LET, DOSE, DOSE-RATE AND OXYGENATION

SHIRLEY HORNSEY

M.R.C., Experimental Radiopathology Unit, Hammersmith Hospital, DuCane Road, London, W. 12, England

Death of the mouse from acute intestinal injury following wholebody irradiation was first attributed by Quastler [12] to damage to the reproductive capacity of the crypt cells of the small intestine. Dr. Vatistas and I postulated that changes in animal sensitivity under various conditions and types of irradiation would reflect changes in sensitivity of these epithelial cells and differences observed in LD_{50} doses in fractionated radiation would give us an indication of one parameter (i.e. D_q) of the cell survival curve [9].

Probit analysis is frequently used for the analysis of animal killing curves. If a straight line can be fitted to data when probits are plotted against some function of dose then the killing curve can be defined by the median lethal dose (LD_{50}) and the slope [5]. The slope is usually considered to be a measure of biological variability, but it may also reflect the statistical distribution of killing events in the stem cell population. If this is so then modifying treatments which might affect the slopes and shapes of cell survival curves might be reflected in changes in slopes of fitted probit lines. An examination of fitted probit lines for a number of different treatments suggests that broadly speaking this is so [2].

A technique developed by Withers and Elkind [13] has enabled us to observe directly the loss of

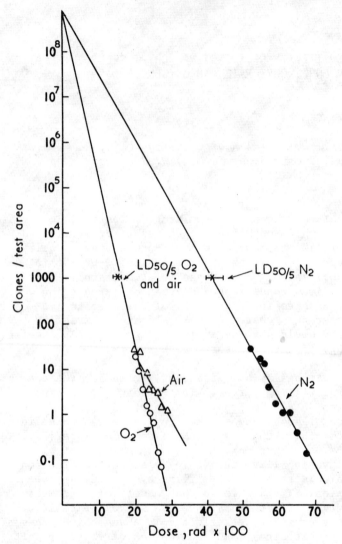

Fig. 1.   Survival of epithelial cells measured by clones arising 12 days
after irradiation of an exteriorised loop of the jejunum of mice
breathing oxygen, nitrogen or air during the irradiation.

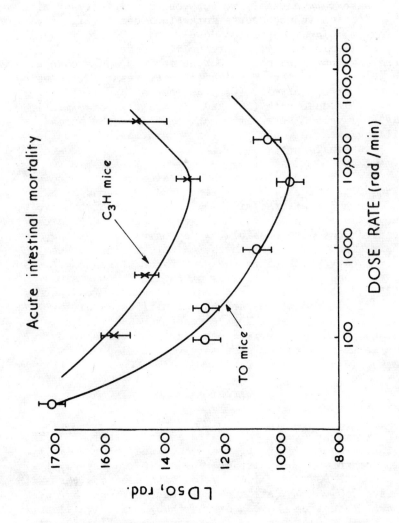

Fig. 2. The change in $LD_{50/5}$ doses of fast electrons delivered at
different dose-rates.

DOSE-RATE

Dose-rate markedly affects the sensitivity of mice to radiation-induced acute intestinal death (Fig. 2). Using two widely separated dose-rates, 100 rad/min and 6 kilorad/min of fast electrons with mice of the TO strain we obtained both a change in LD_{50} and a change in the slope of the animal killing curves [6, 2]. Using another strain of mice (C_3H) but not such a large difference in dose-rate (500 rad/min and 6 kilorad/min) the LD_{50} values were different. So, from the animal killing data we would expect a separation between the cell survival curves.

Cell survival curves were obtained after irradiation of C_3H mice with fast electrons delivered at 500 rad/min and 6 kilorad/min. The separation of the two curves is 150 to 300 rads over the range within which observations were possible, which compares with the separation by 140 rads in the animal killing curves. Curves extrapolating to the same value at zero dose give a good fit to both sets of data. The D_0 values (125 rad for 6 kilorad/min radiation and 160 rad for 500 rad/min radiation) are not significantly different (Fig. 3). If the $LD_{50}/5$ doses for C_3H mice are marked on the appropriate cell survival curve, however, the marks fall at the same survival level on both curves (Fig. 3) [8].

LET

We might expect that, with an increase in LET, the values of both D_0 and D_q would decrease. For animals exposed to wholebody irradiation, D_2-D_1, a presumptive measure of D_q, had a lower value with neutrons than with X-rays [10]. The cell survival curve measured by the clonal technique shows a small, though not significant, change in slope when fast electrons (D_0, 125 rad) are compared with fast neutrons (D_0, 110 rad). If the LD_{50} doses after neutron irradiation and fast electron irradiation are marked on the extrapolated clone survival curves then, as was the case also with the dose-rate comparison and the oxygen and nitrogen data, the marks

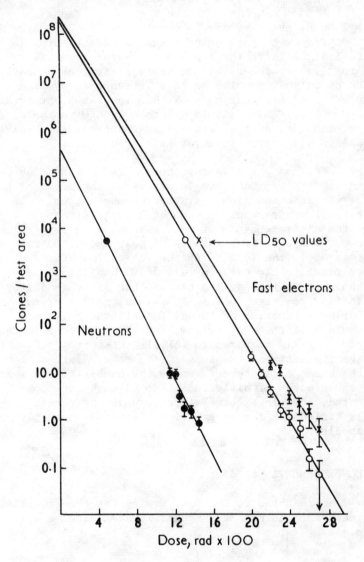

Fig. 3. Survival of jejunal epithelial cells after fast electrons at
6 kilorad/min or 500 rad/min or after fast neutrons.

fall at the same survival level on both curves (Fig. 3).

The RBE obtained from a comparison of LD_{50} doses is 2.7 and from a comparison of doses to reduce surviving epithelial cells to the 1 clone/test area level is 1.7. A comparison of the D_0 values gives a ratio of sensitivities of only 1.14. The small difference in D_0 values observed suggests that most of the high "RBE" obtained for the $LD_{50}/5$ end-point is due to a change in the size of the shoulder of the cell survival curve after neutron irradiation compared to lower LET irradiation.

These data strongly support a direct connection between loss of reproductive integrity of the cells of the small intestine and the death of the mouse from acute intestinal syndrome after wholebody irradiation. Whatever the ultimate cause of death-shock, electrolyte inbalance, dehydration – this is closely and proportionately related to the loss of epithelial cells. Perhaps the close relationship between cell death and animal death is apparent in this system because the steps in differentiation from stem cell to functional cell are few. The primary function of the differentiated cell is to maintain an intact epithelium, and the breakdown in the supply of cells required to fulfill this primary function causes the death of the animal. In other systems such as the heomopoetic system, where the number of steps in and the process of differentiation is much more complicated, the close correlation between the number of cells killed and the probability of animal death may not be so clear.

ACKNOWLEDGEMENTS

I am indebted to Dr. D.K. Bewley for the radiation dosimetry and to Mr. M.J. Hedges for technical assistance.

SUMMARY

Cell survival curves have been obtained from observations of clones arising in a denuded area of

intestinal epithelium after irradiation of an exterior-
ized loop of the jejunum with fast neutrons (D_0 110),
fast electrons at 6 kilorad/min (D_0 125 rad) and 500 rad/
min (D_0 160 rad) in mice breathing O_2 during irradiation;
in mice breathing nitrogen during irradiation with fast
electrons at 15 kilorad/min (D_0, 306) and breathing air
during irradiation with fast electrons at 6 kilorad/min
(D_0, 268). The $LD_{50}/5$ doses for animals given wholebody
irradiation under these various conditions fit on the extrapolated survival curves at the same survival level on
all curves.

REFERENCES

1.   ALPER, T. and HORNSEY, S., *Brit. J. Radiol.*, *41*,
      375, 1968.

2.   ALPER, T., HORNSEY, S., PIKE, M.C. and SMITH, P.,
      In: Effects of Radiation on Cellular Proliferation
      and Differentiation, *I.A.E.A.*, Vienna, p. 515,
      1968.

3.   BARENDSEN, G.W., In: *The Initial Effects of Ion-
      izing Radiation on Cells*, Academic Press, ed.
      Harris, R.J.C., p. 183, 1961.

4.   ELKIND, M.M., SWAIN, R.W., ALESCIO, T., SUTTON, H.
      and MOSES, W.B.,   *Cellular Radiation Biology*,
      The Williams and Wilkins Co., Baltimore and Mary-
      land, p. 442, 1965.

5.   FINNEY, D.J.,   *Probit Analysis*, Cambridge Univ-
      ersity press, 2nd Edit., 1962.

6.   HORNSEY, S. and ALPER, T., *Nature*, *210*, 212, 1966.

7.   HORNSEY, SHIRLEY, *Int. J. Radiat. Biol.*, *18*, 539,
      1970 (a).

8.   HORNSEY, SHIRLEY, *Brit. J. Radiol.*, *43*, 802,
      1970 (b).

9.   HORNSEY, S. and VATISTAS, S., *Brit. J. Radiol.*, *36*,
      795, 1963.

10. HORNSEY, S., VATISTAS, S., BEWLEY, D.K. and PARNELL,
     C.J., *Brit. J. Radiol.*, *38*, 878, 1965.

11. HORNSEY, S. and SILINI, G., *Int. J. Radiat. Biol.*,
     4, 135, 1961.

12. QUASTLER, H., *Radiation Res.*, *4*, 303, 1956.

QUANTITATIVE STUDIES OF CELL POPULATION KINETICS DURING THE ACUTE REACTION IN THE SMALL INTESTINE OF MICE FOLLOWING WHOLE-BODY IRRADIATION

FINN DEVIK

Statens Institutt for Strålehygiene, Medisinsk Seksjon, and Institutt for Generell Og Eksperimentell Patologi, Universitetet i Oslo, Rikshospitalet, Oslo 1, Norway

INTRODUCTION

In the study of the biology of tumours, cell population kinetics has been of increasing importance in providing background material for a better understanding of homeostasis and growth as the balance between cell production and cell loss, and of the mode of action of irradiation and chemotherapeutics. In tumours, however, such studies are met with considerable technical difficulties.

The epithelial cells in a crypt of the small intestine can be regarded as a cell population which is well defined and delimited, where cell population kinetic studies have provided much basic information, both under normal conditions, and after injury, e.g. X-irradiation.

The intestinal crypt is therefore well suited for quantitative studies on a cell population, and it has been chosen as the subject for the present studies on changes following an increasing degree of injury by X-irradiation, until total destruction or elimination of the cell population.

761

MATERIALS AND METHODS

Male and female mice, 2-3 months old, were given whole body X-irradiation with the following doses: 200, 350, 700, 900, 1000, 1200, 1400, 1700, 2000 and 2400 R. Sections were made of the distal part of the jejunum after time intervals varying from one hour to seven days after irradiation, and in each mouse cell counts were made in 10 crypts sectioned longitudinally. Details on materials and methods are given elsewhere [2].

The following parameters were recorded: Number of epithelial cells, dead cells with pyknotic nuclei, misoses, and Paneth cells, all per longitudinal section of one crypt. The relative number of crypts was also determined after some dose levels. Mitotic rate and migration of cells to the villi were studied in some animals, by arresting mitoses with vinblastine, and by the use of tritiated thymidine.

RESULTS

Fig. 1 shows the number of cells per crypt section as a function of radiation dose and time. Each point represents the average value from four or more mice. It should be noted that the variations in the total *number of cells in a crypt* is more pronounced than is apparent from these curves, which refer to a two-dimensional system instead of the three dimensions of the whole crypt.

After 350 R and higher doses a decrease is observed within hours. The decrease is more pronounced and lasts longer with higher doses. Regeneration with a compensatory overshoot is observed after doses up to and including 1000 R, but following 1200 R the mice died before regeneration was observed. This latter dose-level seems to be critical to these mice with respect to intestinal death after whole body irradiation.

Dead cells with pyknotic and fragmented nuclei appear suddenly about two hours after irradiation, as

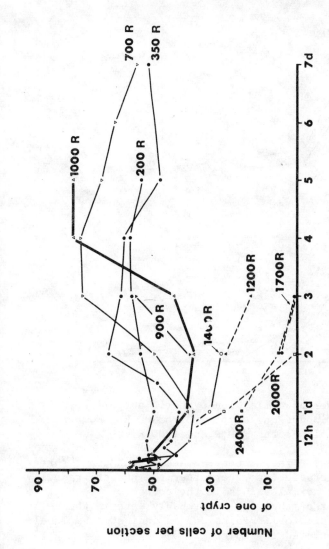

Fig. 1. Number of cells per section of one crypt.
200 - 2400 R.

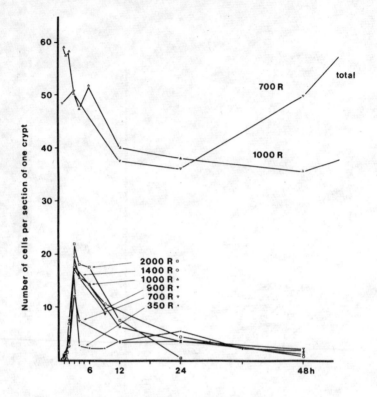

Fig. 2.   Number of cells with pyknotic nuclei per
          section of one crypt 200 - 2400 R.   Number
          of cells after 700 R and 1000 R.

shown in Fig. 2.   The number reaches a peak about three
hours after irradiation; thereafter the number gradually
falls to near normal values in the course of one half to
one day.   Most of these cells probably were in the S-
phase at the time of irradiation, as indicated by labelling with tritiated thymidine [1, 3].

DISCUSSION

     Withers and Elkind [4] reported observations on sur-

vival curves of intestinal epithelial cells after local
irradiation of the intestine *in vivo* with heavy doses.
They calculated D_{37} to be about 100 rads. Later and more
extended experiments [5] have yielded similar, though
somewhat higher values. Although they describe cell survival curves with high extrapolation numbers, it seems at
first difficult to bridge their results with the data obtained in the present experiments.

In Fig. 3 their survival curves have been extrapolated, assuming that the number of cells irradiated was
3.7×10^7 cells [2]. Differences due to different strains
of mice are likely to be small when a semilogarithmic
graph is used, and there is reason to consider that the
same applies to local versus whole-body irradiation with
respect to the number of cells in the intestinal epithelium.

According to the graph, a dose of 1000 R would kill
all but 0,2 - 0,6% of the proliferative crypt cells.
However, the total cell number of the crypts never dropped
below about 30% of the normal, until proliferation again
became evident.

The initial loss of cells can be accounted for by
the observed cell death, and by the loss from the crypts
due to migration to the villi [2]. In addition, cell
production at first stopped and then was slowed down for
some time.

It is reasonable to assume that some lethally injured cells may stay alive for a while, and also divide,
thus preventing a further drop in the cell number for
some time. In the meantime, reproduction of viable cells
proceeds at an increasing rate, with a shortened cell
generation time.

Assuming a surviving fraction of 0,4%, eight cell
divisions are required to bring the cell number up to
100%. Taking the estimated cell generation times into
account, a theoretical curve reaches 100% rather close to
the observed time when the repopulation of the crypts
have reached normal values.

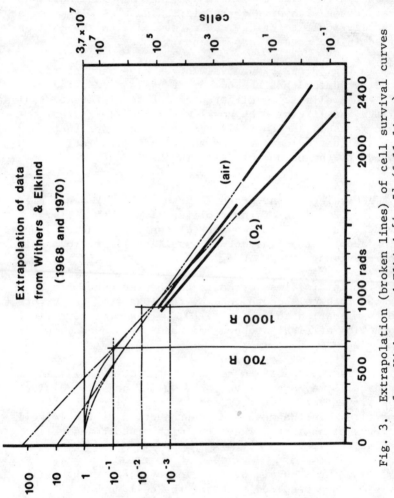

Fig. 3. Extrapolation (broken lines) of cell survival curves
from Withers and Elkind [4, 5] (full lines).

After 700 R there also seems to be a fairly good agreement between the estimated surviving fraction of cells, and the number of cell generations required to bring the number of cells back to normal values.

The data presented may thus be considered as compatible with an exponential cell survival curve with a high extrapolation number and a D_{37} of around 100 rads or somewhat more.

The number of crypts is also of interest in this connection. Assuming that a crypt on the average contains 500 cells, all or nearly all of which are capable of proliferation, the number of crypts would not be expected to decrease until the probability of survival after irradiation dropped below 1:500. In the present experiments a decrease was observed 3 days after 1200 R and higher doses, not after 1000 R and lower doses.

From the extrapolated curves of Withers and Elkind [4, 5] the surviving fraction after 1000 R is estimated to be higher than 1:500, and after 1200 R less than 1:1000, which on the present assumptions is in agreement with the fraction of surviving cells indicated by the extrapolation in Fig. 3.

Therefore, two different lines of reasoning indicate that the present experimental data may agree quite well with the exponential cell survival curves obtained with considerably higher doses.

It may also be pointed out, referring to Fig. 4, that the number of cell generations required to bring the cell number back to normal values can be used to determine the surviving fraction of cells. In this way, *in vivo* cell survival curves may be constructed after doses which are low, compared to the relatively high doses used to obtain such curves by counting of cell colonies. The better the account of cell loss and cell production can be kept, the greater the accuracy is expected to be.

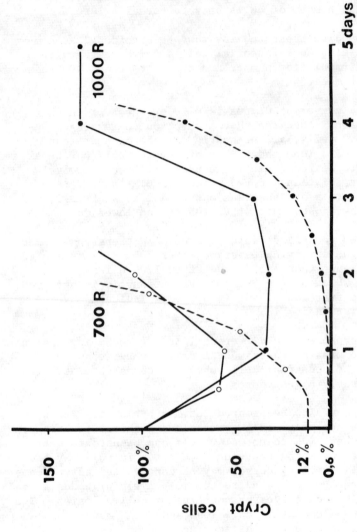

Fig. 4. Cell number in crypts after 700 R and 1000 R, as percentage of normal values (full lines), and hypothetical repopulation in crypts (broken lines).

SUMMARY

The cells of an intestinal crypt may be regarded as a population which may be useful in model studies on the reaction of a rapidly proliferating cell population, to X-irradiation, as well as to cytotoxic agents. Quantitative data after whole-body X-irradiation may be considered compatible with exponential cell survival curves.

REFERENCES

1. DEVIK, F., Symposium on the: Effects of Radiation on Cellular Proliferation and Differentiation, p. 531, *International Atomic Energy Agency*, Vienna, 1968.

2. DEVIK, F., *Acta radiol. Ther. Phys. Biol. 10*,130, 1971.

3. SHERMAN, F.G. and QUASTLER, H., *Exp. Cell Res., 19,* 343, 1960.

4. WITHERS, H.R. and ELKIND, M.M., *Radiology, 91,* 998, 1968.

5. WITHERS, H.R. and ELKIND, M.M., *Int. J. Rad. Biol., 17,* 261, 1970.

EFFECTS OF SPLIT DOSE PARTIAL ABDOMINAL IRRADIATION ON S AND M CELLS IN THE MOUSE DUODENAL CRYPT EPITHELIUM*

JANIE LESHER AND S. LESHER

*Cell and Radiation Biology Laboratories, Allegheny
General Hospital, 320 East North Avenue,
Pittsburgh, Pennsylvania 15212, U.S.A.*

Radiation therapists treating human tumours frequently utilize multiple fractionated exposures directly
to the tumor in an effort to kill the maximum number of
tumor cells with minimum damage to the adjacent normal
tissues. Since little is known about the cellular effects of either partial-body or fractionated exposures,
a series of experiments was designed to study the effects
of single-dose, two dose and three dose exposures on the
proliferative cells of the mouse duodenal crypt epithelium. In these studies the upper half of the mouse was
shielded and the lower half, including the entire intestine and closely associated organs were irradiated.

Results of the single-dose, partial abdominal,
x-irradiation experiments [1] show that the sequence of
changes in the proliferative cells of the duodenal crypt
epithelium are the same as those produced by whole-body
exposures [2] but the degree of change is different;
e.g., duration of G_2 block, time and extent of overshoot
in number of cells in S and M, cell cycle timing, etc.
After 300 R the G_2 block is 3 hours, 5 hours after 600 R
and 8 hours after 900 R partial abdominal irradiation as

*Supported in part by grants #1 PO2 CA10438 and
5 TOL CA05184 from the National Cancer Institute National
Institutes of Health.

compared to 4, 6, and 10 hours respectively following
single-dose, whole-body exposures.

Experiments reported in this paper deal with the
effects of two 300 R partial abdominal exposures separated by 6, 12, 24, 48, and 96 hours on the ability of
the proliferative cells of the duodenal crypt epithelium
to synthesize DNA and divide.

In each of the five experimental groups two mice
were injected (I.P.) with 50 µCi of ^{3}HTdR at 1, 2, 3, 4,
5, 6, 7, 8, 9, 12, 16, 20, 24, 36, 48, 60, 72, 84, and
96 hours after the second dose and sacrificed 30 minutes
after injection. Tissue samples from the upper small
intestine distal to the duodenal flexure were removed,
fixed in cold carnoys (3:1), and crypt squash autoradiographs prepared. From these autoradiographs an estimate
of the number of cells in S (LN/crypt) and M (MF/crypt)
was obtained by counting all labeled nuclei and mitotic
figures in 20 crypts from each mouse. Percent labeled
mitotic figure (PLM) curves 24 hours after the second
dose were obtained for each experimental group. These
data will be referred to, but not discussed in detail.

Repair of radiation damage and the re-establish-
ment of a new steady-state proliferative population with
a high degree of reproductive integrity occurs at all
sublethal dose levels in the intestinal cell renewal
system. Recovery time is dose dependent but it must be
sufficient to eliminate severely damaged cells and to
repopulate the "stem cell" compartments with cells
capable of repeated divisions. Previous experiments,
both whole-body [2-4] and partial body [1] single dose
exposures, show that cells in all phases of the cell
cycle (G_1, S, G_2, M) are affected by radiation. Following a single partial abdominal 300 R exposure most cells
in mitosis at time of irradiation complete division.
Cells in G_2 and those which move into G_2 from S are
blocked ($\sim$ 3 hours). The rate of DNA synthesis on a per
cell basis is not measurably affected. However, the
number of cells in S drops rapidly during the first
six hours after exposure. This reduction in number of
LN/crypt is due to the movement of 4n cells into G_2 and
the blockage of cells moving from G_1 into S.

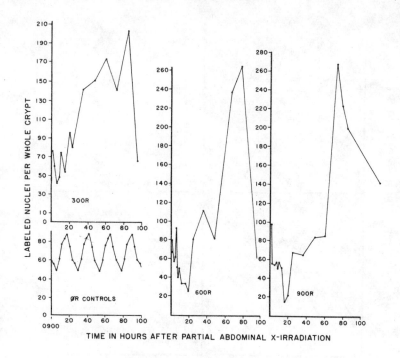

Fig. 1. Number of LN/crypt after single-dose, partial abdominal
X-irradiation at various times after exposure.

Recovery is mediated through two compensatory phenomena, namely, an increase in the absolute size of the
proliferative population combined with an acceleration of
the generation cycle. At the height of recovery the
entire crypt is composed of rapidly cycling cells. Since
the pre-synthesis phase (G_1) is very short, most of the
cells are in S, G_2 and M. Cell production increases by
factors of 3 to 4 above normal.

The pattern of change in the numbers of LN/crypt
and MF/crypt after the second of two 300 R X-ray doses is
similar to that produced by single exposures. However,
there are significant quantitative differences between
the two dose and single-dose series and between the experimental groups within the two dose series. The later

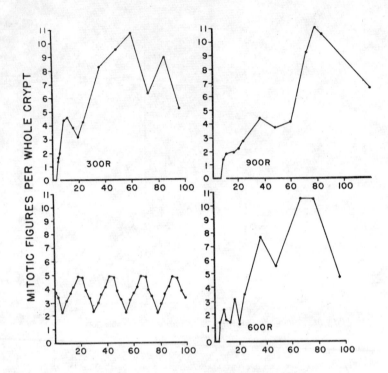

Fig. 2. Number of MF/crypt after single-dose, partial abdominal
X-irradiation at various times after exposure.

differences are related to the time interval between
doses, and involve the degree of change and times at
which they occur, e.g., length of G_2 block, overshoot in
LN/crypt and MF/crypt (comparison of Figs. 1 and 2 with
3 and 4).

If the interval between the first and second dose
is short (6 hours or less) distribution of cells in G_1,
S, G_2 and M will be considerably altered. This is due
primarily to the accumulation of cells in G_2 (as a result of the G_2 block) and a reduction in number of cells
in S (due to the movement of S cells into G_2 and the
retardation or complete block of cells in G_1. The number of cells in G_1 changes very little. At the time the
second 300 R dose is given (six hours after the first

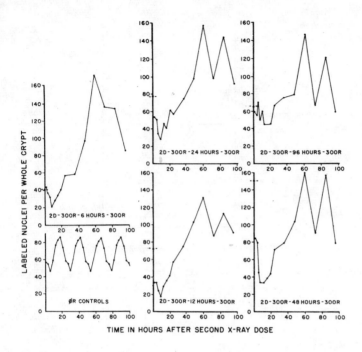

Fig. 3.   Number of LN/crypt after the second 300 R X-irradiation
          dose at various times after exposure.

300 R dose) the number of LN/crypt has already been reduced by the first dose to 41 per crypt (Fig. 3) and the
MF/crypt reduced to 2. (Fig. 4). Since the first 300 R
dose kills about 10-15% of the total proliferative population (primarily in G_2 and M) the remaining population
at six hours after exposure would be approximately 25%
in G_1 over 40% in S, 30% in G_2 and less than 2% in M.
If G_2 is a highly sensitive phase the second 300 R dose
should kill 30 to 35% of the remaining population. An
examination of the LN/crypt and MF/crypt curves (Figs.
3 and 4) tends to support this hypothesis in that the
peak overshoot occurs at 72 hours rather than at 60
hours, as it does in the other split-dose experimental
series. In addition the overshoot is much lower than
that produced by either 300 R or 600 R single-dose,

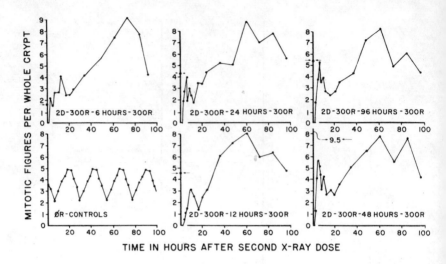

Fig. 4. Number of MF/crypt after the second 300 R X-irradiation
         dose at various times after exposure.

partial abdominal exposures (Figs. 1 and 2). However,
the shape of the LN/crypt and MF/crypt curves closely
resemble the single dose curves. The reduced overshoot
can probably be explained on the basis that the remaining population after the first dose has been reduced,
that many of remaining cells carry residual unrepaired
damage and that repair of damage might be further inhibited by the second dose.

Twelve hours after the first 300 R dose the crypts
contain, on the average, 72 LN/crypt and 4 mitotic figures. PLM curves starting at this time show that many
cells have difficulty with mitosis since a 100% plateau
is not reached and the slopes of the first rising arm
and the first descending arms are not as steep as they
become after severely damaged cells are eliminated from
the proliferative population [4]; e.g., 24 and 48 hours
after 300 R. Many of these cells will not complete
division and will die (> 10%). The ratio of cells in
G_1, S, G_2 and M is much different from that found at six
hours as now about 35% are in G_1, 50% in S, 15% in G_2 and

approximately 3% in M. Giving the second 300 R dose at
12 hours produces a 4 hour G_2 block. Six hours after the
second 300 R the number of cells in S are reduced to
24 LN/crypt and 1.4 MF/crypt. This reduction is partly
due to the second G_2 and G_1 blocks and partly due to the
redistribution of cells around the cell cycle as a result
of the first dose. Cells which accumulated in G_2 following the first dose may now be back in G_2 hence the number
of cells in S and M may be reduced. The overshoot in
LN/crypt and MF/crypt now occurs at 60 hours, falls at
72 hours, rises again at 84 hours and is again reduced
at 96 hours. Apparently, by the third day a new highly
viable proliferative population has been established,
the proliferative rate is now sensitive to diurnal factors
[5], and a new steady-state cell population is being
established.

A large number of cells accumulates in G_2 and to a
lesser degree in G_1 following the first 300 R dose because of the G_1 and G_2 blocks. This cellular component
makes up a significant proportion of the cells in the
proliferative compartment (> 50%). If they continue to
move as partially synchronized cohorts, the sensitivity
of the total population to irradiation could be profound-
ly effected depending on which phase they are in when
they receive the second dose. In fact, the partial synchronization and redistribution of cells probably has
considerable effect on the results of the 6 and 12 hour
two dose series.

As the cells which make up the proliferative populations go through repeated cycles they gradually become redistributed throughout the four phases of the
cell cycle, assume more nearly their original ratios, and
again become asynchronous. When this occurs the reaction
to the second dose should closely resemble the single
dose 300 R response. Curves from the experimental groups
in which the two 300 R doses are separated by 24, 48, and
96 hours respectively show that as the interval between
doses increases the pattern and magnitude of change in
number of LN/crypt and MF/crypt becomes similar to that
produced by a single 300 R exposure.

When the two doses are separated by 48 hours the proliferative cell population is at the peak productive level. The cell cycle is less than eight hours with an S period of approximately 6 hours and $G_2 + M + G_1$ of no more than 2 hours. Most of the cells in the proliferative compartment are now in S (149 - LN/crypt) and M (9.5 - MF/crypt) while the number of cells in G_2 and G_1 are at a low level (G_2 is <30 minutes in a high proportion of cells at this time). It is surprising, in view of the fact that cells in S are thought to be radio-resistant that the number of cells in S fall to a very low level in six hours. This could occur only if it is assumed that the proliferative population was partially synchronized, that most of the S cells were in the latter half of S at the time of the second dose and that movement of cells into S from G_1 was seriously impaired. However, since the overshoot does not occur until 60 hours after the second dose and the peak is not significantly different from that produced in the 24 and 96 hour series a large number of S cells must have been heavily damaged by the second dose and are not capable of continued division.

It would appear that by 96 hours after the first dose the distribution of cells in G_1, S, G_2 and M is approaching normal. When the second 300 R dose is separated from the first by 96 hours the LN/crypt and MF/crypt curves (Figs. 3 and 4) are similar to those produced by a single 300 R partial abdominal exposure both in pattern and magnitude of change.

The diurnal factors [5] which produce fluctuations in number of LN/crypt and MF/crypt with highs at 300 and lows at 1500 is also evident as shown in Figs. 3 and 4 when the two 300 R doses are separated by 24, 48 and 96 hours. Although these points are out of phase they are on the rising portion of the diurnal curve when high and on the descending segment when low.

SUMMARY

One hundred day old C57Bl mice were divided randomly into 5 experimental series and given 2 X-ray doses of

300 R each (total dose 600 R) separated by 6, 12, 24, 48, and 96 hours. The number of cells in S (LN/crypt) and M (MF/crypt) were determined at various times after the second dose following the injection of ^{3}HTdR for each of the 5 experimental groups.

Qualitatively the changes following the second 300 R exposure are similar to single dose effect, namely an immediate blockage of cells in G_2 and G_1 leading to a reduction in number of cells in S and M followed by an overshoot of control levels and a gradual return to control values. Quantitatively there are significant differences in degree of change and time of occurrence. The evidence suggests that some of these differences are due to partial synchronization of cells as a result of the early accumulation of large numbers of cells in G_2 and G_1. This, due to the differences in phase sensitivity, affects the degree of damage and the rate of repair and recovery. When the interval between doses is extended, the proliferative population is gradually redistributed between G_1, S, G_2 and M becoming asynchronous. Early damage is repaired and the effect of the second dose then becomes similar qualitatively and quantitatively to a single 300 R dose.

REFERENCES

1.   LESHER, J., Effects of single-dose, partial abdominal irradiation on cell proliferation in the mouse duodenal epithelium, *Rad. Res.*, (in press), 1971.

2.   LESHER, J and LESHER, S., Effects of single-dose, whole-body, ^{60}Co Gamma irradiation on DNA synthesis and mitosis in the mouse duodenal epithelium, ^{60}Co gamma irradiation on DNA synthesis and mitosis in the mouse duodenal epithelium, *Rad. Res.*, (in press) 1970.

3.   LESHER, S., Compensatory reactions in intestinal crypt cells after 300 roentgens of Cobalt-60 Gamma irradiation, *Rad. Res.*, *32*, 510-519, 1967.

4.   LESHER, S. and BAUMAN, J., Recovery of reproductive
     activity and the maintenance of structural integrity
     in the intestinal epithelium of the mouse after
     single-dose whole-body ^{60}Co Gamma-ray exposures,
     *International Atomic Energy Agency Symposium, Effects
     of Radiation on Cellular Proliferation and Differ-
     entiation*, held in Monaco, pp. 507–513, 1968.

5.   SIGDESTAD, C.P., BAUMAN, J. and LESHER, S., Diurnal
     Fluctuations in the number of cells in mitosis and
     DNA synthesis in the jejunum of the mouse, *Exp. Cell
     Res.*, *58*, 159–162, 1969.

CELL POPULATION KINETICS IN INTESTINAL EPITHELIUM AFTER X-IRRADIATION IN NORMAL AND GERM FREE RATS*

H. GALJAARD, W. VAN DER MEER and N.J. DE BOTH

Dept. Cell Biology, Medical Faculty, Rotterdam, The Netherlands

The effects of X-irradiation on the intestinal epithelium from conventional and germ free rats has been studied to obtain information about the regulation mechanisms involved in cell proliferation and -differentiation in cell renewal systems. Intestinal epithelium has the advantage that the various functional stages (proliferative- non dividing maturing- and functional cell compartments) can be related to the morphological localisation of the cells along the crypt and villus. In previous studies on rat intestine [6] combined autoradiography after ^{3}H-thymidine and quantitative microchemical analyses on various dissected cell compartments have been carried out to relate changes in cell population dynamics after low radiation doses to certain biochemical parameters. It was found that during recovery from various doses of X-radiation (200–700 R) a temporary increase in the pool of proliferating crypt cells occurs at the expense of the number of non-dividing maturing crypt cells. The increase in proliferative activity independently of the radiation dose always starts between 36–48 hours after irradiation and the effect was found to be accompanied by a decrease in the activity of certain enzymes (i.e., aliphatic esterases) normally present in the maturing crypt cell compartment.

---

*Experiments on germ free rats could be carried out through the cooperation of the Radiobiological Institute TNO, Rijswijk, The Netherlands.

In a model of rat intestinal crypt Cairnie *et al.*
[4, 5] described that the proliferative cell compartment
is localized from the bottom of the crypt up to cell position 10. From cell position 10-18 a "cut-off" region is
present where an increasing number of non proliferative
cells are produced; from cell position 18-35 only non dividing maturing cells are present.

The question has been raised what regulation factors
are involved in the cessation of proliferation once the
cell arrives in the "cut-off" region of the crypt and in
this respect a possible role of certain "enzyme activity
gradients" along the crypt has been suggested [5]. It
has been demonstrated that a displacement of this "cut-
off" region towards the mouth of the crypt is possible
under certain experimental conditions. After partial
resection of rat jejunum, after two months a displacement of the "cut-off" region towards the top of the
crypts was observed in the remaining part of the ileum [10] and a humoral factor was suggested to be responsible for this initiation of increased proliferative activity [11]. A temporary displacement of the "cut-off"
region up to the top of the crypt was also found during
repopulation after X-irradiation [6]. The time of onset
of this displacement (36-48 hours after irradiation) corresponds remarkably with the turnover time of the intestinal epithelium.

To investigate if like in some other cell renewal
systems the cell proliferation in the intestinal crypt is
regulated via the functional cells on the villus, combined
autoradiography after ^{3}H-thymidine incorporation and
microchemical analysis of certain enzyme activities
in isolated crypts or parts of these were carried out on
irradiated conventional and germ free rats*; the latter
being supposed to have a longer turnover time of the
villous cells [1, 8, 12]. If the villi were involved in
the regulation of cell proliferation in the crypt one
would expect that after irradiation in germ free rats the
displacement of the "cut-off" region in the crypt and the
simultaneous decrease in esterase activity of the upper
half of the crypt would occur later than in conventional

animals. In the case that cell proliferation is regulated within the crypt no differences between germfree and conventional animals are to be expected.

MATERIAL AND METHODS

Twenty-two germ free Wistar rats and the same number of conventional animals were irradiated (whole body) with 700 R and subsequently sacrificed at 12-24 hours intervals from 24 to 204 hours after irradiation. Before sacrifice all animals together with non-irradiated controls were intravenously injected with ^{3}H-thymidine and after 30 min. a segment of duodenum was dissected. Cryostat sections were prepared for autoradiography after a histochemical staining for non specific esterase activity had been carried out. Details of the techniques have been published elsewhere [6]. After autoradiography in 50 longitudinally cut crypts the total number of cells per crypt column was counted, the percentage of labelled cells and their position in the crypts were scored. The results for conventional and germ free animals at various time intervals after irradiation were compared.

The migration rate was determined by investigating the position of the leading edge of labelled cells along the crypt and villus at various time intervals (12-72 hours) after ^{3}H-thymidine incorporation and the number of villus cells were counted in 50-100 longitudinally cut villous columns.

From each animal cryostat sections were frozen-dried, various cell compartments were dissected under the microscope, the fragments were weighed on a quartz fiber balance and the non specific esterase activity was determined quantitatively on the microscale according to procedures described earlier [6].

RESULTS

Migration rate

Both in conventional and germ free rats at 12 hours after their last DNA synthesis, the crypt cells reached the crypt-villus junction; this indicates a similar migration rate in the crypt for both types of animals. Also during migration along the villus no significant difference in migration rate could be detected. 24 hours after their last DNA synthesis, in germ free rats cell position 27 (from the basis of the villus) was reached and in conventional rats position 28.

After 36 hours in conventional animals labelled cells were present up to cell position 63 and in the germ free up to position 55. As the mean number of villus cells in conventional rats was 76, the turn over time of the epithelium could be determined to be about 45 hours. However, in the germ free rats the mean number of villus cells was 95 and labelled cells did not reach the tips of the villi before 60 hours after ^{3}H-thymidine incorporation. The villus transit time thus seems to be about *15 hours* longer in germ free rats than in the conventional animals.

Proliferation pool after irradiation

The results of the autoradiographic studies at various time intervals after irradiation are illustrated in Table 1 and Fig. 1. The total number of crypt cells was

Table 1. Percentage of ^{3}H-thymidine Labelled Crypt Cells After 700 R Irradiation in Normal and Germ Free Rats

	Control	24	36	48	60	72	84	96	120	168	204
				Hours after Irradiation							
Normal	27	12	22	47	52	54	50	44	35	35	–
Germ free	25	6	14	23	43	51	58	53	34	–	28

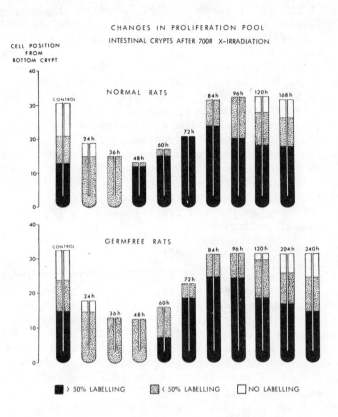

CHANGES IN PROLIFERATION POOL
INTESTINAL CRYPTS AFTER 700R X-IRRADIATION

CELL POSITION FROM BOTTOM CRYPT

NORMAL RATS

GERMFREE RATS

■ > 50% LABELLING   ▨ < 50% LABELLING   ☐ NO LABELLING

found to be identical (31 cells) in germ free and conventional rats and the percentage of labelled cells only
showed a slight difference; the "cut-off" region in the conventional rats was localized between cell position 14-25 and
in the germ free between 13-21. The localisation of the
proliferating cell compartment has been based on the distribution of cell positions for which a labelling percentage
of 50 or higher was found; this figure was considered to
be indicative for a completely proliferating cell population [3, 4, 5, 7, 9, 13]. The effect of X-irradiation
on the displacement of the "cut-off" region in the crypt
is clearly different in conventional and germ free animals.

After 700 R the total percentage of labelled crypt cells,
after an initial decrease, in conventional rats shows a
marked increase above control values at 48 hours after irradiation; in the germ free this increase occurs later, between 60-72 hours after irradiation (Table 1).   In Fig. 1
is illustrated that after irradiation also the localisation in the crypt of the proliferating cell compartment
and the "cut-off" region is different for the two types of
animals.   The extension of the proliferating pool and the
displacement of the "cut-off" region toward the top of the
crypt in the *conventional* rats occurs from *48 hours* after
irradiation and in the *germ free* between *60-72 hours*.   In
both types of animals repopulation of the crypt is completed after 84 hours but nevertheless a displacement of
the "cut-off" region remains present during a period up to
10 days after irradiation.

Enzyme activity after irradiation

In previous work it has been demonstrated that the
esterase activity in isolated crypts can be considered as
indicative for the presence of non-dividing maturing crypt
cells [6].   In the proliferating cell compartment the esterase activity is nearly absent (about 2.0 µmol liberated
naphthol/mg dry weight); from the "cut-off" region towards
the top of the crypt the activity increases to about 10.0
µmol and a further increase is found once the cell arrives
at the base of the villus (30 µmol).   In the case of a displacement of the "cut-off" region towards the villus the
number of non-dividing crypt cells will decrease with a
simultaneous decrease in esterase activity in the crypt.
In Table 2 is shown that after irradiation both in conventional and germ free rats the esterase activity in the
crypts decreases to values corresponding to a completely
proliferating cell compartment without maturing cells
($\sim$ 2.0 µmol).   However, there is a difference in the time
of onset of this effect; in *conventional rats* this is *36-48
hours* after irradiation and in the *germfree* after *60 hours*.
Furthermore it is clear from Table 2 that a decreased esterase activity in the crypt results in a decrease in enzyme activity of the villus cells which in turn might explain some features of the functional disturbances in the
gastrointestinal radiation syndrome [2, 6, 14].

Table 2. Non-specific Esterase Activity in Intestinal
Crypts and Villi from Irradiated Normal and Germ Free Rats*

Hours After 700 R	Normal		Germ free	
	Crypt	Villus	Crypt	Villus
Control	6.3	29.4	7.0	35.0
24	6.0	29.8	6.8	33.1
36	3.4	20.7	5.7	29.3
48	2.3	13.8	4.6	26.8
60	1.8	11.6	2.2	22.7
72	1.2	7.4	1.4	15.4
84	1.4	10.5	1.9	11.9
96	1.8	14.9	2.6	17.4
120	3.7	18.4	4.0	26.2
168	4.0	23.4	5.4	32.5
240	5.3	23.1	5.6	34.2
288	-	-	6.9	34.9

*Enzyme activity is expressed in μmols liberated
naphtol/mg dry weight/ 20 min. Values are the mean of
20 samples from 2-4 rats each.

CONCLUSIONS AND SUMMARY

1.   The transit time of epithelial cells on intestinal
villi in conventional rats is about 36 hours and in germ
free animals about 48 hours; the transit time in the
crypt (12 hours) shows no difference.

2.   Autoradiographic studies after ^{3}H-thymidine incorporation showed that after X-irradiation a temporary increase in the pool of proliferating cells occurs in the
intestinal crypts starting in conventional rats between
36-48 hours and in germ free animals between 60-72 hours.

3.   Quantitative microchemical analyses of non specific esterase activity in isolated crypts demonstrated that after irradiation a decrease in the pool of non-dividing maturing crypt cells starts in conventional rats between 36-48 hours and in germfree animals 12 hours later.

4.   These findings suggest that cell proliferation in the crypt is regulated by an as yet unknown information from the villus and not by information present within the crypt.

5.   Changes in crypt cell population kinetics result in a decreased activity of certain enzymes in the villus which in turn will lead to functional disturbances of the intestine.

REFERENCES

1.   ABRAMS, G., BAUER, H. and PRINZ, H., *Lab. Invest.*, *12*, 355, 1963.

2.   BOND, V., *J. Clin. Nutr.*, *12*, 194, 1963.

3.   BOND, V., FLIEDNER, R. and ARCHAMBEAU, J.,   *Mammalian Radiation Lethality*, Ac. Press, N.Y., 1965.

4.   CAIRNIE, A., LAMERTON, L. and STEEL, G., *Exp. Cell Res.*, *39*, 528, 1965.

5.   CAIRNIE, et al., ibid., *39*, 539, 1965.

6.   GALJAARD, H. and BOOTSMA, D., *Exp. Cell Res.*, *58*, 79, 1969.

7.   LESHER, S., FRY, R. and KOHN, H., *Exp. Cell Res.*, *24*, 334, 1961.

8.   LESHER, S., *Rad. Res.*, *32*, 510, 1967.

9.   LESHER, S. and SACHER, G., *Nature*, *202*, 884, 1964.

10.   LORAN, M. and CROCKER, T., *J. Cell Biol.*, *19*, 285, 1963.

11. LORAN, M. and CARBONE, J., Monographs on Nuclear
     Medicine and Biology, Nr. *1*, 25, Gastroenterology
     Radiation Injury, *Excerpta Medica*, 1966.

12. MATSAZUWA, T. and WILSON, R., *Rad. Res.*, *25*, 15,
     1965.

13. QUASTER, H. and SHERMAN, F., *Exp. Cell Res.*, *17*, 428,
     1959.

14. REDGRAVE, T. and SIMMONDS, W., *Gastroenterolgy*, *52*,
     54, 1967.

SURVIVAL AND MUTATIONAL RESPONSE OF SPERMATOGONIA OF THE MOUSE IN RELATION TO A NEW CONCEPT OF SPERMATOGONIAL STEM-CELL RENEWAL*

E.F. OAKBERG

Biology Division, Oak Ridge National Laboratory, Oak Ridge, Tennessee, U.S.A.

INRODUCTION

Description of the stages of the cycle of the seminiferous epithelium has made possible the accurate identification of cells, determination of cell lineages, quantitation of cells, and elucidation of cell development times in spermatogenesis [7, 9]. The regularity of spermatogenesis held forth the hope that the true stem cell and its point of differentiation could be determined.

It was immediately clear that the stem cell of the seminiferous epithelium was a type-A spermatogonium, which by a series of divisions plus differentiation, gave rise to an unlimited number of intermediate spermatogonia that were irreversibly committed to the production of more mature cell types [7, 9, 2]. Some type-A cells fail to differentiate, and become the stem cells for the next multiplicative cycle. This process has been termed stem-cell renewal.

Models for spermatogonial stem-cell renewal have been proposed on the basis of spermatogonial counts [1, 2] on the combination of ^{3}H-thymidine labeling with spermato-

*Research sponsored by the U.S. Atomic Energy Commission under contract with the Union Carbide Corporation.

gonial counts [8, 14, 5] and on the use of cell morphology in conjunction with cell counts in tubule whole-
mounts [3, 4]. All these models satisfy the numerical
data, but none of them conclusively solves the problem of
the basic kinetics of stem-cell renewal and differentiation.

The currently most widely-accepted model is that proposed by Clermont and Bustos-Obregon [3] as the result of
a study of tubule whole mounts in the rat. They were
able to identify five classes of type-A spermatogonia.
Type A_1-A_4 are analogous to those described by Monesi [8]
for the mouse, and the fifth type, the A_0, is considered
to be a "reserve stem cell". This revised model of stem-
cell renewal separates the type-A spermatogonia into two
groups. One group, comprised of A_1-A_4 cells, is involved
in the four mitotic peaks of spermatogonial multipli-
cation, and is renewed by derivation of A_1 cells from the
A_4 spermatogonia [3]. The other group, the A_0, function
as reserve stem cells, and repopulate the testis after insults by noxious agents, such as radiation.

The present experiments were designed to test for
the presence of A_0 spermatogonia in the mouse, and for
the possiblility that they are the active stem cells from
which A_1 spermatogonia are derived. Independently,
Huckins [6] has used ^{3}H-thymidine labeling of tubule
whole mounts in a similar study in the rat. The present
data and those of Huckins [6] suggest that the isolated
A_0 is the active stem cell in both mouse and rat, and the
designation A_S (A stem) has been proposed for these cells.

MATERIALS AND METHODS

Three experiments were performed: 1) a morphological
classification and enumeration of type A spermatogonia at
all stages of the cycle, 2) a long-term labeling experiment to trace the progression of labeled A_S spermatogonia
through two cycles of the seminiferous epithelium, and 3)
a combination of long term labeling with irradiation.

Adult $(101 \times C3H)F_1$ hybrid mice, 12 weeks old, were given intraperitoneal injection of 12.5 µCi of ^{3}H-thymidine at 5 hour intervals for a total of 6 injections. This regimen was chosen on the basis of the duration of the cell cycle and S as determined by Monesi [8]. Mice were killed at intervals from one hour to 15 days after injection.

A second group of mice was given ^{3}H-thymidine injections as above, and irradiated 24 hours later with single doses of 100, 500, and 1000 R X-rays, and the first 500 R fraction of a divided 1000 R exposure. Irradiation was performed with a G.E. Maximar operated at 250 kv, 15 MA, inherent filtration of 3 mm Al, H.V.L. 0.4 mm Cu, 63 R/ minute. Mice were killed at intervals ranging from 12 hours to 17 days after irradiation.

For morphological studies, testes were fixed in Zenker-formol, sectioned at 5 µ, and stained with PAS and Ehrlich's hematoxylin.

^{3}H-thymidine labeled testes were fixed in Orth's, sectioned at 3µ, deparaffinized, hydrated, stained in PAS, allowed to air-dry, dipped in Kodak NTB_2 liquid emulsion diluted 1:1 with a 0.1% solution of Dreft, and exposed at 4°C for 4 weeks. Autoradiographs were developed in D_{19} at 17°C, fixed, and stained with Ehrlich's hematoxylin.

RESULTS

Five classes of type spermatogonia, analogous to those described by Clermont and Bustos-Obregon [3] for the rat, could be identified in the mouse. It has been suggested [12, 6] that the designation A_S, in recognition of stem-cell function, is preferable to the designation A_0 [3] for the most primitive spermatogonial type. A_1, A_2, A_3, and A_4 spermatogonia are comparable to those described for the mouse [8] and rat [3].

A_S spermatogonia occur as single isolated cells [6]. They divide to form either more isolated cells, or to form pairs. Pair formation appears to be the initial step in the differentiation of more advanced cell types.

A_S spermatogonia divide at all stages of the cycle, but
most frequently at stages IX-I, and least often at stages
VI-VIII. Mitotic peaks as observed for A_1-A_4 spermatogonia do not occur. Formation of chains of spermatogonia
increases at stages IX-I (Table 1), and these chains

Table 1. Mean Number of the Different Classes of A spermatogonia per 5μ Section at each Stage of the Cycle of
the Seminiferous Epithelium, and of In Spermatogonia at
Stage 3. (From [12]).

Stage of the cycle	Spermatogonial types			
	A_S**	A_1	A_2- A_4	In
I	1.30	0.02	4.59*	
II	1.12	0.15	5.54*	
III	1.00	0.38		9.32
IV	1.2	0.28		
V	1.08	0.76		
VI	1.03	1.01		
VII	0.95	1.14		
VIII	0.88	1.32		
IX	0.84	2.47	0.05	
X	1.30	2.09	0.23	
XI	1.17	0.73	2.11*	
XII	1.53	0.21	3.09*	

    *Corrected totals. One half the number of telo-
phases subtracted to correct for cells that already have
divided.
    **This also includes "paired" and "aligned" a sper-
matogonia with morphological characteristics of the isolated A_S. An accurate distinction cannot be made in sectioned material.

transform into spermatogonia A_1 at stages I-VIII. In sections, "pairs" and chains usually are not revealed, and
the A_S population given in Fig. 1 is thereby over-estimated.

Fig. 1. Proposed model of stem-cell renewal in the mouse

Cell type   Stage of the cycle of the
                                   seminiferous epithelium

A_s all stages

A paired

A aligned   X-I

A_1 chains   II-IX

A_2 IX-XI

A_3 XI-I

A_4 I-II

In   II-IV

B   IV-VI

primary spermatocyte   VI - -

Spermatogonia A_1 arise from the A "aligned" cells, and are characterized by larger, light staining round nuclei, and prominent nucleoli. These cells increase in frequency concomitant with decrease in A "aligned" spermatogonia at stages I-VIII (Table 1), and divide at stage IX to form spermatogonia A_2.

An increasing number of clumps of heterochromatin on the nuclear membrane characterize the evolution of A_2 into A_4 spermatogonia. It is not possible to separate A_2, A_3, or A_4 accurately on purely morphological bases. They can be identified, however, by a combination of nuclear morphology, division sequence, and stage of the cycle of the seminiferous epithelium in which they occur. A_2 cells first appear in stage IX, and by division in stage XI give rise to the A_3 type. A_3 spermatogonia persist from stage XI to stage I, where they divide to form type A_4 cells. A_4 spermatogonia then divide in late II to

form intermediate spermatogonia according to the model of
Monesi [8]. There is no evidence for the formation of
either A_1 or A_S spermatogonia by A_4 cells. This is indicated by the lack of an increase of either A_1 or A_S types
immediately after the division of A_4 cells in II (Table 1).

Labeling with repeated ^{3}H-thymdine injections coupled
with observations over long time intervals support the
conclusion that the A_S spermatogonia are the active stem
cells, and that they have a much longer cycle time than
do spermatogonia A_1-A_4. As a result, not all A_S spermatogonia were labeled by repeated injections over a 30-hour
period, but those cells which did incorporate ^{3}H-thymid-
ine maintained label for long time intervals (Table 2).
If the model of Clermont and Bustos-Obregon were correct,
cells at stages III-VI at 10 days would not. be labeled,
since original mean grain counts of 11.7 per nucleus
should have been diluted by 2^4. The heavily labeled
spermatogonia eventually divide, these divisions appear
normal, and they occur at any stage of the cycle. They
thus fit the assumed characteristics of the A_S population.
By 15 days, all heavily labeled cells were gone, suggesting that all spermatogonia divide at least once every two
cycles of the seminiferous epithelium. This supports our
hypothesis that divisions are constantly occurring among
the A_S spermatogonia. Thus the long-term labeling fails
to support the reserve stem cell concept of the A_0 spermatogonium.

For some time, we have been aware of the fact that
the A spermatogonia of the mouse are heterogeneous in regard to sensitivity to radiation induced cell killing,
and that both very resistant and highly sensitive cells
occur [11]. Classification of surviving spermatogonia 72
hours after 100 R indicated survival of 58% for A_S, 22%
for A_1, and 5% for A_2-A_4 cell types. The question might
be raised if this is the result of nuclear morphology or
of "chain" formation. The "chains" show many characteristics of syncytia and it is entirely possible that a
lethal event in one cell could thereby be amplified. Previous observations have indicated that surviving spermatogonia came from all stages of the cycle of the seminiferous epithelium. Also, repopulation kinetics after doses

Table 2. Frequency of Labeled A Spermatogonia 1 hour to 15 Days after the Final Injection of ^{3}H-thymidine (From [12]).

Stage	1 hour	3 days	6 days	10 days
I	0.892	0.608 (VIII-X)	0.037 (IV-VI)	0.060 (XI-XII)
II	0.890	0.537 (X-XI)	0.043 (VI-VII)	0.082 (XII-I)
III	0.214	0.600 (XI)	0.115 (VII)	0.188 (I)
IV	0.095	0.333 (XI-XII)	0.048 (VII-VIII)	0.196 (I-II)
V	0.048	0.412 (XII-I)	0.045 (VIII-IX)	0.174 (II-III)
VI	0.032	0.556 (I)	0.023 (IX-X)	0.135 (III-IV)
VII	0.028	0.431 (II-III)	0.286 (X-XI)	0.035 (IV-VI)
VIII	0.275	0.314 (III-IV)	0.531 (XI-XII)	0.041 (VI-VII)
IX	0.660	0.133 (IV-VI)	0.558 (XII-I)	0.039 (VII-VIII)
X	0.757	0.121 (VI)	0.435 (I)	0.044 (VIII)
XI	0.748	0.100 (VI-VII)	0.458 (I-III)	0.026 (VIII-IX)
XII	0.781	0.261 (VII-VIII)	0.112 (III-IV)	0.060 (X-XI)

Roman numerals in parentheses indicate the stage of the cycle of the seminiferous epithelium at which labeling occurred.

of $\sim$ 100 R suggested that surviving cells were already
"programmed", i.e., they differentiated in perfect synchrony with spermatocytes and spermatids characteristic
of the different tubule stages. These results would be
expected if the stem cell is radiation resistant, and if
differentiation is initiated one cycle of the seminiferous epithelium earlier than previously thought. The
concept of the A_s spermatogonium as the stem cell, and
that one cell cycle is required for evolution of A_1 spermatogonia from A_s agrees with the observed radiation response.

Derivation of differentiating spermatogonia from a
stem cell population rather than from a re-cycling of
more differentiated elements also changes the base-line
for evaluation of the relationship between differential
cell survival and genetic effects. Accordingly, mice
were labeled by repeated injection of ^{3}H-thymidine, and
irradiated 24 hrs later. Doses selected were 100 and 500
R, which should be on the linear portion of the mutation
rate curve, a single exposure of 1000 R, which gives reduced mutation frequency, and a 1000 R exposure divided
into two 500 R fractions given 24 hrs apart which gives
an enhanced frequency of mutation [15]. Data on frequency of labeled cells given in Table 3 show fluctuations
prior to 8.5 days which can be interpreted as movement of
cells from A_s into more differentiated elements. At 8.5
days, one cycle of the seminiferous epithelium has been
completed, and cells of the renewing compartment are in
the same stages as at the time of irradiation. Labeling at
100 and 500 R was the same, suggesting a similar qualitative composition of the A spermatogonia. At 1000 R, survival of labeled cells was drastically reduced, and at
500 + 500 R, it was enhanced. Confidence in the values
at 8.5 days is strengthened by the observation that labeling in all groups dropped by one order of magnitude by 17
days.

DISCUSSION

The following model of stem-cell renewal (Fig. 1) has been constructed on the basis of the results of Huckins [6] on the rat, and of Oakberg [12] on the mouse. A_s "singles" are indicated as the active stem cells. They replenish themselves by division and also form "pairs". A certain probability of pair formation occurs at each division. The pairs evolve into chains of A spermatogonia by division at stages IX-I of the cycle of the seminiferous epithelium. These A chains transform into spermatogonia A_1 at stages II-VIII, and the A_1 cells divide at stage IX to form A_2 spermatogonia. The division of A_2 to form A_3 at stage XI, of A_3 at I to form A_4, and of A_4 to form In (intermediate) spermatogonia at stage III occurs according to the model of Monesi [8]. In agreement with Monesi [8] there was no evidence of formation of A_1 spermatogonia from the A_4 type, since number of A_1 spermatogonia did not increase immediately after the A_4 divisions in II (Table 1). Furthermore, chains of A spermatogonia were present at stages XII-I, prior to the division of A_4. Finally, only 70% of the divisions at stage IX were labeled 5 days after ^{3}H-thymidine, whereas according to the model of Clermont and Bustos-Obregon [3] one would have expected 100% labeling.

From the above model of stem-cell renewal, it is clear that highly sensitive spermatogonial types are not contributors to the stem-cell pool, and are of minor importance in estimates of overall genetic damage. All long term mutation frequencies in spermatogonia will be based on the A_s cell. The data of Table 3 show that qualitatively, the spermatogonial population surviving 100 and 500 R (linear portion of the mutation curve) is the same, and furthermore, that the kinetics of both irradiated and control groups was similar for the 8.5 to 17 day interval. Thus we have more confidence that extrapolation of the linear portion of the mutation rate curve will not under-estimate the effect of low doses. Thus "humped" dose-rate curves as those given by Oftedal [13] would depend upon sampling transient cell types in later stages of development, and would represent a relatively unimportant contribution to the total genetic effect.

Table 3. Frequency of Labeled A Spermatogonia Surviving
X-irradiation

Time after X-ray	Con- trol	100	500	1000	500 + 500*
12 hrs	0.600	0.349	0.343	0.229	0.387
72 hrs	0.159	0.474	0.557	0.557	0.593
5 d.	0.134	0.467	0.629	0.590	0.598
8.5 d.	0.078	0.156	0.163	0.024	0.391
17 d.	0.007	0.016	0.017	0.002	0.031

*Fractions given 24 hrs apart.

It was necessary to follow labeling for one full
cycle of the seminferous epithelium (8.5 days) to demonstrate differences in the population of cells surviving
different radiation treatments. This was necessitated by
continued differentiation and degeneration of labeled
cells throughout one cycle, after which label was restricted primarily to the slowly dividing A_s spermatogonia. That these differences were real was supported by
observation 8.5 days later (at 17 days), when labeling in
all groups, including controls, dropped by one order of
magnitude (Table 3). This suggests that normal A_s kinetics had been established by 8.5 days, and that there
was no fundamental change in the kinetics of A_s cells in
the irradiated testis.

The relevance of the above observations (Table 3) to
observed mutation frequency cannot be definately stated.
It is remarkable, however, that doses on the straight
line portion of the mutation curve showed equal labeling
(i.e., qualitatively the same), the single 1000 R exposure showed a very low frequency of labeled cells, and
the 500 + 500 hour exposure showed the highest amount of
labeling. These differences are roughly comparable to
the mutation rate data of Russell [15] and suggest that
the population of cells labeled in this experiment may be

those in which mutations were preferentially induced. Though at first glance this may appear to be selection of cells with inherent differences in sensitivity, it is equally likely that selection operates by changing the frequency of cells which have the capacity to repair pre-mutational damage.

The enhanced effect of two 500 R exposures 24 hours apart has been attributed to synchronization by the first radiation exposure. In our earlier work [10] we had demonstrated that most A spermatogonia were in interphase 24 hours after 500 R, presumably supporting the hypothesis of synchronization. It is now clear that this could also arise from survival of A_S spermatogonia, most of which normally are in interphase. This does not deny the hypothesis of synchronization, however, since it still could operate within the A_S spermatogonia. The data of Table 3 demonstrate that the second 500 R exposure also has a selective effect in that proportionally more un-labeled cells are killed. This effect could also be a factor in the enhanced effectiveness of the 500 + 500 R dose in mutation induction.

It was observed that pairs and chains of cells dropped to very low frequency 5 days after 100 R, and disappeared entirely with higher doses. New formation of paired cells may give new insight into the high sensitivity of certain A spermatogonia, since the pairs of A_S, and the "chains" of A_1 appear to be syncytia. This alters our concept of effective target size, for degeneration of the entire chain occurs if one cell is killed.

The total A population in controls does not constitute the proper baseline for estimating differential cell survival and cell kinetics of irradiated spermatogonia. For example, with doses of over 100 R, A_S cells are the sole survivors, and determination of the mitotic index would be made on cells with an inherently long cell cycle, and the effect of differential cell survival and effects on mitosis would be confounded.

The concept of a mixture of cell cycle times in dividing cell populations is not new, and the implications
for radiobiologists have been discussed by Webster and
Davidson [16] on the basis of studies in *V. faba*. The
data given here extend this observation to the extent
that a long cell cycle is characteristic of the stem
spermatogonium, i.e., the cell primarily involved in both
fertility and genetic effects in mammals.

REFERENCES

1.   CLERMONT, Y. and LEBLOND, C.P., *Am. J. Anat.*, *93*,
      475, 1953.

2.   CLERMONT, Y., *Am. J. Anat.*, *111*, 111, 1962.

3.   CLERMONT, Y. and BUSTOS-OBREGON, E., *Am. J. Anat.*,
      122, 237, 1968.

4.   DYM, M., *Anat. Rec.*, *160*, 342, 1968.

5.   HILSCHER, W., *Arch. Anat. Microscop. Morphol. Exp.*,
      56 (Suppl. No. 3, 4), 75, 1968.

6.   HUCKINS, C. *Anat. Rec.*, *169*, 533, 1971.

7.   LEBLOND, C.P. and CLERMONT, Y., *Am. J. Anat.*, *90*,
      167, 1952.

8.   MONESI, V., *J. Cell Biol.*, *14*, 1, 1962.

9.   OAKBERG, E.F., *Am. J. Anat.*, *99*, 391, 1956.

10.   OAKBERG, E.F., *Jap. J. Genet.*, *40*, 119, 1964.

11.   OAKBERG, E.F., Exc. Med. Inf. Congr., Ser. No. 184,
      Prog. in Endocrinol., *1070*, 1968.

12.   OAKBERG, E.F., *Anat. Rec.*, *169*, 515, 1971.

13. OFTEDAL, P., *Genetics, 49*, 181, 1964.

14. ROOIJ, D.G. DE and KRAMER, M.F., *Zellforsch, 85*, 206, 1968.

15. RUSSELL, W.L., *Proc. Nat. Acad. Sci., 48*, 1724, 1962.

16. WEBSTER, P.L. and DAVIDSON, D., *J. Cell Biol., 39*, 332, 1968.

CELL POPULATION KINETICS IN THE SEMINIFEROUS EPITHELIUM UNDER CONTINUOUS LOW DOSE RATE IRRADIATION*

JACOB I. FABRIKANT #

*Department of Radiological Science,
The John Hopkins University,
Baltimore, Maryland 21205, U.S.A.*

There is evidence that the testis is the most sensitive tissue in the mouse to continuous γ-irradiation at very low dose rates [6-11]. Brown and his colleagues [1, 2] found dose rate dependent damage at 2 to 20 R/day; at 2 R/day, rats and mice maintained reproduction for 10 generations or more. At only a little in excess of 2 R/day, there was continuous serious depletion of cell population in the germinal epithelium with subsequent sterilization [4]. Oakberg and Clark [9, 10] reported that 0.009 R/min or less is near the threshold for recovery processes permitting maintenance of the mouse spermatogonial population, but to total doses greater than 300 R, a dose rate of 0.001 R/min resulted in the spermatogonial population reaching an equilibrium at 80% of normal. With dogs, Casarett [3] found no evidence of deleterious changes in sperm production or fertility below 0.6 R/week, but progressive failure at 3.0 R/week (0.6 R/day). The following studies examine cellular response and cell population kinetics during spermatogenesis in 6-week-old C57BL mice under continuous exposure (cesium-137 γ-irradiation) at 1.8 rads/day for up to 15 weeks, to determine the extent to which the spermatogonial cell population accumulates damage under con-

---

*Work Supported by CH Contract No. AT(11-1)-3013 m from the United States Energy Commission.

#Present address: Professor and Head, Department of Radiology, The University of Connecticut, Farmington, Connecticut 06032, U.S.A.

tinuous low dose rate irradiation affecting cell proliferation, and thus the speed and efficiency of regeneration.

CELL TYPE DISTRIBUTION

There was little change in the cell distribution
pattern during the 15 weeks of irradiation, in spite
of prolonged exposure to an accumulated dose of 200 rads
(Fig. 1). After 6 weeks of exposure, there was an increase in degenerative forms of type B (B) and intermediate (In) cells, respectively. This was much less
apparent in the type A (A) population. There was an increase in TdR-^{3}H labeled degenerate forms in these tubu-
lar stages, suggesting that cells were undergoing interphase death, and that cell death did not necessarily depend on an intervening mitosis (Fig. 2). Furthermore,
a decrease in the proportion of resting primary spermatocytes (RPS) was seen at 6-10 weeks, and this would be
expected as a consequence of the reduction of B cells
seen at that time. The In cell population also was reduced at 6 weeks, but to a lesser degree than B cells.
This again indicated that In spermatogonia were less
sensitive to continuous irradiation than B cells, and
that the reduction of RPS at 6-10 weeks was due primary to a reduction of the B spermatogonia, but also,
to the decrease in proliferating In cells which maintain the B cell population. By 15 weeks, the cell distribution pattern returned to normal levels, with little
appreciable change in the cell population structures between irradiated and control animals.

CELL PROLIFERATION

Normally, TdR-^{3}H labeling indicates were $\sim$30%,
$\sim$63%, and $\sim$50% in A, In and B cells in Stages I, III
and V, respectively (Fig. 3). At 1 day of irradiation,
there was an increase in labeling in all three cell
classes, followed by a fall by 1 week, another rise
at 6-10 weeks, and then return to normal values by
15 weeks. The increased labeling at 6-10 weeks appears

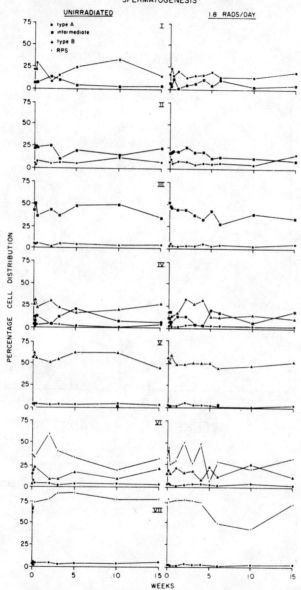

Fig. 1. Cell type distribution in premeiotic stages of spermatogenesis under continuous low dose rate irradiation at 1.8 rads/day.

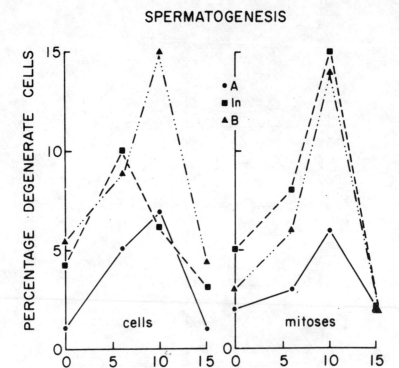

Fig. 2. Distribution of degenerate interphase and dividing spermatogonia
under continuous irradiation at 1.8 rads/day.

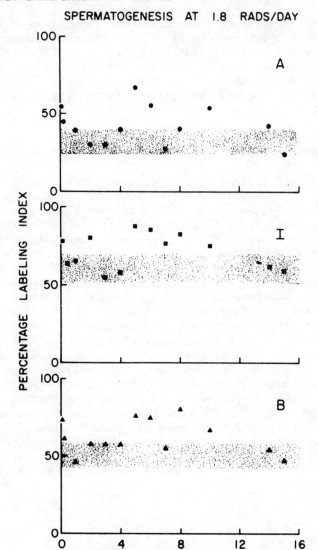

Fig. 3.   Percentage labeling indices in type A, intermediate and type B
spermatogonia under continuous exposure at 1.8 rads/day.
Shaded area - normal range.

to be a response to some cellular depopulation at this
time with an attempt to alter the cell kinetics to compensate for cellular radiation death. By 15 weeks, these
data, together with defferential cell type distributions,
indicated that the new steady state of cell proliferation
was established and the cell population structure returned
to a normal pattern.

CELL CYCLE OF SPERMATOGONIA

(Table 1) in normal 13-week-old mice, the $\tilde{T}_C$ were
34 hr, 32 hr and 34 hr for A, In and B spermatogonia
respectively, based on labeled mitosis data. The $\tilde{T}_{g2}+$
m/2 periods were 3 hr in each class, and $\tilde{T}_C$ values did
not change appreciably. There was a lengthening of the
G_2 + M/2 complex period in each class associated with a
greater spread in these values, and with decrease in the
number of cells synthesizing DNA in early prophase.
This was compensated for by a concomitant decrease in
$\tilde{T}_s$ by approximately the same duration ($\sim$3-4 hr), so that
no significant change occurred in $\tilde{T}_{g\,1+m/2}$. While the
overall $\tilde{T}_C$ did not change appreciably, the effect of
continuous irradiation was a delay in the flow of cells
from the premitotic compartment into cell division,
i.e., through G_2 and early prophase, a decrease in $\tilde{T}_s$,
and possibly a greater spread of the distribution of
cell cycle times. The data indicate that G_2-prophase
delays of up to 8 hr or more may have occurred, that continuous irradiation affected the early prophase cells
more than the G_2 cells, and that the flow of cells
through the $G_1 \rightarrow S \rightarrow G_2$ portion of the cell cycle was least
disturbed.

DISCUSSION

An increased *rate of cell proliferation* was apparently an importnat homeostatic mechanism to compensate
for the loss of cells due to radiation. The changes
were seen earliest in A cells -- at $\sim$4-6 weeks, and
slightly later in In cells -- $\sim$6-8 weeks, and later in
B cells -- $\sim$8-10 weeks. The extent to which these changes

were due to a true shortening of $\tilde{T}_C$ or to the introduction of a reserve cell population is not yet fully resolved. However, from percentage labeled mitosis curves so far obtained, a change in the spread in the cell cycle durations, particularly among the type subpopulations, does appear to play a part. Under continuous irradiation, the $\tilde{T}_C$ remained relatively unchanged, but there is an increase in $\tilde{T}_{g2}$ associated with a reduction in $\tilde{T}_S$. Therefore, any lengthening of $\tilde{T}_C$ by direct radiation effect, such as a G_2-delay, was more than compensated by normal homeostatic processes in the tissues.

TABLE 1. Spermatogonial Cell Cycle Parameters (hr) under Continuous Irradiation at 1.8 Rads/ Day for 15 Weeks.

Phase	Unirradiated			Irradiated		
	A	In	B	A	In	B
$T_{g2} + m/2$	3	3	3	8	7	5
T_S	22	23	25	18	19	22
$T_{g1} + m/2$	9	6	6	8	7	8
T_C	34	32	34	34	33	35

The *production of degenerate cells*, and particularly labeled degenerate cells, increased during the initial 6-8 weeks under irradiation, indicating the effect at this very low dose rate was to increase the rate of cell death in the proliferative compartment. This was most evident in the more mature forms, *B* cells primarily and *In* cells, respectively. By 15 weeks, the cell population structure returned to control values, and the number of degenerate cells in each subcompartment decreased, so that any cell killing by direct radiation effect was compensated by normal homeostatic control mechanisms. This could be due, in part, to a selection process associated with a decreased radiosensitivity among surviving cells, and in part, a decreased birth rate of new spermatogonia.

Thus far, there appears to be no appreciable *recruitment of nondividing cells* into the proliferative compartment, but this is presently under investigation.

The *shortening of T_S* under irradiation may represent an important effect on replicating cells, and in part, the limiting event leading to the breakdown of factors regulating spermatogonial cell reproduction. Lamerton [5] has suggested that at dose rates > 2 rads/day, spermatogonia are very sensitive to radiation death, and the main reason for this low tolerance to continuous irradiation could be the lack of any compensatory mechanisms. Without a decrease in $\tilde{T}_C$ combined with more divisions per maturation sequence, there could be no effective increased rate of spermatogonial cell production to compensate for cellular depopulation under continuous irradiation. It may be that the seminiferous epithelium cannot compensate to any appreciable degree by changing its patterns of the kinetics of the cell cycle and cell populations even at such low dose rates, thereby leading to progressive deterioration of the system.

SUMMARY

Under continuous irradiation, cell renewal during spermatogenesis in the mouse could achieve a near-steady state of cell population at a dose rate of 1.8 rads/day or less for at least 15 weeks by limited mechanisms of compensatory cell proliferation. Changes in the patterns of spermatogonial cell population kinetics indicated there was some reserve of proliferative capacity, but the extent to which these changes were due to decreasing the $\tilde{T}_C$ of a precursor subpopulation in the *A* cell compartment, or the bringing-in of a potentially proliferative dormant cell population, is not, as yet, clearly understood.

REFERENCES

1. BROWN, S.O., *Genetics*, *50*, 1101, 1964.

2. BROWN, S.O., KRISE, G.M., PACE, H.B., and de BOER, J., In: *Effects of Ionizing Radiation on the Reproductive System*, W.D. Carlson and F.X. Gassner, eds. p. 103, Macmillan, New York, 1964.

3. CASARETT, G.W., In: *Effects of Ionizing Radiation on the Reproductive System*, W.D. Carlson and F.X. Gassner, eds., p. 127, Macmillan, New York, 1964.

4. de BOER, J., In: *Effects of Ionizing Radiation on the Reproductive System*, W.D. Carlson and F.X. Gassner, eds., p.59, Macmillan, New York, 1964.

5. LAMERTON, L.F., In: *Radiation Research*, G. Silini, ed., p. 964, North-Holland, Amsterdam, 1967.

6. MONESI, V., *Radiation Res.*, *17*, 809, 1962.

7. NEARY, G.J., MUNSON, R.J., nad MOLE, R.H., *Chronic Radiation Hazards*, Pergamon Press, London, 1957.

8. OAKBERG, E.F., *Radiat. Res.*, *2*, 396, 1955.

9. OAKBERG, E.F., and CLARK, E., *J. Cell. Comp. Physiol.*, *58*, (Suppl. 1). 173, 1961.

10. OAKBERG, E.F., nad CLARK, E., In: *Effects of Ionizing Radiation on the Reproductive System*, W.D. Carlson and F.X. Gassner, eds., p. 127, Macmillan, New York, 1964.

11. RUSSELL, W.L., *J. Cell Comp. Physiol.*, *58*, (Suppl. 1), 183, 1961.

CELL POPULATION KINETICS OF ERYTHROPOIETIC CELLS
IN RESPONSE TO RADIATION

N.M. BLACKETT

*Biophysics Department, Institute of Cancer Research,
Sutton, Surrey, England*

A great amount of work has been carried out on the
effect of radiation on haemopoietic tissue but there is
still considerable uncertainty as to the changes in cell
kinetics that are produced. In this paper an attempt has
been made to review what is known and to put this in the
context of what is required in order to have a comprehensive understanding of the response of this tissue to
radiation.

Considering first of all acute irradiation, one
would like to know the radiosensitivity of the different
cell types, that is one would like to know the dose survival curves for cells in the various stages of maturation
from the stem cell to the mature functional cell in the
circulation for each of the cell lines comprising haemopoietic tissue. In actual fact survival curves have only
been obtained for the stem cells and little is known
about the sensitivity of other stages of maturation except that the more mature non-proliferating stages are
resistant to radiation and are not significantly affected
by doses below a few thousand rads.

The reason for this situation is that stem cells can
be measured because they give rise to discrete clones of
cells in the spleen when transplanted into heavily irradiated recipients. It is therefore a quite straight-
forward matter to determine the survival of these cells

following irradiation by determining the reduction in the
number of spleen colonies as a result of irradiating the
injected bone marrow cells. This was first done by
McCulloch and Till (1961) and has been repeated many
times since.

The D_0 values obtained are mainly in the range 80 -
110 rads and are similar to other types of cells growing
in vivo such as lymphocytes producing antibody [7] or a
graft versus host reaction [3]. Survival curves for
cells grown *in vitro* are more variable ranging from 70 -
200 rads many of these however are cell lines derived
from tumour tissue.

Another method that has been used to obtain survival
curves *in vivo* is to hypertransfuse animals with red
blood cells and then wait several days until the marrow
is almost devoid of recognisable erythroid cells. These
animals are then irradiated and the ability to respond to
a standard dose of erythropoietin is measured by determining the incorporation of ^{59}Fe into red blood cells two
to three days later [8].

This is an indirect method since the measurement
will be affected by changes in the proportion of cells
which are induced to differentiate, the dose of erythropoietin, the capacity of the induced cells to produce
haemoglobin synthesizing cells and the kinetics of radioactive iron distribution within the animal. Should any
of these factors differ as between irradiated and the unirradiated control animals the slope of the survival curve
will be affected. In spite of all these possible influences it would seem likely that the survival curve for
large doses of erythropoietin gives a reasonable estimate
of the sensitivity to radiation of the unrecognised cells
which respond to erythropoietin. The work of Byron and
Lajtha [8] indicates the need to use high doses of erythropoietin and thus favours a D_0 of about 90 rads for these
cells obtained with a dose of 10 units of erythropoietin
per mouse [13]. Porteous et al. however favoured the
lower value of about 70 rads which they obtained with 1
unit of erythropoietin because they considered that
skipped cell divisions might make the high dose value
incorrect.

It was thought at first that cells responding to
erythropoietin in hypertransfused mice were the stem
cells. However there is now considerable evidence that
these cells are more numerous than the stem cells and so
must be considered as a separate population. This conclusion does not exclude the possibility that stem cells
may also respond directly to erythropoietin as is indicated by the recent work of Guzman and Lajtha [9].

The difficulty in measuring the survival of cells
which have commenced differentiation arises from the fact
that cells irradiated while they are at one stage of maturation will not die until after one or more cell divisions
by which time they may well have reached a later stage of
maturation. So the number of cells in a particular stage
will depend on the sensitivity of cells in an earlier
stage and also on the number of cell generations before
the cells die and have been removed from the population,
as well as on the rate of cell maturation. It is to be
expected that cells become more resistant to radiation as
they approach the stage of maturation where proliferation
ceases, since some cells which have lost their reproductive integrity may be able to go through the required
number of divisions without dying and become mature cells.

For acute irradiation the killing of maturing cells
is not of great importance as far as survival is concerned
since there are sufficient numbers of mature functional
cells to tide the animal over until mature cells are obtained by differentiation from the surviving stem cells.
However the cell kinetics of the maturing cells is of importance because the number of mature cells produced depends on the number of cell generations during maturation
as well as on the recovery of the stem cell population.

Following acute irradiation it is generally found
that the stem cell numbers decrease for one or more days
before recovery begins. This decrease is an effect over
and above that produced by the irradiation of the cells
themselves since the transplantation of cells allows sufficient time for cells which have lost their reproductive
integrity to die. Furthermore it is observed not only
following irradiation Blackett et al (1964), Silini et al

[15], Guzman and Lajtha [9] but also following the transplantation of unirradiated cells into heavily irradiated
recipients, Schooley [14], Lahiri and van Putten [11] and
Kretchmar and Conover [10] but was not observed by
McCulloch et al [12].

It has been suggested that this dip is due to a depletion of stem cells as a result of the differentiation
of stem cells into maturing cells and Dr. Lahiri is dealing with this suggestion in this symposium.

Consideration of the dip and the recovery is of some
interest in the light of what is known about the cell
kinetics of the stem cells.

In the normal animal the number of stem cells remains
constant as a result of a balance between the rate at
which these cells are produced (P) and the rate at which
they are lost (L) through differentiation into the maturing stages, as illustrated in Fig. 1. Following irradiation a proportion of the stem cells loose their reproductive integrity and these are the "doomed cells" shown
in Fig. 1.

According to orthodox radiobiological thinking these
doomed cells will not die until they have undergone one or
more cell divisions and consequently depletion of the stem
cells will be spread over several days since the evidence
from tritiated thymidine suicide experiments is that stem
cells have a mean cell cycle time in excess of 30 hours
(since Bruce et al [1] have shown that only 80% of the
stem cells have passed through DNA synthesis in the space
of 24 hours).

The removal of doomed cells will not influence the
colony forming cells directly since these cells have retained their reproductivity integrity but will influence
the time at which the stimulus for increased cell proliferation occurs, if this stimulus is dependent on the
size of the stem cell population as is generally assumed.
Consequently after irradiation one would not expect an
early onset of increased proliferation or an early recovery.

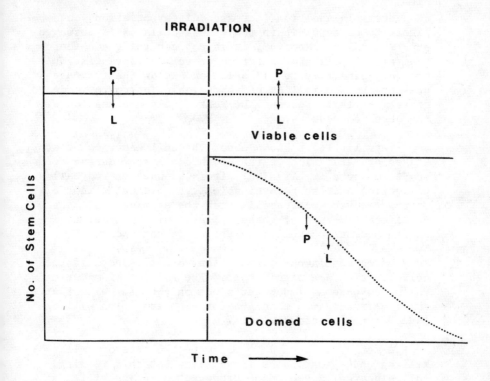

Fig. 1.   Illustration of the influence of cell proliferation (P) and cell
          loss (L) on the number of viable and 'doomed' stem cells follow-
          ing irradiation.

The fact that cell proliferation has been shown to
be increased 1 day after a dose of only 200R [15] and that
recovery is observed as early as two days by some workers
[10] is not in agreement with the above expectation.

This difficulty can be overcome if the stem cells
undergo intermitotic death or if radiation stimulates
cell proliferation directly. Either of these will lead
to a more rapid loss of stem cells and an early recovery
of the viable stem cells as a result of the increased
proliferation (Fig. 1). Alternatively radiation might
stimulate cell differentiation which would also lead to a
more rapid loss of the doomed cells and hence an earlier

recovery. In addition increased differentiation would be
likely to cause a dip in the viable cells as is observed
experimentally. However, it is not generally considered
that either cell proliferation or cell differentiation
are very sensitive to radiation and so on the evidence at
present the possibility of appreciable intermitotic death
of stem cells is perhaps the most likely explanation of
the observed results.

Very little is known about the cell kinetics of other
stages of maturation of the erythroid system during recovery from acute irradiation. It is known that red cell
production and the recognisable erythroid cells in the
marrow recover more rapidly than the stem cells, but the
proliferation rate of these cells, their maturation time
and the number of cell generations is not known.

Under continuous irradiation, other aspects of the
cell kinetics are significant. The killing of maturing
cells now becomes important since only those cells that
survive irradiation throughout their maturation will become mature functional cells.

A method is needed to estimate the rate of cell
killing under continuous irradiation but this is difficult since cells are being produced and being killed at
the same time and this is equally true for the stem cells
as for the maturing cells. One attempt to estimate the
rate of cell killing of stem cells was by terminating the
irradiation and then measuring the rate of increase in
the stem cell population, on the assumption that the initial increase would be due to cells that would otherwise
have been killed had the irradiation continued. This
gave the somewhat large value of about 30% of the cells
being killed each day for a dose rate of 45 rads/day [4].

In spite of the uncertainty about the rate of cell
killing it has been possible to obtain some information
about the cell kinetics of the maturing cells under continuous irradiation. Tarbutt [16] has shown that the
rate of entry of cells into the proerythroblast stage of
maturation is reduced to about one quarter of normal in
rats irradiated at 45 rads/day. Since red cell production

remains normal in these animals, except perhaps for a
temporary slight decrease during the first few weeks of
irradiation, it is evident that the maturing cells must
undergo at least two extra cell generations so as to allow a normal output of mature cells when the flow into
the proerythroblast is reduced by a factor of 4. In
actual fact there are probably more than two extra cell
generations since it is also necessary to compensate for
the cells which die as they mature. From the rate of decrease of labelled proerythroblasts following injection
of ^{55}Fe it would appear that it is an increase in the
maturation time rather than an increase in the rate of
cell generations.

It has also been shown that the stem cells are
severely depleted and are proliferating more rapidly than
normal [5]. This response occurs in animals that are not
anaemic and so the response is not due to increased production of erythropoietin. Indeed the response to anemia
is quite different [16].

It would seem therefore that the whole of the erythroid system responds to irradiation and not just the stem
cells. What control mechanisms are operating is uncertain. Does the increased proliferation of the stem cells
depend on a stimulus resulting from the depletion in their
own cell numbers, or depletion of some other stage of
maturation or some other effect. What causes the increased maturation of the recognisable cells?

A more detailed knowledge of the cell kinetics and
how it changes after acute irradiation and after the
start of continuous irradiation would seem likely to provide answers to these questions.

Information about the other cell lines of haemopoietic tissue would seem at present to be insufficient
to give any clear indication as to how they respond to
stress.

REFERENCES

1. BRUCE, W.R., MECKER, B.E. and VALERIOTE, F.A.,
   J. Nat. Cancer Inst., *37*, 233, 1966.

2. BLACKETT, N.M., ROYLANCE, P.J. and ADAMS, K., *Brit.
   J. Haematol.*, *10*, 453.

3. BLACKETT, N.M., *Int. J. Radiation Biol.*, *9*, 323,
   1965.

4. BLACKETT, N.M., *Int. Atomic Energy Agency Publication*, *119*, 1967.

5. BLACKETT, N.M., *J. Nat. Cancer Inst.*, *41*, 909, 1968.

6. BYRON, J.W. and LAJTHA, L.G., *Brit. J. Haematol.*,
   15, 47, 1968.

7. CELADA, F. and CARTER, R., *J. Immunol.*, *89*, 161,
   1962.

8. GURNEY, C.W., DEGOWIN, R., HOFSTRA, D. and BYRON, J.,
   *Application of Erythropoietin to Biological Investi-
   gation in Erythropoiesis*, Eds. Jacobsen and Doyle,
   p. 151, Grune and Stratton, 1962.

9. GUZMAN, E. and LAJTHA, L.G., *Cell and Tissue Kinet.*,
   3, 91, 1970.

10. KRETCHMAR, A.L. and CONOVER, W.R., *P.S.E.M.Biol.*,
    129, 218, 1968.

11. LAHIRI, S.K. and van PUTTEN, L.M., *Cell & Tissue
    Kinetics*, *2*, 21, 1969.

12. McCULLOCH, E.A. and TILL, J.E., *Radiation Res.*, *22*,
    383, 1964.

13. PORTEOUS, D.D., TSO, S.C., HIRASHIMA, K. and LAJTHA,
    L.G., *Nature*, *206*, 204, 1965.

14. SCHOOLEY, J.C., *J. Cell Physiol.*, *68*, 249, 1966.

15. SILINI, G., ELLI, R., SYRACUSA, G. and POZZI, L.V.,
     Cell & Tissue Kinet., *1*, 111, 1968.

16. TARBUTT, R.G., *Brit. J. Harmatol.*, *16*, 9, 1969.

17. TILL, J.E. and McCULLOCH, E.A., *Radiation Res.*, *14*,
     213, 1961.

18. TWENTYMAN, P.R. and BLACKETT, N.M., *J. Nat. Cancer
     Inst.*, *44*, 117, 1970.

DIFFERENTIATION OF HAEMOPOIETIC PRECURSOR CELLS DURING RECOVERY IN RADIATION DEPLETED ANIMALS

S.K. LAHIRI*

Rotterdam Medical Faculty, Rotterdam, The Netherlands

and

Radiobiological Institute TNO, Rijswijk, Z.H., The Netherlands

Haemopoietic precursor cells in a normal animal are in a dynamic equilibrium between self-replication and differentiation. Their rate of production is equal to the rate of loss by death or differentiation. When an animal is irradiated, this equilibrium is disturbed, and the surviving precursor cells are in new conditions where some of the mature blood cells and many immature blast cells have been destroyed. Somewhat similar conditions exist in animals which have been lethally irradiated and given haemopoietic cell injection.

Though the haemopoietic precursor cells, or the so-called multipotent stem cells have not been morphologically identified, the spleen colony assay technique of Till and McCulloch has made it possible to make both quantitative and qualitative studies of them. The fact that some spleen colonies contain mixtures of erythroid, myeloid and megakaryocytic population and on replantation produce new colonies proves that the technique deals with multipotent cells, which can self-replicate and differen-

*Present address of correspondence: Dr. S.K. Lahiri, Postfach 365, 517 Jülich 1, Germany.

tiate. Hence a study of the kinetics of colony forming
units gives us some insight in the behaviour of stem
cells. All our studies reported here, deal with colony
forming units.

There is reason to believe that changes in the environmental condition can modify the growth pattern of haemopoietic precursor cells. Six weeks after 600 R, when
the CFU level is back to normal or at a supranormal level,
a second dose of 600 R cannot suppress endogenous colony
formation as effectively as the first dose did [2].
Though 800 rads given to normal mice reduces the background endogenous spleen colony count to less than one,
this dose given to a mouse which was administered 450 rads
2 weeks ago, leaves a higher background colony number.
This is in spite of the fact that 2 weeks after 450 rads,
the CFU content in spleen and femur is below normal level.
Since there is no evidence that a rapidly proliferating
cell population is radioresistant, this would suggest
that in conditions where there is rapid self-replication,
the precursor cells are less susceptible to differential
stimuli. Erythropoietin injection in polycythaemic recipients increases colony formation after a haemopoetic
cell transplant [16]. Injection of endotoxin has been
found to accelerate repopulation after irradiation [18].
Further reference in the literature supports this idea.
In polycythaemic irradiated mice, the growth pattern of
injected CFU is different from that of normal irradiated
animals [15]. There is a difference in the radiation
sensitivity of bone marrow as assayed by leucocyte response to endotoxin or by Fe^{59} uptake [8]. Bled or
erythropoietin injected recipients of bone marrow cells
respond less to endotoxin induced leucocytosis [7]. All
these would suggest a modified behaviour by the stem cell
under changed conditions.

In rats suffering from chronic anaemia, the cycle
times of repopulating haemopoietic precursor cells are
significantly modified [1].

We are interested in the growth kinetics of precursor cells in irradiated mice. A continuing loss of colony forming units from the femur during the first 24

hours after sublethal irradiation has been observed [6, 19] and similar results have been reported by using erythropoietin sensitivity as indicator [3]. After this initial dip the precursor cells start proliferating. A similar phenomenon has been found in the spleen CFU content [11]. Although part of this initial loss has been attributed to loss in transplantability, this alone can not explain the total effect [4].

Similarly, early loss of colony forming units that could be recovered from the spleen of irradiated and bone marrow or spleen cell injected mice has been reported [12, 14, 15, 16].

Qualitatively similar conditions prevail in the sublethally irradiated and in the heavily irradiated and haemopoietic cell injected animals, although some differences are observed in the distribution of cells in the two cases. In injected animals more CFU are found in the spleen than in a femur, and during repopulation, the spleen CFU content is always more than that in the femur. After sometime, the spleen CFU content reached the supranormal levels and only after that gradually returns to normal (Fig. 1). The femur CFU content does not attain supranormal levels but gradually rises to the normal value. In sublethally irradiated animals, where the surviving endogenous cells are allowed to repopulate the haemopoietic tissues, the femur CFU content remains at a higher level than that of the spleen for some time; then the spleen CFU content surges ahead and overshoots. However, this difference between exogenous and endogenous systems should not affect our examination of the kinetic behaviour of repopulating haemopoietic precursor cells. We therefore used the spleen CFU population of irradiated and bone marrow cell injected mice for our study.

Referring to Fig. 1, we find that the growth of CFU content in the spleen after injection can be divided into three phases: (i) the fall during the first 24 - 48 hours; (ii) the near exponential growth following this dip; and (iii) the return to normal from the overshoot. A similar picture has been obtained in mice given 450 rads of irradiation, although the growth rate is different.

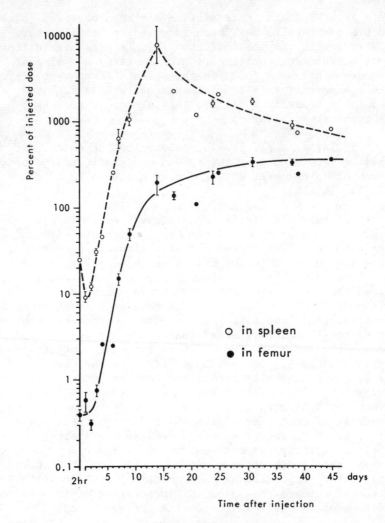

Fig. 1. Swiss mice: Growth of injected CFU.

There is much controversy concerning implications of
the early dip in the injected CFU in phase (i). One explanation suggests a loss of transplantability, but it
has been shown that this alone cannot account for the dip
[11]. A cell loss by the spleen resulting in shrinkage
of its size, and consequent loss in its CFU content has

also been suggested as an explanation. However, cellular
loss by the spleen has been found to be dispropotion-
ately higher than CFU loss [12]. Suggestions have also
been made [9] that an appreciable number of CFU (presumably migrating from the homing sites) can be found in the
circulation by 24 - 48 hours after injection, though our
own findings have been to the contrary [12].

We examined the roles of the spleen and the rest of
the body as contributors of circulating CFU. Irradiated
mice were given bone marrow cell injections. Two hours
later, they were divided in groups and one of these was
given 800 rads total body irradiation with the spleen exteriorised and shielded; in another group the spleen was
exteriorised and irradiated while the rest of the body
was shielded. A third group, with the spleen exteriorised and given whole body sham-irradiation, served as
controls. CFU levels in femur, spleen and blood of these
three groups 2 hours and 24 hours after the second irradiation can be seen in Table 1. It was found from

Table 1. Redistribution of CFU in Irradiated and Bone
Marrow Injected Mice After Partial Body Irradiation
(pooled results from 5 donors and 5 - 10 recipients)

	Treatment	CFU distribution 2 hours after treatment			CFU distribution 24 hours after treatment		
		CFU/ spleen	CFU/ femur	CFU/ ml blood	CFU/ spleen	CFU/ femur	CFU/ ml blood
EXP. I	Sham controls	900	30.4	20	228	21	8
	TBR with spleen shielded	982	0	12	230	1.5	0
EXP. II	Sham controls	750	26.3	18	420	13	7
	Spleen irradiation with rest of body shielded	139	28.5	10.5	165.3	29	3.5

spleen shielding experiments that only a small fraction
of the CFU which had settled in the spleen, would migrate
to femur. After 24 hours no CFU could be detected in
blood. Moreover, the spleen irradiation with body shielding data show that the rest of the body contributes to
the circulating CFU, and some of these settle in the
spleen. It may therefore be assumed that the net loss or
gain of CFU by the spleen during this period is not appreciable because some CFU also migrate to the spleen
from the rest of the body.

Failure to prove otherwise has given us more confidence in the hypothesis that the early dip in the CFU content of the spleen in irradiated and injected mice is
largely due to differentiation of a fraction of the CFU
to non-CFU. By analogy we think that differentiation
plays a role in the early loss of CFU in spleen and femur of sublethally irradiated mice as well. This means
that a fraction of the haemopoietic precursor cells loses
its self-replicating ability during this period.

The exponential part of the CFU growth curve shows a
CFU population doubling every 22 hours. This increase is
only possible if self-replication produces more precursor
cells than are lost by death or differentiation.

Frindel, et al. [5] found a generation time of 8.5
hours for normal mouse bone marrow cells. Their method
deals with cells in cycle, and since cycling stem cells
comprise only a small fraction of bone marrow cells, this
value cannot be accepted as applicable to stem cells.
But at least for an exponentially growing CFU population,
vinblastine studies [20] indicate a cycle time much shorter than 22 hours for most of the CFU. The long doubling
time is a result of some loss by differentiation, which
is evident from the fact that the CFU can end up as a
macroscopic colony by 8 - 9 days.

In phase (iii) of the CFU growth the elevated CFU
content of the recipient's spleen is found to come down
from the high level   A logical explanation for this decline is that more and more CFU are becoming non-CFU.
This a supported by retransplantation experiments, the

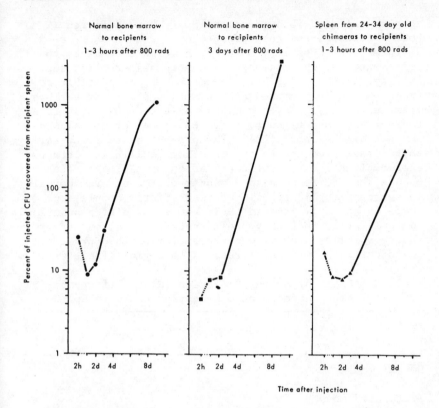

Fig. 2. Growth in spleen of injected CFU under different conditions.

results of which are shown in Fig. 2. In new hosts the
dip continues till at least 3 days, and each CFU can
produce fewer daughter CFU than normal.

In Fig. 2 the effects of the host's condition can
be seen. In recipients, which were injected three days
after irradiation, not only is the dip absent, but for
each CFU injected, 9 days later the spleen contains significantly larger numbers of CFU than normal.

Previous studies [12] have shown that the CFU population is not homogenous, because CFU from different

sources injected into identical hosts have different 2
hour f factors, and they produce different numbers of
daughter CFU. Possibly some CFU have more tendency to
differentiate, while others have more self-replicating
ability. It has also been found that it is possible to
produce a change in the early kinetics of CFU by various
treatments [13]. Erythropoietin injection has been found
to increase the CFU content of the spleen of normal mice
but not of the femur [10]. The present studies suggest
that irradiation upsets the existing equilibrium between
self-replication and differentiation of CFU. As a consequence the CFU respond in a manner different from normal.
Though self-replication is necessary for repopulation,
there is an early loss in their number by differentiation,
and only after that they proliferate. Again, an overshoot is followed by more differentiation than proliferation until the CFU level returns to normal (Table 2).

Table 2. Ratio of Self-replication (S) to Differentiation (D) Among Haemopoietic Precursor Cells in Spleen

	$\frac{S}{D}$
Normal mouse	1
Irradiated mouse	
(i) early after irradiation	< 1
(ii) during recovery of precursor cell population	> 1
(iii) during decline to normal level following peak	< 1

SUMMARY

Cell transplantation and spleen colony formation
have been used to study the kinetics of growth of haemopoietic cells in irradiated mice. Before the haemopoietic colony forming cell population starts growing, it
suffers a loss in number, at least partly by differenti-

ation. During the rapid growth phase, there is more self-replication than differentiation. An overshoot, which occurs in the spleen but not in the femur, is followed by more differentiation than self-replication.

ACKNOWLEDGEMENT

The studies were performed in collaboration with Dr. L.M. van Putten, M.D., of the Radiobiological Institute TNO, Rijswijk (Z.H.), the Netherlands. The technical assistance of Mrs. E. Koning is gratefully acknowledged.

REFERENCES

1. BLACKETT, N.M., In: *Effects of Radiation on Cellular Proliferation and Differentiation*, IAEA, Vienna, p. 235, 1968.

2. BOOGS, D.R., Marsh, J.C., Chervenick, P.K., Cartwright, G.E. and Wintrobe, M.M., *J. Exp. Med., 126*, 871, 1967.

3. BYRON, J.W. and LAJTHA, L.G., *Brit. J. Haemat., 15*, 47, 1968.

4. FRED, S.S. and SMITH, W.W., *Proc. Soc. Exp. Biol. Med., 128*, 364, 1968.

5. FRINDEL, E., TUBIANA, M. and VASSORT, F., *Nature, 214*, 1017, 1967.

6. HANKS, G.M. and AINSWORTH, E.G., *Nature, 215*, 20, 1967.

7. HELLMAN, S. and GRATE, H.E., *Nature, 216*, 65, 1967.

8. HELLMAN, S., GRATE, H.E. and CHAFFEY, J.T., *Blood, 34*, 141, 1969.

9. KRETCHMAR, A.L. and CONOVER, W.R., *Proc. Soc. Exp. Biol. Med., 131*, 703, 1969.

10. KUBANEK, B., TYLER, W.S., FERRARI, L., PORCELLINI, A.,
     HOWARD, D. and STOHLMAN, F. JR., *Proc. Soc. Exp.
     Biol. Med.*, *127*, 770, 1968.

11. LAHIRI, S.K., KEIZER, H.J. and van PUTTEN, L.M.,
     Cell Tissue Kinet., *3*, 355, 1970.

12. LAHIRI, S.K. and van PUTTEN, L.M., *Cell Tissue Kinet.*
     2, 21, 1969a.

13. LAHIRI, S.K. and van PUTTEN, L.M., In: *Radiation In-
     duced Cancer*, IAEA, Vienna, p. 107, 1969b.

14. McCOLLOCH, E.A. and TILL, J.E., *Radiation Research*,
     22, 383, 1964.

15. POZZI, L.V. and SILINI, G., In: *Effects of Radiation
     on Cellular Proliferation and Differentiation*, IAEA,
     Vienna, p. 139, 1968.

16. SCHOOLEY, J.C., *J. Cell Physiol.*, *68*, 249, 1966.

17. SMITH, W.W., ALDERMAN, I.M. and GILLESPIE, R.E.,
     Am. J. Physiol., *192*, 549, 1958.

18. SMITH, W.W., MARSTON, R.Q. and CORNFIELD, J., *Blood*,
     14, 737, 1959.

19. SMITH, W.W., WILSON, S.M. and FRED, S.S., *J. Nat.
     Cancer Inst.*, *40*, 847, 1968.

20. VALERIOTE, F.A. and BRUCE, W.R., *J. Nat. Cancer Inst.*,
     38, 393, 1967.

PATTERNS OF RECOVERY AND REPOPULATION IN IRRADIATED SKIN

J. DENEKAMP

Medical Physics Department, Royal Postgraduate Medical School, Hammersmith Hospital, London, W. 12, England

Because skin tolerance is the limiting factor in orthovoltage radiotherapy and skin is an easily accessible tissue, it has often been used in radiation experiments as a model normal tissue. It is in fact a complex tissue, consisting of a renewing population of cells in the epidermis and a mixed population of non-renewing or slowly renewing cells of several types in the dermis. After a dose of radiation several waves of gross damage are seen. An initial wave of erythema occurs in the first few days, which might be associated with changes in the capillary permeability. This is followed at about one to four weeks by a second wave of erythema, leading to desquamation and ulceration, which may be attributed to depletion of the stem cells of the basal layer of the epidermis. In some species, a *late reaction* is observed [9] in which desquamation and necrosis is again seen after appropriate doses, and this may result from fibrosis and damage to the vascular system in the dermis, possibly with secondary death of epithelial cells caused by starvation. Despite the complexity of the radiation response, not surprising in view of the complexity of the tissue, it can be expressed quantitatively. This has been done (a) in terms of the average reaction (scored on an arbitrary scale) over any stated period of time, e.g.8-30 days and (b) by the survival of epithelial clones *in vivo*.

The gross skin reactions have been used by clinicians for many years but recently they have been used

quantitatively in pigs [10], mice [2, 11] and rats [8].
The exact timing of the appearance of radiation damage
varies from species to species, but the rate at which the
damage appears does not vary with dose. When larger
doses are given, the damage is more severe and healing
occurs later. This is consistent with a response caused
mainly by cell killing. The time at which desquamation
occurs depends on the turnover time of the basal layer,
but the extent of desquamation and the time at which it
is healed depends on the number of surviving cells and
the rate at which they can repopulate. The time of
appearance of the gross reactions correlates well with
the turnover time of the basal layer and the thickness of
the differentiated layers in the few instances where
these have been measured, e.g. the skin reactions appear
at about 8 days in mouse epidermis having a cell cycle
time of $4\frac{1}{2}$ days, but at approximately 4-5 days in plucked
epidermis where the cycle time is reduced to 2 days [13].

The average skin reaction over a given time period
can be determined for a range of doses and can be used to
construct a dose response curve. When a set of dose response curves is obtained with different fractionation
intervals, the dose required when given in two fractions
(D_2) can be compared with that required in a single dose
(D_1) to produce the same level of injury. The additional
dose (D_2-D_1) is that necessary to compensate for the intracellular repair of sublethal injury and for increase
in cell numbers due to repopulation.

Withers [15] developed a method of estimating the
survival of epithelial cells *in vivo* by the regrowth of
visible clones in irradiated test areas. The areas are
defined and isolated from the surrounding epidermis by a
moat of heavily irradiated cells. The size of the initial population is not known with any certainty, but
islands of various sizes can be irradiated with doses
that allow some, but not all, areas to regrow as a visible clone, and the ratio of their areas can be used
to obtain several decades of a cell survival curve (Fig.
1). Because of the problem of shielding small areas of
skin during the moat formation, all clone experiments
have been performed on plucked epidermis [7, 15]. When

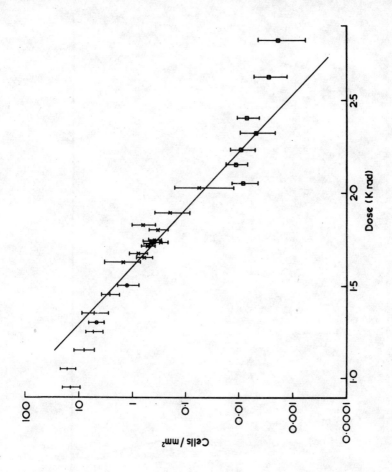

Fig. 1.   Survival of ephithelial cells following a single dose of X-rays,
estimated by using the Withers *in vivo* cloning technique (Emery
et al., Radiation Research, 1970).

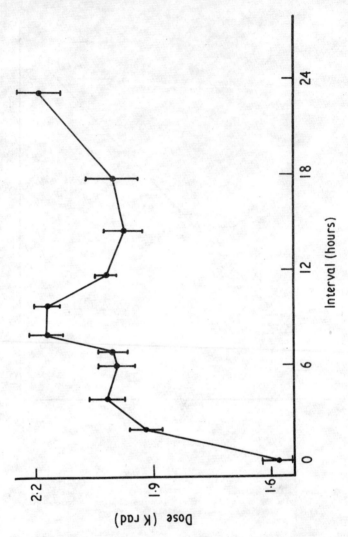

Fig. 2. Total X-ray dose given as two fractions, required to give one
surviving epithelial cell per mm², as a function of time after
the initial dose of 900 rads. (Emery et al., Radiation Research, 1970).

the radiation is given in more than one fraction, the doses to produce selected survival levels can be compared (as for the gross skin reactions). The values of (D_2-D_1) necessary to counteract repair and repopulation are very similar when estimated by the clone technique or from skin reactions.

The time course of recovery in epidermal cells in the first hours following a dose of radiation is similar to that found by Elkind and many other workers for cells *in vitro* [6]. There is prompt repair of sublethal injury in skin within 6 hours as evidenced by a D_2-D_1 of approximately 500 rads when tested by either technique. In the clone experiments (Fig. 2) an inflection occurs in the recovery curve at 7 hours both in the experiments by Withers [15] and by Emery et al. [7]. The significance of this inflection is not understood. In both systems there is a suggestion of a trough after eight hours but the value of D_2-D_1 at 24 hours is closely similar to that at 8 hours after irradiation with X-rays or electrons.

In order to test for repopulation rates, the intervals between fractions were extended out to 21 days [7, 2]. During the first three days, a cyclic variation in response was noted in the gross skin reaction results. The peaks and troughs were approximately 13-17 hours apart with an amplitude of 500-1000 rads (Fig. 3). This cyclic response may be a result of the selection of a synchronous population in the most resistant parts of the cell cycle, which would later move through the phases showing variations in sensitivity. A similar cyclic response to radiation has been found by Kallman [14] for 30-day death and for tumour cure experiments.

In the clone experiments and those using gross skin reactions, the dose increment D_2-D_1 increased with longer time intervals, an additional 580 rads being needed between day 1 and day 21 (Fig. 4). This increment is equivalent to approximately 30 rads per day, a value closely similar to those found for pig skin [10], rat skin [8] and for patient skin in radiotherapy [5]. Using $D_0 = 130$ rads from the clone experiments [7], this gives an estimate of the generation time of the

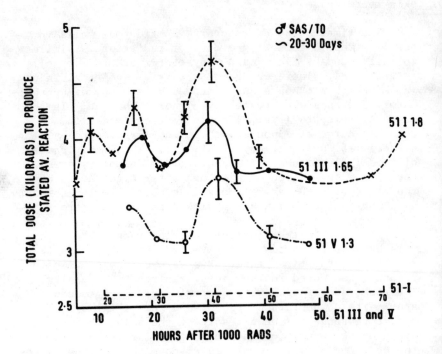

Fig. 3. Total dose to produce the stated levels of skin reaction as a
         function of time after the first dose of 1000 rads. One level
         of reaction from each of three experiments is shown. The time
         axis has been adjusted for experiment 51-1, in order to super-
         impose the peaks and trough. (Denekamp et al., Radiation Re-
         search, 1969).

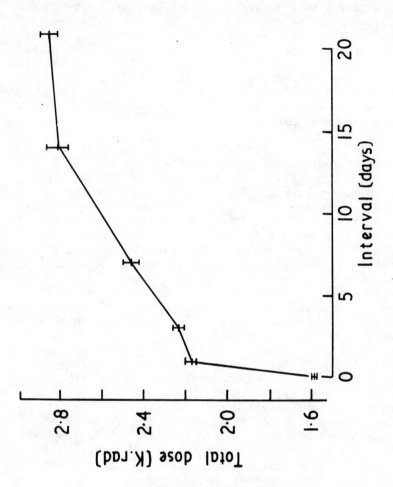

Fig. 4. Total dose required to produce one cell surviving per mm² in the skin clone experiments. A dose increment of 550 rads is needed within 24 hours. A further 580 rads is needed between day 1 and day 21. (Emery et al., Radiation Research, 1970).

basal layer of 2-3 days. By a similar procedure Withers
[15] obtained an estimate of 22 hours from his experiments. It is obvious therefore that the effect of repopulation between doses is small in skin, relative to
the repair of sublethal injury. Thus extending the time
over which a fractionated course of radiotherapy is
given would need a relatively small adjustment of dose,
but a change in the number of fractions would require a
much larger adjustment.

In principle, repopulation rates can also be measured by conventional cell proliferation kinetic techniques, using radioactive tracers and autoradiography.
In practice these techniques are difficult to use on
tissues which have long cell cycle times, and particularly on epithelial tissues, where many sections are
needed to provide sufficient basal layer cells for microscopic counting. However, the unirradiated skin of a number of species has been investigated; the wide range of
turnover times quoted by different workers, e.g. 6½ -
45 days for human skin is an indication of the difficulties involved in such measurements. Furthermore,
the proliferation parameters may change with physiological status or with site in any one animal. In mice
the cycle time has been found to be 12 hours in the hair
follicle [4, 12] during the growth phase, 47 hours in
interfollicular epidermis after plucking and 110 hours
in undisturbed epidermis [13]. The problems involved
in using tracer techniques are even greater when the
tissue under investigation has been perturbed by radiation. Some of the available techniques cannot be used
because a steady state condition does not exist. Many
of the cells that will contribute to the measurements
will be lethally injured and doomed to die; these cells
may behave differently from true survivors. Consequently
there is little direct kinetic information on irradiated skin. Griem and his colleagues have studied
changes in the hair matrix population and these are reported in the following paper. Devik [3] has shown
little change in the cell cycle time in an irradiated
area 5 days after 2700 rads, but a considerable shortening of T_C at the edge of the irradiated field. A
similar result was reported by Hegazy [13]. Brown [1]

has shown a 15-30% decrease in T_c after 500-1000 rads to the buccal epithelium in hamsters. In addition to the technical problems in using tracer techniques to measure repopulation, there is little known about the time at which the homeostatic mechanisms would operate in response to radiation damage. In general, the kinetic data, and that derived from split-dose experiments suggest that repopulation between fractions in radiotherapy is not of major importance relative to intracellular repair of sublethal injury.

SUMMARY

The patterns of repair and repopulation of epidermal cells are very similar both qualitatively and quantitatively when measured by gross skin reactions or an *in vivo* cloning technique. A dose increment of about 500 rads is needed in the first 8 hours to counteract repair of sublethal injury; over 2 to 3 weeks after irradiation, only 30 rads per day are needed to counteract repopulation.

REFERENCES

1. BROWN, J.M., *Radiation Res.*, 43, 627-653, 1970.

2. DENEKAMP, J., BALL, M.M. and FOWLER, J.F., *Radiation Res.*, 37, 361, 1969.

3. DEVIK, F., *Int. J. Radiation Biol.*, 5, 59, 1962.

4. CATTANEO, S.M., QUASTLER, H. and SHERMAN, F.G., *Nature*, 190, 923, 1961.

5. COHEN, L., *Brit. J. Radiol.*, 41, 522, 1968.

6. ELKIND, M.M. and SUTTON, H., *Radiation Res.*, 13, 556, 1960.

7.   EMERY, E.W., DENEKAMP, J., FIELD, S.B. and BALL, M.M., *Radiation Res.*, *41*, 450, 1970.

8.   FIELD, S.B., JONES, T. and THOMLINSON, R.H., *Brit. J. Radiol.*, *41*, 597, 1968.

9.   FIELD, S.B., *Radiology*, *92*, 381, 1969.

10. FOWLER, J.F., MORGAN, R.L., SILVESTER, J.A., BEWLEY, D.K. and TURNER, B.A., *Brit. J. Radiol.*, *36*, 188, 1963.

11. FOWLER , J.F., KRAGT, K., ELLIS, R.E., LINDOP, P.J. and BERRY, R.J., *Int. J. Radiation Biol.*, *9*, 241, 1965.

12. GRIEM, M.L., *Nature*, *210*, 213, 1966.

13. HEGAZY, M.A.H. and FOWLER, J.F., in preparation, 1970. See also HEGAZY, M.A.H., Ph.D. Thesis, London, 1969.

14. KALLMAN, R.F., *National Cancer Institute Monograph*, *24*, 205, 1966.

15. WITHERS, H.R., *Radiation Res.*, *32*, 227, 1967.

SOME STUDIES OF THE X-RAY EFFECTS ON RESTING HAIR CELL POPULATIONS

M.L. GRIEM, F.D. MALKINSON,* R. MARIANOVIC AND D. KESSLER

Department of Radiology and the Department of Medicine (Section of Dermatology), Pritzker School of Medicine, University of Chicago and the Argonne Cancer Research Hospital (operated by the University of Chicago for the United States Atomic Energy Commission), the Section of Dermatology and the Department of Medicine, Presbyterian-St. Luke's Hospital; and the Departments of Medicine and Dermatology, the University of Illinois College of Medicine, Chicago, Illinois, U.S.A.

In the planning of treatment for patients with malignant disease, one of the problems the radiotherapist would like to solve concerns the responsiveness of both proliferating and non-proliferating cell populations to ionizing radiation. We have found that the hair matrix cells, which keratinize to form the hair shafts, provide a most useful test system because of the wide variations in their metabolism from states of complete proliferative inactivity (the resting or telogen hair) to states of extremely high mitotic activity (growing or anagen hair). Later in this program another paper by Fry and co-workers will present some aspects of this proliferating activity in greater detail.

We would like to discuss some of our work dealing with the resting phase of the hair cycle and its response to ionizing radiation as measured by several different techniques.

---

*This investigation was supported in part by a grant from the Environment control Administration, C.P.E.H.S., U.S.P.H.S. EC00084-07.

The first series of studies consisted of irradiating
animals in the telogen phase of the hair cycle, following
which radiation damage was measured by impaired incorporation of tritium-labelled serine into keratin [1].   In all
experiments, a two centimeter area on the flank of the
mouse was irradiated with 45 kV X-rays with two millime-
ters aluminum filtration, at a focal skin distance of
11.5 centimeters. The exposure dose rate was 400 rads
per minute. The technique produced a tissue penetration of 1.2 centimeters half value depth. In these experiments, the unirradiated contralateral flank served
as the control site for each animal.

Mice, CF #1 female, were prepared by plucking hairs
to induce anagen. They were then observed during anagen
for uniformity of regrowth and allowed to continue into
telogen 18 days later. On the 21st day, graded doses of
radiation were given to the right flanks of separate
groups of mice. Zero to 12 days after irradiation, hairs
were again plucked to induce a growing coat, and tritiated serine was injected intraperitoneally four days
after plucking. When the newly growing hairs had entered
the telogen phase of the cycle, samples were plucked from
control and irradiated sites. The hairs were weighed and
combusted in oxygen using the Schöniger technique. The
tritiated water from combustion samples was then assayed
for radioactivity in a liquid scintillation spectrometer.
Control and irradiated samples were compared for tritium
incorporation on a weight basis. The resulting data
(Table 1) revealed decreasing incorporation of tritiated
serine with increasing doses of radiation during telogen.
There appeared to be no repair of radiation injury from
six hours to twelve days after irradiation, as measured
by tritiated serine incorporation into newly growing hairs
four days after plucking (Table 2). Further studies with
this hair indicator system showed that anagen hairs were
more sensitive to irradiation than telogen hairs [1].

The second series of experiments on the resting hair
population is an analysis of the hair density following
graded doses of X-ray radiation. The animals were
plucked and irradiated 22 days later when the follicles
were in telogen. Three weeks afterwards, during the same

Table 1. Reduced Levels of ^{3}H-DL-Serine in Subsequent "Generation" of Mouse Hair Following Irradiation in Telogen

Dose (rads)	Animals	Intervals between irradiation & plucking	DPM/ mg C (control)	DPM/ mg X (Radiated)	X/C (%)	Standard Error of the mean
500	8	Nil	236	192	86	7.16
1000	9	Nil	246	130	57	5.75
1500	6	Nil	268	83	39	7.07

Tabel 2. Reduced Levels of ^{3}H-DL-Serine in Subsequent "Generation" of Mouse Hair Following Irradiation with 1000 Rads in Telogen

Animals	Intervals between irradiation & plucking	DPM/ mg C (control side)	DPM/ mg X (radiated)	X/C (%)	Standard error of the mean
20	6 hours	209	149	71	3.80
20	12 hours	154	116	75	3.80
17	24 hours	76	50	66	2.33
8	4 days	117	89	76	7.16
13	8 days	286	186	65	3.46
19	12 days	239	160	66	4.01

telogen period, the animals were shaved on both control and irradiated sides and photographed on a Zeiss photomicroscope using bright field epi-immuniation. After the initial set of photographs were taken, the mice were observed for anagen regrowth. When this first regrowth

period was completed and the follicles were again in telogen (six to nine weeks after irradiation) the animals were
shaved and rephotographed.

Fig. 1 shows a dose response curve generated by computer in a non-linear regression analysis for the expression $S = 1 - (1 - e^{-D/D_0})^n$. The parameters n and D_0 were
derived from this analysis and the curves which best fit
these parameters were then drawn. The first count remained at 100% (survival equals 1) and showed no telogen
hair loss for the first three weeks immediately followig
irradiation. The new cycle that began four to five weeks
after irradiation may have been spontaneous or partially
induced by shaving. Hair survival after this first post-
irradiation growth cycle is shown in Fig. 1. A steady
slope for the constructed curve cannot be obtained by our
technique because the skin begins to ulcerate at doses
above 2200 rads. Therefore, only the shoulder of the survival curve has been determined experimentally; computer
analysis was necessary to evaluate the available data and
project the parameters n and D_0.

Fig. 2 presents a computer-analyzed dose response
curve utilizing pooled data from several experiments to
show the reaction of the 14 day anagen coat to graded
doses of X-ray irradiation. By comparing this figure to
the previous one, one can conclude that the telogen follicle is less sensitive to low kilovoltage X-rays than
the anagen follicle.

In a third series of experiments, mouse telogen
hairs were irradiated with doses of 1500 to 2500 rads,
and the lengths of later generations of awl-type hairs
were carefully measured [2]. Three to ten months later,
hairs from irradiated sites were 27% to 33% shorter than
those plucked from control areas. Fifteen months after
irradiation, several mice were given tritiated thymidine
and biopsies from irradiated and control sites were
studied. Per cent labelled mitosis curves revealed no
change in the cell generation cycle of 11 1/2 to 12 hours.
On the other hand, there was a decrease in the mitotic
index from 1.5 in the control sites to 0.7 in the irradiated areas.

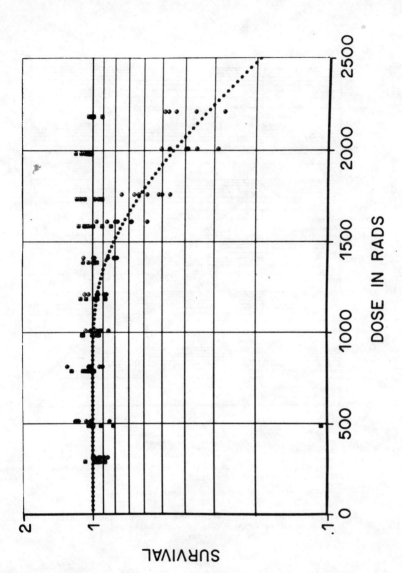

Fig. 1. Dose-response curve showing hair density in the second telogen phase following irradiation in telogen phase.

Computer derived parameters: D_0 – 492 ± 54 rads, n – 34 ± 14, D_q – 1741 ± 371 rad .

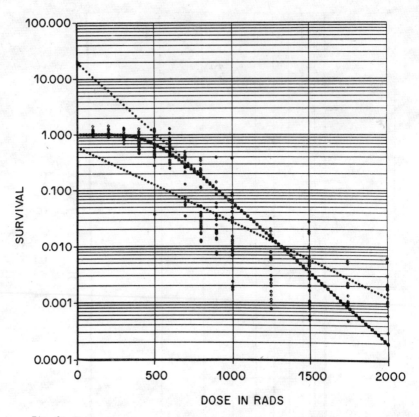

Fig. 2. Dose-response curve showing hair density in the first telogen phase
         following irradiation in anagen.

         Computer derived parameters for steep slope: D_0 - 174 ± 14 rads,
         n - 20 ± 5, D_q - 516 ± 84 rads.

         An attempt was made to search for a 2nd population of cells: for
         shallow slope: n - 0.6 ± 1.3, D_0 - 324 ± 147 rads.

From our studies of telogen or resting hairs, we can draw several conclusions concerning this non-proliferating cell population:

1.   No recovery in the reduced uptake of tritiated serine was demonstrable in telogen hairs up to 12 days post-irradiation, indicating a lack of repair in the resting cell population.

2.   Data on survival of hair, post-irradiation, revealed significantly lowered radiosensitivity in telogen, as compared to anagen hair populations. This was reflected in a broader shoulder and a higher D_q in the telogen survival curve.

3.   Observations of the body coat made almost one year after irradiation in the telogen with 2000 to 2500 rads revealed persistently reduced hair lengths and slower hair regrowth after plucking. Per cent labelled mitosis curves showed no change in proliferative cell cycle times, but mitotic index determinations suggested permanent reductions in hair matrix cell populations.

4.   We feel that the above observations may have important implications for radiation responses of non-proliferating cell populations in radiotherapeutic situations.

Our X-ray studies on non-proliferating telogen hair in mice have shown: (a) no recovery during the non-proliferating period, (b) reduced radiosensitivity with a broader shoulder on the survival curve in the resting phase, and (c) late changes with retarded regrowth and reduced hair length in telogen.

ACKNOWLEDGMENT

We gratefully acknowledge the assistance of Dr. Irving Lerch in performing the computer analyses.

REFERENCES

1.   MALKINSON, F.D. and GRIEM, M.L., *Radiation Res.*, *33*, 554, 1968.

2.   MALKINSON, F.D., GRIEM, M.L. and MARIANOVIC, R., *Radiation Res.*, (in press.)

STUDY OF CELL PROLIFERATION OF THE HAIR FOLLICLE

R.J.M. FRY, C.L. WEBER, W.E. KISIELESKI, M.L. GRIEM*
and F.D. MALKINSON**

*Division of Biological and Medical Research,
Argonne National Laboratory, Argonne, Illinois,
60439, U.S.A.*

and

*Departments of Radiology and Medicine, University of
Chicago, Chicago, Illinois, U.S.A.*

INTRODUCTION

The hair follicle provides a suitable test system
for a number of studies on cell proliferation, differentiation and intermittent growth [10, 2, 5, 6]. The
latter characteristic makes it possible to study radiation effects in active and inactive proliferative cell
populations [8, 11]. Plucking produces an injury which

_____

*Department of Radiology, Argonne Cancer Research
Hospital.†

**Department of Medicine (Section of Dermatology),
University of Chicago, Department of Medicine (Section
of Dermatology), Presbyterian-St. Luke's Hospital, Department of Medicine (Section of Dermatology), University of Illinois, College of Medicine, Chicago, Illinois.

†This investigation was supported by the U.S. Atomic
Energy Commission and in part by the United States
Public Health Service Research Grant #EC-00084-7, Environ-
mental Control Administration, CPEHS.

is suitable for the study of tissue response to injury
as the response appears to be reproducible and similar
in different animals and similar in some respects to
spontaneously occurring intermittent growth [3, 12]. It
is therefore possible to study the cell kinetics of the
cell population during the repopulation phase after
injury and compare this with the normal growth cycle.
This paper is concerned with the study of the growth
induced by plucking and the suitablity of squash preparations and combustion--liquid scintillation counting
methods for such studies. Two further questions were
asked: 1. What is the precise length of the induced
anagen and is it the same for all the hair types? 2.
Does the cell cycle alter with impending cessation of
growth?

METHODS AND MATERIALS

All the studies have been carried out on CF_1/Anl
female mice of 82-86 days of age. In the study of the
growth cycle after single plucking, mice were injected
with ^{3}HTdR (0.5uCi/g, 0.36 Ci/mM) at 3, 6, 10, 16, 17,
18, 19 and 20 days and sacrificed at one hour later.
Small pieces of skin with newly grown hair were fixed
in cold acid alcohol for about 24 hours, transferred
to 70% alcohol and eventually brought through graded
alcohols to water, hydrolyzed in 1 N HCl at 60° for
10 mins. Tissues were kept in Feulgen reagent overnight
in the dark. Individual hair follicles were dissected
out in 45% acetic acid. In some experiments hairs of
the four types were identified and selected [9]. Squash
preparations for autoradiographs were made.

The total number of labeled cells and mitoses were
determined on samples of the hair types for each of the
time intervals. For the Fraction Mitoses Labeled curve
near the end of the induced anagen, mice were injected
at appropriate times so that sacrifices were from 1 to
36 hours later and 16 days after plucking. The fraction
of mitoses labeled was determined for 100 or more mitoses
on samples from 2 or 3 mice for each time interval.
Samples for assay of tritium content were collected in

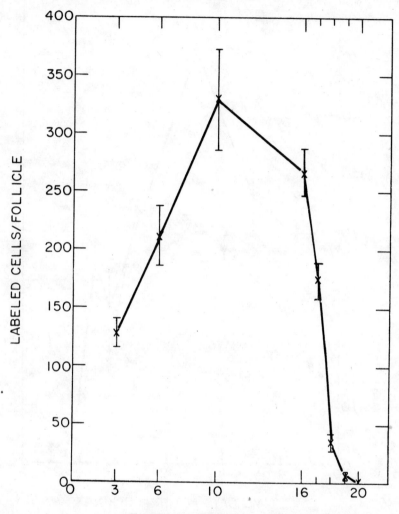

Fig. 1. The mean number of labeled nuclei per follicle one hour after the
injection of ^{3}HTdR as a function of time after plucking. Samples
of follicles included all hair types and were not balanced for
hair type nor were the means weighted. The standard errors of the
means are indicated. Data for three mice were used for each interval except day 17 when the number of mice was four.

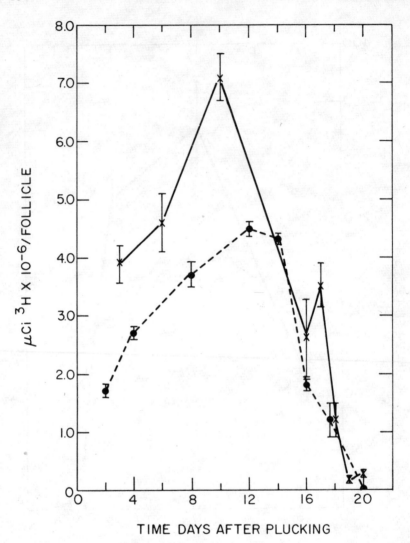

Fig. 2.   The mean tritium content per follicle one hour after injection of
³HTdR on the various days after plucking. Single plucking: x---x,
Double plucking: ●---●. Standard errors of the means are indicated.

groups of 20 and 40 follicles without regard to the
hair type but in another experiment duplicate samples of
10 monotrich, 20 awl, 30 auchene and 40 zigzag were
taken 14 days after plucking. The samples were combusted in a flask, which was then connected to a cold
trap. The water containing the tritium is sublimed into
a scintillation vial and 15 ml of liquid scintillator
(toluene containing 21% absolute ethyl alcohol, 0.4%
PPO and 0.005% POPOP) was added and the samples counted
in a Beckman LS-100.

RESULTS AND DISCUSSION

The proliferative activity, indicated by the number
of labeled matrix cells during the induced growth cycle,
is shown in Fig. 1. During the first 10 days after
plucking, the number of initially labeled cells increases.
From the microscopic appearances this increase is due to
an expanding proliferative population with concomitant
differentiation for production of hair.

In the early part of the growth phase the follicles
can only be divided into large and small and it is only
12-14 days after plucking that the distinction between
zigzag and auchene is clear. It is difficult to determine the total proliferative cell population on squash
preparations and therefore the labeling index and the
fraction of the population of the follicle in cycle.
Between 16 and 18 days the number of cells in DNA synthesis (S) decreases rapidly. Despite intra-and inter-
animal variations, in particular the marked difference
in population size between the large and small follicles, there is a reduction in the number of labeled
cells per follicle by a factor of about 10 in a time
equal to about 4 cell cycles. The results for the
uptake of ^{3}HTdR per follicle on various days of the
induced anagen, not surprisingly, show the same pattern
(Fig. 2) as the labeled nuclei per follicle. Although
there was no evidence of spontaneous anagen in the mice
an admixture of induced anagen and spontaneous changes
might have occurred during the experimental period. As
an induced anagen is followed by telogen, an investigation

TABLE 1. Proliferative Activity of Hair Types

Hair Type	Labeled Cells per follicle			Mitoses per follicle	
	Days after plucking				
	10	16	17	10	16
Zigzag		189±21	153±77		12±1
Auchene	149±18	255±37		15±2	15±3
Awl	284±44	255±50	210±158	19±4	
Monotrich	505±164	451±66		39±8	29±6

TABLE 2. ^{3}H Content 1 hr after ^{3}HTdR on Day 14

Hair Type	Sample size*	μCi ^{3}H $\times$ 10^{-6}/follicle			Mean±S.D.
		1	2	3	
Zigzag	40	2.78	2.52	3.92	3.05±0.77
		2.96	2.11	4.01	
Auchene	30	4.07	3.59	5.00	4.48±1.30
		4.07	3.32	6.84	
Awl	20	5.33	5.16	6.22	5.58±0.50
		5.22	5.39	6.16	
Monotrich	10	11.61	7.51	11.97	10.15±2.07
		8.32	9.15	12.32	

*No. of follicles combusted together in samples from 3 CF_1/Anl mice.

of the proliferative activity after a second plucking may be more satisfactory [10]. We determined the uptake of ^{3}HTdR on various days of anagen induced by plucking 24 days after an initial plucking. The results in Fig. 2 show that the pattern of proliferation and the duration

of the induced anagen is similar to that following a
single plucking.

The uptake of ^{3}HTdR and the number of initially
labeled cells for the four hair types are shown in Tables
1 and 2. The least numerous, the monotrich, has about
twice the number of proliferative cells than the most
numerous, the zigzag. It would be interesting to determine whether or not this difference in proliferative cell
population was reflected in changes in the relative frequency of the hair types after irradiation.

The duration of the cell cycle of the matrix cells
16-17 days after plucking was found to be 11-12 hours,
which is similar to that for cells at 8 days, 10 days
[7] and 10-11 days [1]. It is clear that the end of induced anagen does not involve a slowing of the cell
cycle but an increase in the number of cells leaving the
cycle and proceeding to differentiation.

We have not yet determined the cell cycle time for
cells in spontaneous anagen, but as the duration of anagen
and the total production of cells are considered to be
similar to those in induced anagen it is unlikely that
the cell cycle time could be much longer than after plucking. Change in cell cycle times do not appear to be an
important mechanism for altering proliferation in this
cell system.

CONCLUSIONS

1. Squash preparations and ^{3}H content assay of individual
hair types are useful and practical methods for the study
of hair follicles.

2. The duration of induced anagen depends on the definition of the growth phase, but it is clear that proliferative activity has ceased in all hair types of 19 days after
plucking. The number of cells in cycle increases for
several days initially and the decrease in proliferation
starts at about 15 days. These results are in fair agreement with those of Moffat [10]. The duration for different hair types appears to be similar.

3. Grouping of follicles into large and small is not
sufficiently precise for some experiments.   a

4. There is no alteration in the cell cycle time during
the initial period of reduction of the number of proliferative cells at the end of induced anagen.

REFERENCES

1.   CATTANEO, S., QUASTLER, H. and SHERMAN, F., *Nature,
      190*, 923, 1961.

2.   CHASE, H.B. and SILVER, A.F., In: *The Biological
      Basis of Medicine*, Eds. Bittar, E.E. and Bittar, N.,
      Academic Press, 1969.

3.   DAVID, L.T., *J. Exper. Zool., 68*, 501, 1934.

4.   DRY, F.W., *J. Genet., 16*, 287, 1926.

5.   EBLING, F.G., In: *The Biological Basis of Medicine*,
      Eds. Bittar, E.E. and N. Bittar, Academic Press,
      1969.

6.   FRY, R.J.M., KESSLER, D., KISIELESKI, W., WEBER,
      C.L., GRIEM, M.L. and MALKINSON, F.D., *Argonne
      National Laboratory Division of Biological and
      Medical Research Annual Report*, ANL-7535, *77*, 1968.

7.   GRIEM, M.L., *Nature, 210*, 213, 1966.

8.   GRIEM, M., MALKINSON, F., MARIANOVIC, R. and KESSLER,
      D., this proceedings.

9.   HUEBNER, L.G. and KISIELESKI, W., *Atompraxis, 16*, 1,
      1970.

10.   MOFFAT, G.H., *J. Anat., 102*, 527, 1968.

11.   POTTEN, C.S. and CHASE, H.B., *Radiat. Res., 42*, 205,
      1970.

12.   SILVER, A.F., CHASE, H.B. and ARSENAULT, C.T., In:
      Advances in Biology of Skin, Ed. W. Montagna, 1969.

INTRODUCTORY REMARKS AND THE ROLE OF SULFHYDRYLS IN THE CELL CYCLE RESPONSE OF MAMMALIAN CELLS TO X RAYS

W.K. SINCLAIR

Division of Biological and Medical Research,
Argonne National Laboratory,
Argonne, Illinois, U.S.A.

I am pleased to welcome you all to this symposium on "Radiation Responses and the Cell Cycle". One of the important aspects of the dependence of the radiation response of mammalian and other cells upon their position in the cell generation cycle is the opportunity it affords us to study, and hopefully eventually to elucidate, the relationship between the radiobiological lesion in cells and the biochemical events relevant to it.

Most of the principal biochemical changes induced in cells by ionizing radiation were known prior to the identification of the main features of the cell generation cycle response in mammalian cells. These include the importance of nuclear damage, the reduction in DNA synthesis, the interference of radiation with biochemical processes controlling energy generation in cells, the potential role of sulfhydryls and even the usefulness of UV studies in helping to explain the damage induced by ionizing radiation.

The development of techniques, mainly of synchronization of cell populations, to study these phenomena as a function of cell cycle position has given new life to many radiobiological studies. In the principal papers to be presented by the invited speakers to this symposium we have attempted to emphasize the biochemical aspects of cell cycle radiation studies. Dr. Peterson

will undertake the difficult task of describing the biochemistry of the cell cycle in order to provide a suitable background for later papers. Dr. Van't Hof will
present his work on energy considerations during the
cell cycle and radiation recovery. Dr. Humphrey will
concentrate on the cell cycle dependence of damage and
repair to DNA as measured by single strand breaks, while
Dr. A. Han will describe some features of the ultraviolet
response in mammalian cells and their relationship to
the X ray response. The final invited paper will discuss
the radiation response of stationary phase mammalian cells
in culture, a subject of increasing importance as a potential model system for tumors and intimately related
to our knowledge of cell cycle dependencies.

Thereafter, there have been included in this symposium a group of selected proffered papers relating to
the general topic of cell cycle responses. We look forward in these papers to amplification of some of the material presented in the invited papers and to new information on the cyclic dependence of various radiation responses.

I wish now to describe briefly some of my own recent studies on the relationship between the concentration of sulfhydryls and the dependence upon the position
of the cell in its generation cycle of lethal damage produced by X radiation. In doing so I shall not attempt
to review all the important work concerning the role of
sulfhydryls in radiobiological damage extending now over
more than twenty years and including such investigators
as Barron [1], Patt [2], Bacq and Alexander [3], Ord and
Stocken [4], and Revesz and his collaborators [5]. The
present situation with regard to the role of sulfhydryls
and the radiation response is too fluid to develop a last-
ing general hypothesis and recent results, or their interpretations, have been conflicting (compare Revesz,
Bergstrand and Modig [5] with Harris, Painter and Hahn
[6]).

My interest in this matter began with my observation [7,8] that cysteamine exerted a differential protective effect on the cell cycle of Chinese hamster cells

(Figure 1), the dose-modifying factor varying from
about 3.3 for resistant late S cells to over 5.0 for
sensitive mitotic or G_2 cells. This observation has
led to a renewed interest in the determination of free
and bound sulfhydryls in mammalian cells as a function
of their position in the cell generation cycle. One
such recent investigation, by Ohara and Terasima (Figure 2), shows that there is direct correlation between
the survival of HeLa cells and the incidence of free
non-protein sulfhydryl at all points during the cell
cycle except during mitosis when both cell sensitivity
and free sulfhydryl concentration are high. There may
be special circumstances that yield such a result during mitosis.

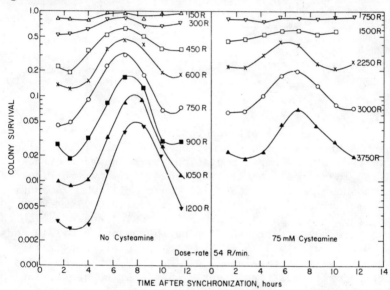

Fig. 1.   Survival of X-irradiated synchronous Chinese hamster cells with
          and without 75mM cysteamine during the cell cycle.

Another approach to the evaluation of the role of
sulfhydryls in controlling radiation damage is by considering the effects upon cells of sulfhydryl-binding agents
such as N-ethylmaleimide [10]. If free sulfhydryl is associated with high cell survival, binding of sulfhydryl

groups should sensitize the cell and presumably this
sensitization should be greatest during the late S
period when the cell is most resistant.

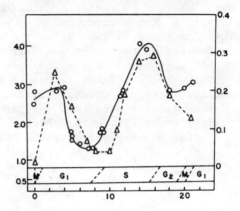

Fig. 2. Changes of non-protein sulfhydryls (NPSH), [left ordinate × 10^{-15}
          moles, O——O] and X-ray survival [right ordinate Δ----Δ] during
          the cell cycle of synchronous HeLa cells.(From Ohara and Terasima [9].)

The survival of synchronized Chinese hamster cells
as measured by colony formation after irradiation with
710 rads of 250 kVp X radiation, as a function of position in the cell generation cycle, is shown in Figure 3.
Also shown is the response of these cells when amounts
of N-ethylmaleimide (NEM) ranging from 0.0025 mM to 0.0075
mM (the latter is the maximum non-toxic concentration that
can be used) are present during the exposure to 710 rads.
Evidently with 0.0075 mM NEM the cells are sensitized
specifically in the late S period only, when the cells
are normally most resistant. Little or no sensitization
is apparent at other stages. More detailed studies
over a broad range of doses also showed that only a
small degree of sensitization occured at other stages.
The sensitization factor for late S cells for 0.0075 mM
NEM is about 1.5 over a wide range of X ray doses.

It is also possible to demonstrate that the effects
of NEM can be counteracted by the addition of free sulfhydryl using cysteamine as the source. In Figure 4 the
effects of 710 rads upon synchronized Chinese hamster

cells are shown together with the effects of 0.0075 mM
present during exposure, 0.1 mM or 1 mM cysteamine (MEA)
present during exposure and varying amounts of MEA present together with 0.0075 mM MEM. These data show that
0.1 mM MEA completely neutralizes the effects of 0.0075
mM NEM, and the cell responds just as if neither agent
were present. The exact amounts involved in this "tit-
ration" depend upon the fact that the medium also contains free non-protein sulfhydryl (about 4.4×10^{-9} μ
moles NPSH/ml according to an assay made for me by J.W.
Harris [11]).

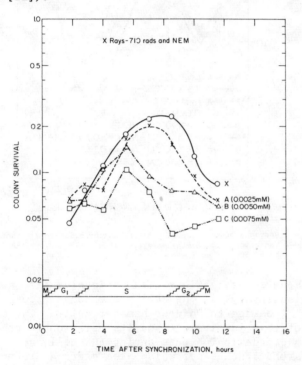

Fig. 3. Responses of synchronous Chinese hamster cells to 710 rads X-
         radiation, with and without N-ethylmaleimide (NEM) present in
         concentrations shown during exposure only.

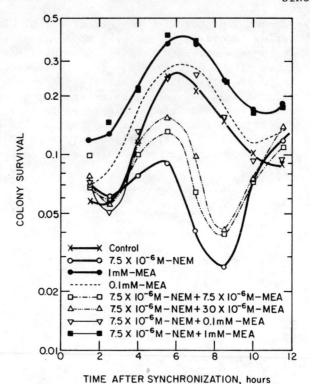

Fig. 4. Response of synchronous Chinese hamster cells to 710 rads X-radiation, with N-ethylmaleimide (NEM), cysteamine (MEA) or both, present during exposure only.

These investigations clearly involve free non-protein sulfhydryl in the cell cycle dependence of X-ray lethal damage to Chinese hamster cells. The exact nature of this involvement and its relation to other changing biochemical events during the cell cycle (such as DNA synthesis), which also exert a profound influence over the radiation response, await further investigation.

SUMMARY

Experiments in synchronized Chinese hamster cells with a sulfhydryl binding agent N-ethylmaleide (NEM) indicate selective sensitization mainly in the resistant late S period. This finding plus the results of additional studies in which the sensitization of NEM is counterbalanced by the protection afforded by cysteamine support the notion that free sulfhydryl, naturally occurring in the cell and varying during the cell cycle, plays an important role in the lethal response to X irradiation.

REFERENCES

1.   BARRON, E.S.G. and FLOOD, V., *J. Gen. Physiol.*, *33*, 229, 1950.

2.   PATT, H.M., TYREE, E.B., STRAUBE, R.L., and SMITH, D.E., *Science*, *110*, 213, 1949.

3.   BACQ, Z.M. and ALEXANDER, P., *Fundamentals of Radiobiology*, Second Edition, Pergamon Press, Oxford, 1961.

4.   ORD, M.G. and STOCKEN, L.A., *Nature*, *20C*, 136, 1963.

5.   REVESZ, L., BERGSTRAND, H. and MODIG, H., *Nature*, (London), *198*, 1275, 1963.

6.   HARRIS, J.W., PAINTER, R.B. and HAHN, G.M., *Int. J. Rad. Biol.*, *15*, 289, 1969.

7.   SINCLAIR, W.K., *Science*, *159*, 442, 1968.

8.   SINCLAIR, W.K., *Rad. Res.*, *39*, 135, 1969.

9.   OHARA, H. and TERASIMA, T., *Exp. Cell Res.*, *58*, 182, 1970.

10.   BRIDGES, B.A., *Nature*, *188*, 415, 1960.

11.   HARRIS, J.W., Laboratory of Radiation Biology,
       University of California Medical Center, San
       Francisco, personal communication.

BIOCHEMICAL EVENTS DURING THE MAMMALIAN CELL CYCLE*

D.F. PETERSEN, E.C. ANDERSON, and R.A. TOBEY

Biomedical Research Group, Los Alamos Scientific Laboratory, University of California, Los Alamos, New Mexico 87544, U.S.A.

INTRODUCTION

The cycling mammalian cell in culture is one of the most important quantitative test objects in modern radiobiology, and the detailed biochemical description of cell culture systems is fundamental both for understanding radiation effects *in vitro* and for designing radiotherapeutic regimes. This brief review is intended to provide a biochemical framework for radiation effects to be discussed in subsequent presentations and represents our view of the pertinent features of cellular behavior in the unperturbed cycle in culture. Radiation effects related to these features are intentionally omitted. Relevance of *in vitro* systems to cellular life processes *in vivo* can be questioned on quantitative grounds, but we take the position that similarities far outweigh the differences, that residual control mechanisms *in vitro* also function *in vivo* and that *in vitro* systems are of fundamental interest in their own right.

Within each generation, all structural and functional components of the cell double under the control of regulatory mechanisms spanning the range from end-product

---

*This work was performed under the auspices of the U.S. Atomic Energy Commission.

feedback inhibition to transcription of specific gene
sequences. It is not within the scope of this paper
to discuss the details of individual biochemical events
(for such discussions, see recent reviews [5,15,16,17])
but, rather, to attempt the assembly of apparently pertinent features in such a way that some perspective concerning the relevance of particular events to cycle traverse and consequently to radiation effects emerges.

GENERAL CELL-CYCLE PHENOMENA

A fundamental characteristic of the cell cycle is
its apparently stochastic nature; that is, the time required for individual cells to pass from birth to division varies from cell to cell (with a coefficient of
variation of some 10 to 20 percent), and this variation
has not been shown to correlate strongly with any other
parameter. It has been suggested by Puck that this variability may have survival value (by distributing cells
into different states in which their susceptibilities
to insults vary); but the primary result for the experi-
mentalist is that all periodic phenomena connected with
the life cycle are rapidly dispersed in synchronized
cultures. This dispersion, whose rate is quantitatively
known from the distribution of generation times, can be
used as an indicator of the degree of association between a periodic phenomenon and the mitotic cycle. Thus,
the coefficient of variation of the volume distribution
of cells in a synchronous culture prepared by mitotic
selection is invariant over the first subsequent cycle.
Since cell density is invariant [2], volume is proportional to mass, and this proves that total mass increase
does *not* share the stochastic properties of generation
times. (Dispersion of volume begins with the second
cycle and results from a dependence of growth rate on
age, the age variability appearing in this population
only after the first division). Coupling, of course,
exists between the division cycle and these other periodic phenomena but is weak and second-order so that a
system perturbed, for example, with respect to average
mass (e.g., by thymidine block) returns only slowly over
a period of several generations to its original state [16].

EVENTS OF G_1

From the standpoint of cell-cycle analysis, G_1 appears least likely to be amenable to temporal description. Whether a cell enters another cycle or becomes temporarily or permanemtly arrested appears to be decided by early G_1. In the event the cell does cycle, the duration of G_1 is subject to a number of influences, largely nutritional, which cause wide variations in comparison with times for traverse of S and G_2 [22].

The existence of cell lines reported to be "G_1-less" [20] suggests that G_1 may indeed be a buffer phase in which deficits in prerequisites for DNA synthesis are made up. Therefore, the time spent in this phase will be determined by the extent to which DNA-related enzymatic activity is carried over from the previous generation [15] or is synthesized immediately after telophase [6,14]. Non-cycling systems which exist in a stationary phase between M and S from which cells are mobilized as needed (e.g., in response to nutritional or traumatic stimulation as in regenerating liver) show a significant G_1 period in which preparations for DNA replication are made. Thus, variability of G_1 [23] may reflect the degree to which the DNA synthetic machinery has kept ready for use and the extent to which controlled biochemical systems are in states compatible with entry into S. If the decision to divide commits a cell to tightly programmed progress through S and M, then the only stopping place for cells which have chosen the option of stasis must be after M and before another S (i.e., G_1 or G_0).

Confluency inhibition is a well documented phenomenon, and cells which stop cycling under conditions of adequate nutrition are arrested in G_1. Tobey and Ley [13,24] have recently reported that Chinese hamster cells grown in suspension culture, when starved for a single specific amino acid, isoleucine, are also arrested in G_1. These cells can be induced to re-enter the cycle by the simple expedient of adding back iso-

leucine and, moreover, re-enter the cycle synchronously.
Control of the cycle by restricting the availability of
a single amino acid suggests the failure to synthesize
a macromolecular component crucial for DNA synthesis, but
the nature of the component is not yet known. Bulk protein synthesis continues, and the component is not critical for survival, since cells remain in a condition
of G_1 arrest for prolonged periods and promptly resume
cycling when given isoleucine. General starvation or
starvation for other specific amino acids, on the other
hand, causes arrest randomly throughout the cycle, and
starved cells promptly begin to die. This system holds
great promise for studying regulation of the initiating
steps in DNA synthesis. However, at present, the reasons
that the G_1 period, which normally contains over half
the cells of an exponentially-growing population, can
become essentially expendable are certainly not clear
nor is the mechanism of specific isoleucine starvation.

EVENTS OF THE S PERIOD

In the classical cell cycle of Howard and Pelc [10],
S is defined as the interval devoted to replication of
the genome. Depending on the system and the concentration of inhibitor chosen, neither RNA nor protein synthesis is required for several hours preceding initiation,
demonstrating that certain requisite steps for initiation
are anticipated well in advance [14]. However, completion of DNA synthesis is prevented if actinomycin or cycloheximide is added early in S, indicating continuing RNA
and protein synthesis requirements [15]. Some workers
have made a clear distinction between requirements for
initiation and continuation of DNA synthesis, but the
kinetic arguments and inhibitor studies do not effect-
tively rule out sequential transcription-regulated initiation over a protracted period. It is clear that
there are multiple initiation sites, that the time of
initiation at each site is closely controlled by a mechanism independent of chromosomal location [21]; that is,
translocation of a segment of DNA from an early to a
late replicating site still results in early replication, and numerous examples of differences in the over-

all kinetics of DNA synthesis -- discontinuous bursts
or relatively smooth increase -- can be found depending on the cell system. Reasons for the dependence of
kinetics on cell type remain unclear in the absence of
definitive experiments on primary material to rest the
hypothesis that smoothing of the kinetic curve results
from extensive rearrangement of karyotype during the
transition from strain to line. In any event, the
translocation experiments make such an explanation unlikely.

If one asks what chemical events appear to be ir-
revocably coupled to duplication of the genome, the
only candidate for which compelling arguments can be
marshalled is histone biosynthesis. Details of this
relationship are not yet clear; for example, evidence
that histone synthesis precedes DNA synthesis has been
obtained under conditions of DNA synthesis inhibition
[7]. In cells synchronized by mitotic selection (biochemically unperturbed), DNA and histone biosynthesis
are coincident [9,19]. These observations could be
reconciled by envisioning a rapid complexing of histone with newly sythesized DNA so that, under conditions of balanced exponential growth, the nonchroma-
tin histone pool is vanishingly small and undemonstra-
ble except by fractionation techniques.

The nature of control exerted by histone association with DNA is at present unknown, but clear that,
under normal circumstances, each replicon is duplicated
only once per cycle. However, Lehman [12] has recently
reported the occurrence of *double* rounds of DNA synthesis without an intervening mitosis as the first step
toward heteroploidy in SV-40 transformed Chinese hamster cells. The double rounds appear to be complete as
judged by karyologic examination. This is a curious
and important observation because the virus appears to
be triggering a complete second round of DNA synthesis.

EVENTS OF THE G_2 PERIOD

Of the observable events in the cycle, by far the
most spectacular is mitosis; therefore, it is not sur-
prizing that mitosis would serve as a useful timing
marker for biochemical events in the terminal portion
of the cell cycle. Employing metabolic inhibitors
which exert more or less specific effects, it has been
possible to locate with a high degree of precision the
final synthesis of RNA and protein required for successful mitosis [22,25]. In our Chinese hamster line,
both events clearly occur in G_2. Doida and Okada [4]
have reached similar conclusions employing L5178-Y cells.
Similar transcriptions and translations, presumably related, probably occur throughout the cycle and, in
principle, each could be worked out in detail. The
limitation of the techniques employing functional assays
and inhibitors with multiple points of actions is that
only terminal points of action can be measured and new
functional or chemically defined markers are the outstanding requirement for further description of cell-
cycle fine structure.

COMMENTS

The idea of regulation was implicit in the original introduction of Howard and Pelc's cell cycle as
a formal concept, and there is still no evidence that
mechanisms for regulation differ substantially as the
cell progresses through the major subdivisions of the
cycle. It is of considerable importance that our experimental attempts to clarify these mechanisms be
guided by an appropriate picture of the logical framework in which the system operates. The picture must,
of necessity, be vague and flexible enough to encompass
the alternatives left open by present knowledge and to
accomodate new information as it becomes available but
at the same time be specific enough to suggest useful
models and tests. Most important, it should steer
thinking in profitable directions and prevent wasting
time on irrelevancies.

Two principal types of regulation are known in cells: "chemical" control governing reaction rates and product concentrations by mass action, and "informational" control originating with gene transcription. The relative importance attached to these modes of control determines in a fundamental way the experimental approach and kinds of questions asked.

A tightly coupled transcription-translation sequence with ultimate control residing in an ordered progression of genes represents one extreme possibility, and one would expect an invariant order of specific biochemical operations (i.e., a-b-c, etc.) between cell birth and division. The original Howard and Pelc model of the cycle as a single closed line would be useful framework, and one could profitably talk about "progress" toward division as a single-valued variable uniquely related to time. Progress would stop with injury to any step and would resume only after appropriate repair. Differentiation, G_1 arrest, etc., would signify a shift to a different pattern of gene transcription and, hence, a different line of development.

At the other extreme, all genes would be continually accessible to transcription but strong positive and negative feedback mediated through chemical kinetics would determine the direction of a cell's development. This model is inherently unattractive, but much biochemistry is demonstrably controlled by chemical mechanisms. The element of randomness and variability resulting from instability of highly fedback systems is attractive when considering such factors as the variability of generation times and loose coupling between growth and division [1]. In a picture based only on this type of control, one might expect that, although a-b-c, etc., must all be accomplished before division, their order might be subject to arbitrary rearrangement (cf. the models of Rahn [18] and Kendall [11]). "Progress" toward division now ceases to be a simple concept, since there is no longer a single track along which progress is made. Inhibition of a single process might delay acquisition

of marker b, but the "following" markers -- c-d --
could be reached, thus giving the cell a biochemical
composition not attainable by normal populations (unbalanced growth). Progress toward division and the
path followed would not resemble the corresponding
quantities for normal cells. In this case, the simple
"one-track" cycle would be of questionable value, and
it would do positive harm if it led to investigation
of imaginary quantities.

All that really seems clear is that both types of
control are used to a sufficient degree to invalidate
both extreme models. On the one hand, the extraordin-
ary capabilities of multi-potential cells and the precision with which complicated operations such as mitosis
are performed can be explained only on the basis of a
highly precise but flexibly programmed supply of information. Genetic specification of major decisions must
be fundamental, but these decisions are implemented by
complex chains of biochemical events and a specific result may be far removed from the initial gene transcription. Clearly, there are numerous cell parameters which
are not rigidly specified in advance. Loose coupling
of growth with division [1] is an outstanding example,
and many of the "housekeeping" operations of the bio-
synthetic machinery (for instance, glycolytic enzymes
and respiratory chain components) appear to have a considerable degree of autonomy [3]. Cells of a considerable size range divide with equal facility, and volume regulation responds differently to environmental
changes than does division [1]. Dispersion of generation times is a related example of a stochastic element in the life cycle.

While we do not know the details, it is clear that
we should avoid thinking in terms of a limited "one-
track" model of the life cycle and not use the concept
of "progress toward division" as some kind of "clock"
which is counting down toward a preordained event.
The most promising alternative appears to be a type
of description in which the "state" of a cell is characterized by its biochemical composition [8] and in
which coupling among the several biochemical systems

is loose enough to permit a variety of "trajectories"
for the cells through the states between birth to division. Slight deviations from the path of minimal
transit time will leave the major "markers" in unal-
tered sequence, but a severe interference (radiation,
chemical blocks) may lead the cell into states far
removed from normal. The time required for recovery
would depend on the path followed, and some "markers"
may not be passed in their normal order. The "biochemical age" of a cell still measures its progress toward
ultimate division, but as growth becomes more "unbalanced"
the simple one-track model becomes less relevant. To
talk in terms of delay and resumption implies return to
the initial trajectory and division via a normal sequence
of biochemical states. This may be misleading; in fact,
even after division the cell may remain in an abnormal
state for an extended period [16]. The time required
for effects of a perturbation to disappear becomes an
important parameter, since it is related to the strength
of the coupling between various biochemical subsystems
of the cell. The concept that some of the cell's activities following perturbation may represent "progress"
while others do not may also be misleading. The direction
of development followed by a perturbed cell is presumably determined by its biochemical state (unless there
is a large stochastic element) so that most of its activities are required (in a sense dictated by composition but not in a teleological sense) and, hence, relevent even though they may, for example, result in the
dividing cell being larger than "normal". By visualizing biochemical states and transition times between
them, rather than a single closed path along which progress must be made, descriptions and hypotheses may
more closely approximate the actual regulatory system
(s) of the cell.

Applying these ideas leads one to regard the classic
G_1, S, and G_2 subdivisions of the life cycle not as specifying a path along which the cell must proceed to division but, rather, as a first approximation to specification of a biochemical state by defining the cell's
DNA content. Additional markers are to be sought not
as points along this line subdividing these phases but,

rather, as other biochemical parameters which must be added to specification of the DNA content to complete the description. Some of these parameters will be so closely related as to permit only very limited combinations to be attained by real cells; others may combine more freely. The former category is clearly more definitive for the normal cell cycle and will constitute a less variable sequence.

Description of the biochemical state of the cell may, therefore, resemble a genetic map in a rather fundamental way. The map inventories the information on which the cell can draw to guide its development; the state description lists those operations completed or in progress. Thus, G_2 comprises all cells which have completed DNA replication and means only that cells in this class have a 4n chromosome content. Additional biochemical parameters must be added to indicate both the exact state and direction in which the cell has been programmed to proceed. Experimental observation of the time required for a given cell to reach division must correspond to a line integral of the time differential, dt, over the path followed. The differential dt is "inexact" in mathematical terminology, and its integral t is not a "property" of the system. The *time* required to complete the cell cycle is similar to the work done or heat absorbed in a thermodynamic system in that it depends on the path followed. Thus, the notion of a chemical or biological "clock" regulating progress through the cycle is misleading in the sense that it directs our attention away from the biochemical state description and contains an implicit assumption of time as an independent, rather than a dependent, variable.

REFERENCES

1.   ANDERSON, E.C., BELL, G.I., PETERSEN, D.F., and TOBEY, R.A., *Biophys. J.*, *9*, 246, 1969.

2.   ANDERSON, E.C., PETERSEN, D.F., and TOBEY, R.A., *Biophys. J.*, *10*, 630, 1970.

3.   BLOMQUIST, C.H., GREGG, C.T., and TOBEY, R.A., *Exp. Cell Res., 66*, 75, 1971.

4.   DOIDA, Y., and OKADA, S., *Radiation Res., 38*, 513, 1969.

5.   EPIFANOVA, O.I., and TERSKIKH, V.V., *Cell Tissue Kinet., 2*, 75, 1969.

6.   GOLD, M., HELLEINER, C.W., and PERCY, M., *Biochim. Biophys. Acta, 80*, 204, 1964.

7.   GURLEY, L.R., and HARDIN, J.M., *Arch. Biochem. Biophys., 136*, 392, 1970.

8.   HAHN, G.M., *Biophys. J., 6*, 275, 1966.

9.   HODGE, L.D., ROBBINS, E., and SCHARFF, M.D., *J. Cell Biol., 40*, 497, 1969.

10. HOWARD, A., and PELC, S.R., *Heridity, 6, Suppl.*, 1, 261, 1953.

11. KENDALL, D.G., *Biometrika, 35*, 316, 1948.

12. LEHMAN, J.M., Ph.D. dissertation, Department of Pathology, University of Pennsylvania 1970.

13. LEY, K.D., and TOBEY, R.A., *J. Cell Biol., 47*, 453, 1970.

14. LITTLEFIELD, J.W., McGOVERN, A.P., and MARGESON, K.B., *Proc. Natl. Acad. Sci. U.S., 49*, 102, 1963.

15. MUELLER, G.C., *Federation Proc., 28*, 1780, 1969.

16. PETERSEN, D.F., TOBEY, R.A., and ANDERSON, E.C., *Federation Proc., 28*, 1771, 1969.

17. PRESCOTT, D.M., *Cancer Res., 28*, 1815, 1968.

18. RAHN, O., *J. Gen. Physiol., 15*, 257, 1931-1932.

19. ROBBINS, E., and BORUN, T.W., *Proc. Natl. Acad. Sci. U.S.*, *57*, 409, 1967.

20. ROBBINS, E., and SCHARFF, M.D., *J. Cell Biol.*, *34*, 684, 1967.

21. STUBBLEFIELD, E., *J. Natl. Cancer Inst.*, *37*, 799, 1966.

22. TOBEY, R.A., ANDERSON, E.C., and PETERSEN, D.F., *Proc. Natl. Acad. Sci. U.S.*, *56*, 1520, 1966.

23. TOBEY, R.A., ANDERSON, E.C., and PETERSEN, D.F., *J. Cell Biol.*, *35*, 53, 1967.

24. TOBEY, R.A., and LEY, K.D., *J. Cell Biol.*, *46*, 151, 1970.

25. TOBEY, R.A., PETERSEN, D.F., ANDERSON, E.C., and PUCK, T.T., *Biophys. J.*, *6*, 567, 1966.

TWO PRINCIPAL POINTS OF CONTROL IN THE MITOTIC CYCLE OF PEA MERISTEM CELLS: ENERGY CONSIDERATIONS, CHARACTERIZATION, AND RADIOSENSITIVITY*

JACK VAN'T HOF

Biology Department, Brookhaven National Laboratory, Upton, New York 11973, U.S.A.

The Howard and Pelc model of the mitotic cycle has constituted the structural framework for most cell population kinetic experiments since its presentation in 1953 [12]. The compartmentalization of the cycle into the G1, S, G2, and M periods and the further insights of Quastler and Sherman [16] have beckoned the cytologist to search for the controlling factors implicit in the segmentation and periodicity of DNA and RNA synthesis and in the mitotic phenomenon. To the radiobiologist this search is made even more tantilizing because of the spectacular effect of ionizing radiation on proliferative cells of all types and one wonders if the controlling factors and the radiosensitive sites are one and the same.

This paper represents an attempt by cell kinetic analysis to demonstrate that the controlling factors and the radiosensitive sites are of the same system. The work is not altogether as complete and comprehensive as one may wish but it does provide a source of direction and sufficient structure to indicate where further and more specific information is necessary.

---

*Research carried out at Brookhaven National Laboratory under the auspices of the U.S. Atomic Energy Commission.

THE EXPERIMENTAL SYSTEM

The biological material used in these experiments is the primary root tip meristem of pea seedlings (*Pisum sativum*, var. Alaska). The procedures for the culture of meristems are published [22-24] and only a brief description is presented here. The terminal 1 to 1.5 cm of the root is excised and aseptically cultured in a completely synthetic medium [31]. The cells measured are located in the root meristem, 40% of which under these conditions are proliferative. Also, because they are tissue constituents and are subjected to anatomical and developmental constraints, their progeny undergo normal differentiation.

Control of DNA synthesis and mitosis of meristematic cells is easily effected nutritionally by the presence or absence of exogenous carbohydrate in the culture medium [24]. To accumulate cells in G1 and G2, the carbohydrate is omitted; to reverse this stationary condition carbohydrate is provided. When continuously supplied 2% sucrose, cell division is asynchronous and the mitotic cycle time is 16-18 hours, of which 7-8 hours are spent in G1, 5-6 hours in S, 1-1.5 hours in G2, and 2-2.5 hours in M [22].

INTRODUCTION TO THE PARAMETERS OF THE SYSTEM

The curves in Fig. 1 (upper) are from meristems starved of carbohydrate for 48 hours and then supplied 2% sucrose and tritiated thymidine (^{3}H-TdR) at time zero. The entry of cells from G1 into S is shown in Fig. 1a (upper). After an initial delay (T_{ds}) the first cells began DNA synthesis, and thereafter cells continued to enter S at a relatively constant rate of 1.7 to 2% per hour. Subtraction of T_{ds} from the time the first ^{3}H-TdR labeled cells divide (Fig. 1b upper) estimated the sum of the durations of S and G2 ($T_S + T_{g2}$). In Fig. 1, (upper) $T_S + T_{g2}$ was approximately 6.8 hours. The mitotic index expressed as percent mitotic figures (Fig. 1c upper) had two waves. The first, preceded by an initial delay of 4 hours (T_{dm}), consisted of G2 cells; the second, which is

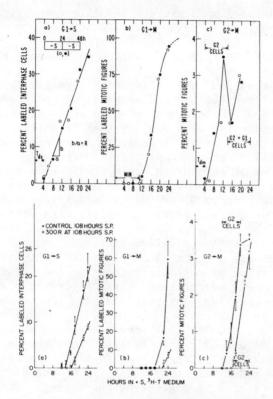

Fig. 1A.   The kinetics of cells in meristems previously starved of carbohydrate for 48 hours and provided medium with 2% sucrose (+S)
and tritiated thymidine at zero hour; a) the entrance of cells
from G1 into the S period; b) the appearance of former G1 cells
in mitosis, MIN, the sum of T_s, T_{g2}, and T_{ds}; c) the mitotic index expressed as per cent mitotic figures. Early mitotic cells
are of G2 origin and provide a measurement of G2 → M (from ref.
[26]).

Fig. 1B.   The kinetics of cells in meristems previously starved of carbohydrate for 108 hours and then exposed to 300 R of gamma rays
at zero hour. The transfer to medium with 2% sucrose and tritiated thymidine was made immediately after exposure. Control,
closed circles; irradiated, open circles. Panels (a), (b) and
(c) are the same as for Figure 1A.

incomplete in Fig. 1c (upper), was composed of mostly G1
cells. The intervening trough, from 14–16 hours, reflected the absence of cells in S during starvation and,

as such, consisted of a mixture of cells that originated from G1 and G2.

LOCALE OF PROPOSED PRINCIPAL CONTROL POINTS (P.C.P.)

The observation that cells which normally divide asynchronously segregated and accumulated preferentially in the G1 and G2 periods when starved of carbohydrate implied the possession of a quality that is unique and not shared by either S or M. Indeed, if it were equally probable for cells to stop at any position in the cycle a certain degree of asynchrony would remain. However, because cell accumulation was nonrandom and because the preference to stop in G1 and G2 was manifested when cell metabolism was low and decreasing [25], significance was attached to the points in G1 and G2 where the cells halted. These loci were called principal control points (P.C.P.) and were postulated to play a significant role in the regulation of cell progression in the mitotic cycle. It should be mentioned that dehydrated plant embryos, which are also characterized by a low metabolic level, also lack cells in S and M [1, 5] and starved paramecium [13] and amoebae [11] likewise accumulate preferentially in G1 and G2 respectively. Since nonrandom accumulation was precipitated by starvation, one may conceive of the P.C.P. as being metabolic blocks not necessarily composed of a single factor but a complex the sum of which regulates the transition of a cell from one cycle period to the next.

The proposal of two P.C.P. requires at least another aspect for consideration. It is that cells accumulated in G1, when induced to enter S by carbohydrate provision, and then immediately starved again, completed DNA synthesis and stopped in G2; they did not accumulate in S [27]. This aspect is important in view of Gelfant's hypothesis that tissues, normally nonproliferative, contain two discrete cell populations, one which arrests in G1 and another that stops in G2 [7-10]. The demonstration that cells of pea root meristems have two P.C.P. was accomplished with the experiment described in Fig. 2. The test consisted of two groups of meristems each handled in the same manner except for ^{3}H-TdR labeling. After 48

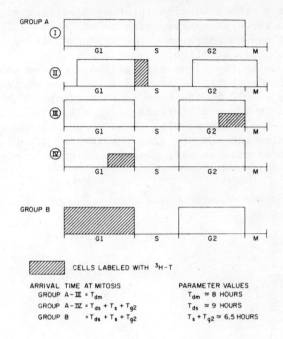

FIGURE 2

Fig. 2.   Schematic representation of experiment used to demonstrate that
cells, once stopped in G1 can also stop in G2. Groups A and B
were starved 48 hours and cells accumulated in G1 and G2 (I);
Group A labeled with tritiated thymidine during an 8 hour sucrose incubation (A-II); A-III and A-IV two alternatives where
the labeled cells in Group A may stop when starved again.
Group B, all cells labeled originated in G1. For further information see text.

hours of starvation, they were provided sucrose for 8
hours to position some cells in S and those of Group A
were labeled with ^{3}H-TdR at that time (Fig. 2, A-II).
Next followed 24 hours of starvation during which the
cells induced to enter S had three alternatives: a) to
remain in S; b) to complete S and stop in G2 (Fig 2,
A-III); or c) to complete one cycle and return to G1
(Fig. 2, A-IV). Alternative "a" may be discarded because
it was previously shown that cells treated in the format
described did not stop in S [27].   To examine the two remaining alternatives both groups were provided sucrose
but only Group B received ^{3}H-TdR. Because cells do not

stop in S, those labeled in Group B originated in Gl and
as such serve as marker cells to which those labeled in
Group A may be compared. The expected arrival time of
labeled cells at mitosis under alternative "b" and "c"
are given in Fig. 2 as well as that for the labeled Gl
cells in Group B. If stopped in Gl, the arrival time at
mitosis should be the same in each group; if the cells
stopped in G2, a difference of $T_S + T_{g2}$ (6.5 hours) would
be observed. The results (Fig. 3) showed that the arrival time was not the same for the two groups. In Group
A, labeled mitoses were observed in greater numbers after

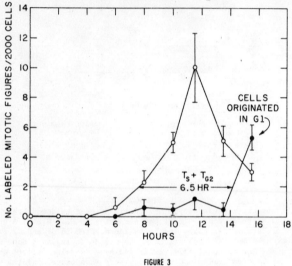

FIGURE 3

Fig. 3.   The results of the experiment represented in Figure 2: open
circles, cells of Group A; closed circles, cells of Group B.

7-8 hours; in Group B, the labeled Gl cells, began to
divide from 14-15 hours. The displacement of the two
ascending portions of the curves was 6.5 hours and equal
to the average $T_S + T_{g2}$ value determined from several experiments. These results were only in agreement with the
concept of two P.C.P. per cell, one located in Gl and
another in G2.

THE UNIDIRECTIONAL CHARACTERISTIC OF THE P.C.P.

Implicit in the observation that cells starved of carbohydrate for as long as 108 hours remained in position, i.e. either in G1 or G2 until carbohydrate was again supplied, is the fact that the P.C.P. are unidirectional and they are always oriented toward mitosis. This characteristic was easily demonstrated for cells in G2. For example, in Fig. 1c (upper) the cells that divided from 4-12 hours had been stationary in G2 for 48 hours, yet when able to resume movement toward mitosis, they did so without commencement of another round of DNA replication. Though chick esophageal cells respond as do pea root cells to starvation and feeding [4], not all cells share the unidirectional characteristic. Amoebae, for instance, when stopped in G2 by starvation, reinitiated DNA synthesis when fed [11].

Like those accumulated in G2, cells that were stationary in G1 also remained fixed in position for the duration of starvation. It was noted in Fig. 1a that cells entered S from G1 in a linear fashion when provided exogenous sucrose. If they had gathered either in early, late, or mid-G1, the respective manner of entry into S would have been nonlinear, concave upward; nonlinear, concave downward; or sigmoidal. At the present state of knowledge, only a rectangular distribution in G1 is in agreement with and explains a linear increase in labeled interphase cells with time.

FUNCTIONAL EXPRESSION OF THE G1 AND G2 P.C.P.

Given the supposition that P.C.P. exist it was necessary to obtain a measurement that expressed either directly or indirectly the functional condition of the P.C.P. When comparing the effect of increasing the duration of starvation it was noted that the initial delays T_{ds} and T_{dm} also increased accordingly but the transit time of S plus G2 remained unchanged (Fig. 4). It was significant that $T_s + T_{g2}$ was independent of carbohydrate starvation for it demonstrated that the effects produced were confined to G1 and G2. Further, since $T_s + T_{g2}$ was

refractory but processes localized in G1 and G2 were affected by starvation it was postulated that T_{ds} and T_{dm}
were functional expressions of the P.C.P.

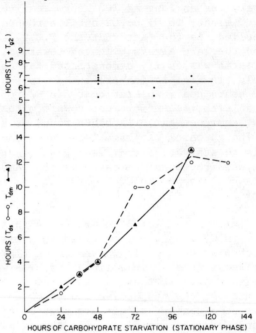

FIGURE 4

Fig. 4.   The influence of carbohydrate starvation on the cell parameters
T_{ds}, T_{dm}, and $T_s + T_{g2}$.

The manner in which T_{ds} and T_{dm} changed with length
of starvation revealed an interesting and important difference between these two parameters. T_{ds} approached a
limit of approximately 12 hours after 96 hours of starvation while T_{dm} showed no signs of limitation even up to
108 hours (Fig. 4). A limit for T_{ds} suggested that it
represented entities of a finite amount the last of which
was depleted after 96 hours. The absence of a limit for
T_{dm}, on the other hand, implied that arrest in G2 may be
indefinite. The net effect of a limited T_{ds} and an un-

limited T_{dm} is that tissues stimulated to proliferate and continuously labeled with ^{3}H-TdR should have mitoses that are unlabeled and when these mitoses are observed is dependent on the difference between the limit of T_{ds} and the extent of T_{dm}. Though not all performed with plant tissue, there are observations in the literature that are consistent with these expectations [5, 15] and included are those of Gelfant [7-10].

METABOLISM AND THE P.C.P.

The dependence of the P.C.P. on energy metabolism was inferred in the observed increase of T_{ds} and T_{dm} with longer durations of carbohydrate starvation (Fig. 4) and further substantiated by experiments with hypoxia and an uncoupler of oxidative phosphorylation, 2,4-dinitrophenol [26, 28]. Cells of starved meristems when supplied sucrose but maintained under hypoxic conditions proceeded neither into S nor into M and only when aerobic conditions were restored did cell progression resume. Similar results obtained with 2,4-dinitrophenol provided additional evidence that the requirements of the P.C.P. in pea can be met only by aerobic metabolism. In this regard, several other experiments performed with plant [1] and animal [17-19] cells have provided corroborative results.

In addition to a high energy dependence the P.C.P. require macromolecular synthesis as well. Using puromycin or cycloheximide to inhibit protein synthesis and actinomycin D to inhibit RNA synthesis it was shown that the transitions G1 → S and G2 → M were dependent on these syntheses [29]. The manner in which the requirements were manifested however, was not the same. The inhibitors of protein synthesis essentially prevented the G1 → S and G2 → M transitions in all cells and extended T_{ds} and T_{dm} indefinitely. Actinomycin D in contrast affected neither T_{ds} nor T_{dm} but reduced the number of cells that made the transition to S. From these results it was concluded that the P.C.P. had an immediate requirement for protein synthesis and a belated dependence on RNA synthesis. Increased starvation time made the RNA requirement more apparent and eventually caused the cells to extend T_{ds} and

T_{dm} when treated with actinomycin D. The effect, however, was never as pronounced as that obtained with the inhibitors of protein synthesis.

RADIOSENSITIVITY OF THE P.C.P.

The final characteristic of the P.C.P. to be discussed is their radiosensitivity. This was made possible by the supposition that T_{ds} and T_{dm} were functional manifestations of the P.C.P. There are three aspects to this characteristic that will be considered. The first is an expression of the radiation effect, the second is the recovery from radiation damage, and the third is the antagonism between recovery activity and preparations for the G1 $\rightarrow$ S and G2 $\rightarrow$ M transitions.

The expression of a radiation effect on the P.C.P. was an increase in T_{ds} and T_{dm} and this effect is demonstrated in Fig. 1a and b (lower). When meristems in the stationary condition were irradiated with 300 R of gamma rays and then supplied sucrose both G1 and G2 cells were delayed in the resumption of cell progression in the cycle. The extension of T_{ds} and T_{dm} by the gamma irradiation and that produced by inhibitors of protein synthesis were similar in that each acted immediately and neither allowed cell advancement toward mitosis. However, once recovery had occurred the irradiated cells that were in G1 traversed S and G2 in 6 hours. The delay induced by irradiation was confined solely to the G1 period and no residual effect was evident in $T_s + T_{g2}$. This observation is not unique to pea cells but also has been noted with mammalian cells [20], and suggested that the transition to S or to M does not occur until recovery of injury was completed [26].

If the recovery events of damaged P.C.P. were responsible for radiation-induced delay, the provision of sufficient time for these processes to be completed free from concurrent demands for resumption of mitotic cycle activities should be indicated by near normal T_{ds} and T_{dm} values when such activities are finally resumed. Experiments performed to test this postulate showed that it was

valid [25, 26, 30] and suggested that the preparations
for the transitions G1 → S and G2 → M and the recovery of
damaged P.C.P. were antagonistic. Antagonism is what is
expected if the P.C.P. and the sites damaged by irradiation were one and the same. Injury to the P.C.P. would
impair preparations for the G1 → S and G2 → M transitions
and this would be reflected in an extended T_{ds} and T_{dm}.

The fact that T_{ds} approached a limit offered an opportunity to test whether the recovery from irradiation
damage and the requirements for the G1 P.C.P. were antagonistic. Because meristems starved for 108 hours have a
maximum T_{ds} of 12 hours (Fig. 4), irradiation and the immediate provision of sucrose should produce one of two
effects: T_{ds} may remain unchanged or it may be further
extended beyond 12 hours. The first result would indicate
the absence of antagonism and the likelihood that T_{ds} was
not a functional expression of P.C.P.; the second would
suggest antagonism and that the preparations for the transition G1 → S and recovery processes were sequential.
The results (Fig. 1a, lower) showed that T_{ds} was prolonged
to 16-17 hours and indicated that the processes of recovery and those for the initiation of DNA synthesis were
antagonistic and may involve the same entities.

Many of the observations made with pea meristem
cells are described for other cell types. For example,
mammalian cells are delayed in both G1 and G2 [6] and experience enhanced recovery if the competition between repair of damage and cycle activities is minimized [3, 14].
The inclusion of eukaryotic and prokaryotic microorganisms
[13, 21] where the antagonistic effects were first described serves as notice to be cautious about the general
applicability of the P.C.P. concept. Perhaps the best
course to take is to insist that a true test of the hypothesis for a given cell type in a given environment must
await development of procedures having the same rigor and
degree of control as that demonstrated with cultured pea
root meristem cells.

SUMMARY

    Cell population kinetic evidence was presented for
the hypothesis that in the mitotic cycle of pea meristem
cells there are two principal control points (P.C.P.),
one in G1 and the other in G2. Some of the metabolic and
biochemical characteristics of the P.C.P. were described
and it was postulated that radiation-induced delay at
G1 $\rightarrow$ S and at G2 $\rightarrow$ M reflected the recovery time of damaged P.C.P.

ACKNOWLEDGEMENTS

    The work of and discussions with Drs. P.L. Webster
and C.J. Kovacs were considerable contributions to the
concepts presented herein.

REFERENCES

1.   AMOORE, J.E., *Proc. Roy. Soc. B, 154*, 109, 1961.

2.   AVANZI, S.A. and D'AMATO, F., *Develop. Biol., 20*,
368, 1969.

3.   BELLI, J.A. and SHELTON, M., *Science, 165*, 490, 1969.

4.   CAMERON, I.L. and CLEFFMAN, G., *J. Cell. Biol., 21*,
169, 1964.

5.   DAVIDSON, D., *Am. J. Botany, 53*, 491, 1966.

6.   ELKIND, M.M. and WHITMORE, G.E., In: *The Radiobiology
of Cultured Mammalian Cells*, Gordon and Breach
Science Publishers Inc., New York, N.Y. 1967.

7.   GELFANT, S., *Exptl. Cell Res., 26*, 395, 1962.

8.   GELFANT, S., *Exptl. Cell. Res., 32*, 521, 1963.

9.   GELFANT, S., *Intern. Rev. Cytol., 14*, 1, 1963.

10.   GELFANT, S., in: *Methods in Cell Physiology* (D.M.
Prescott, ed.), p. 359, Academic Press, Inc., New
York, N.Y. 1966

11. GOLDSTEIN, L. and PRESCOTT, D.M., in: *The Control of Nuclear Activity* (L. Goldstein, ed.), p.3, Prentice-Hall, Inc., Englewood Cliffs, N.J. 1967.

12. HOWARD, A. and PELC, S.R., *Heredity, 6,* Suppl., 261, 1953.

13. Kimball, R.F., *J. Cell. Comp. Physiol., 58,* Suppl. 1, 163, 1961.

14. PHILLIPS, R.A. and TOLMACH L.J., *Radiation Res., 29,* 413, 1966.

15. POST, J. and HOFFMAN, J., *Exptl. Cell Res., 57,* 111, 1969.

16. QUASTLER, H. and SHERMAN, F., *Exptl. Cell Res., 17,* 420, 1959.

17. ROBBINS, E. and MORRILL, G.A., *J. Cell Biol., 43,* 629, 1969.

18. ROONEY, D.W. and WILER, J.J., *Exptl. Cell Res., 48,* 649 1968.

19. SCAIFE, J.F. and BROHEE, H., *Can. J. Biochem., 47,* 237, 1969.

20. SINCLAIR, W.K., in: *Radiation Research 1966* (G. Silini, ed.), p. 607, North Holland Publishing Co., Amsterdam, 1967.

21. STAPLETON, G.E., BILLEN, D. and HOLLAENDER, A., *J. Cell. Comp. Physiol., 41,* 345, 1953.

22. VAN'T HOF, J., *J. Cell Biol., 27,* 179, 1965.

23. VAN'T HOF, J., *Am. J. Botany, 53,* 970, 1966.

24. VAN'T HOF, J., *J. Cell Biol., 37,* 773, 1968.

25. VAN'T HOF, J., *Radiation Res., 32,* 792, 1967.

26. VAN'T HOF, J., *Radiation Res.*, *41*, 538, 1970.

27. VAN'T HOF, J., *Exptl. Cell Res.*, *61*, 173, 1970.

28. WEBSTER, P.L. and VAN'T HOF, J., *Exptl. Cell Res.*, *55*, 88, 1969.

29. WEBSTER, P.L. and VAN'T HOF, J., *Am. J. Botany*, *57*, 130, 1970.

30. WEBSTER, P.L. and VAN'T HOF, J., *Radiation Botany*, *10*, 145, 1970.

31. WHITE, P.R., In: *A Handbook of Plant Tissue Culture*, Cattel and Co., Inc., Lancaster, Pa., 1943.

DAMAGE AND REPAIR IN DNA AS RELATED TO THE CELL CYCLE

R.M. HUMPHREY

Section of Cellular Studies, Department of Physics, The University of Texas, M.D. Anderson Hospital and Tumor Institute at Houston, 6723 Bertner Avenue, Houston Texas 77025, U.S.A.

INTRODUCTION

Over the last 10 years many studies have been carried out on the cell age dependent response of mammalian cells to both ultraviolet and ionizing radiations,[10]. However, the exact cause of this phenomenon has not, as yet, been completely determined.

Two explanations which have been advanced are (a) that a given dose of radiation might produce a different amount of damage in a critical target molecule, and (b) qualitative or quantitative differences in repair capability depending on the position of the cell in the division cycle [2].

The purpose of my part of the discussion today will be to present data which bear on these two subjects. In order to do this we have used alkaline sucrose gradients, as originally described by McGrath and Williams [7] to measure the changes in sedimentation characteristics of the DNA from control and irradiated cells. Some of the specific questions which have been investigated are : (a) What is the influence of the stage of the mammalian cell cycle on the yield and rejoining of single strand breaks (SSB)?; (b) Is the rejoining process in mammalian cells enzymatic in nature?; (c) Is there a requirement for synthesis of DNA, RNA, or protein in the rejoining of SSB mammalian cells?

MATERIALS AND METHODS

Most of our present experiments have been carried out with the Chinese hamster ovary (CHO) cell line [11]. The methods of synchronizing cells, irradiation, lysing technique and centrifugation technique have been reported in detail [1].

To label the DNA cells were incubated in medium containing ^{3}H-TdR (0.5 μ/ml, 1.9 Ci/mM) for 15 to 18 hours. At this time cells were synchronized by the excess TdR technique [8]. The response of cells in S phase was determined 1 hour after washing out the excess TdR at which time about 90 to 100 percent of the cells were in DNA synthesis. To obtain mitotic cells, [3], the synchronized cultures were incubated for 5 hours. Colcemid (0.06 μg/ml) was added to the medium and incubation was continued for 2 hours. Cells arrested in metaphase were collected by gentle agitation of the culture vessel. The mitotic index of such a population of cells was usually greater than 95 percent. Subsequent experiments have been conducted on mitotic cells, without the use of colcemid arrest, with no significant difference in results.

RESULTS AND DISCUSSION

Effect of temperature on single strand rejoining

Several studies have indicated that the rejoining of SSB is enzymatic in nature. To test this possibility we have examined the effects of low temperature and KCN on rejoining of SSB. Incubation at low temperature, even up to 4 hours failed to show any rejoining. These data confirm those of Sawada and Okada [9]. However when the chilled, irradiated cells were returned to 37° C and incubated for 30 minutes the sedimentation profile showed a shift to a higher MW distribution. A similar effect by 10^{-3} M KCN has also been reported [2]. Other workers have not found such an effect using a specific inhibator of oxidative phophorylation, dinitrophenol [9]. These data suggest that the rejoining of SSB in the

DNA of mammalian cells is an enzymatic process having
an optimal temperature in the range of 37° C and a
requirement for an active oxidative metabolism.

Influence of cell cycle on yield of SSB

We also have obtained data concerning the yield of
SSB per rad from the DNA of synchronized CHO cells and
these are in agreement with several investigators [5, 9].
The data is given in Table 1 and is the average between
30 and 40 determinations. The data from Table 1 indicate
that the number of SSB per rad is uniform throughout
these phases of the cell cycle, and thus the yield of damage is independent of the cells position in the division
cycle. A further conclusion from these data is that the

Table 1. The yield of single strand breaks as a function
of cell age for CHO cells.

Phase of division cycle	Breaks per gm/rad*
Asynchronous	2.05×10^{12}
S Phase	1.91×10^{12}
Mitosis	2.05×10^{12}

* Calculations based on the relationship of: $B/gm/rad$
$= N \left[\frac{1}{MW_i} - \frac{1}{MW_c} \right]$ where N is Avogadro's number, MW_i is the
number average molecular weight of the DNA from irradiated
cells and MW_c is unirradiated controls.

the age dependent radiation response of mammalian cells
is not the result of fluctuation of break damage during
different phases of the division cycle. However, it is
possible that other DNA lesions, such as base damage,
might differ in yield during the cycle and correlate with
changes in the age response function.

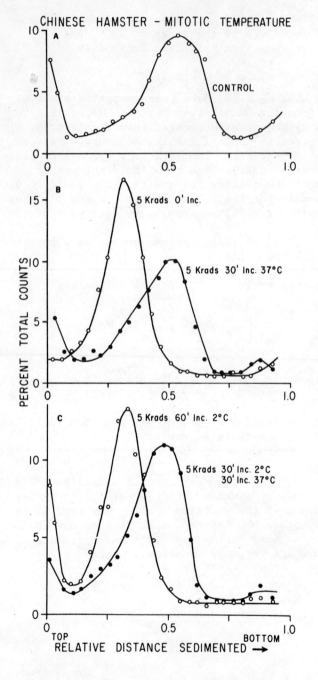

CHINESE HAMSTER - MITOTIC TEMPERATURE

A

CONTROL

B

5 Krads 0' Inc.

5 Krads 30' Inc. 37°C

PERCENT TOTAL COUNTS

C

5 Krads 60' Inc. 2°C

5 Krads 30' Inc. 2°C
30' Inc. 37°C

TOP   BOTTOM
RELATIVE DISTANCE SEDIMENTED ➔

Fig. 1. Sedimentation profiles of DNA from mitotic cells. Following irradiation cells were incubated at 2° C or 37°C
or first at 2° C then shifted to 37° C.

Influence of the division cycle on DNA break rejoining

If we accept the conclusion that the DNA rejoining process is an enzyme mediated procedure, then it followed that cells of different resistance to X-rays like mitotic cell compared to S phase cells, might also differ with respect to their capability to carry out the reaction. My colleague, Dr. Paul Lohman [6] and ourselves [1] first reported that cells in all phases of the division cycle had the capability of rejoining SSB, but rather surprising at the time was the finding that mitotic cells retained this function. Fig.1. We have since confirmed this observation in numerous experiments with hamster cells of different origin.

Sawada and Okada in a recent publication [9] have also observed DNA break rejoining in mitotic cells of rodent origin, namely the L5178Y mouse leukemic cell. It is, as yet, too early to predict that the mitotic phase cells of all mammalian cell types have this capability. However, it is clear that the data from several laboratories support the conclusion that the DNA rejoining process probably enzymatic in nature, is present and functional during all phases of the division cycle including mitosis. Thus, the special morphological features of chromosomal DNA and its associated proteins during mitosis do not preclude the action of enzymes necessary to complete the rejoining process.

We have continued our work on DNA break rejoining by performing experiments to determine the rate of rejoining during the M and S phases of the cycle. In these experiments synchronized populations were irradiated (5,000 rads) and incubated in normal growth medium for different periods of time. At the end of the incubation period cells were lysed and centrifuged on alkaline sucrose gradients as described earlier. As reported by Lett *et al.* [5] the rejoining process for mammalian cells is a rather rapid one as can be seen from the data of Fig. 2. Five minutes of incubation after irradiation results in a significant shift of the DNA profile to a higher MW (Fig. 2, panel B). Furthermore, the process was essentially complete within 15 minutes, (Fig. 2, panel C). Data for

mitotic cells are presented in Fig. 3. From these profiles one can observe a shift in the DNA distribution to
the heavier side, but the time required is significantly
increased.

To quantitate the rate of rejoining from these data
we have plotted the percent of breaks remaining in the
DNA after incubation. It is apparent that the rate of
SSB rejoining is greatly reduced in the mitotic cells.
The S phase cells undergo SSB rejoining at a rate of 5 to
6 times faster than cells in mitosis. However, another
important feature is that, in both cases, the percent of
breaks remaining falls very close to the same level within 60 minutes. Therefore, mitotic cells, even if forced
to remain in mitosis, eventually succeed in the repair of
the majority of SSB. Since the technique of alkaline sucrose gradients does not have the resolution necessary to
allow precise measurements in the range of 1 to 10 percent remaining damage, it is impossible to determine if
all of the breaks are rejoined.

SUMMARY

We have drawn the following conclusions from these
data: (a) the yield of breaks is uniform throughout the
division cycle and therefore difference in quantity of
this lesion cannot account for fluctuation in cycle sensitivity; (b) the process resulting in the rejoining of
single strand breaks is enzymatic in nature; (c) cells in
all stages of the division cycle have the capability of
rejoining breaks and the extensive synthesis of DNA, RNA
or protein is not required. Therefore, the enzymes
necessary for this process are present and functional at
all times in the division cycle; (d) S phase cells can
rejoin breaks at a faster rate than cells in mitosis but
the end result is that nearly all breaks are resealed in
both phases of the cycle. Although, it is probable that
single strand breaks and their repair have biological significance, their role in determining radiation response
is not established.

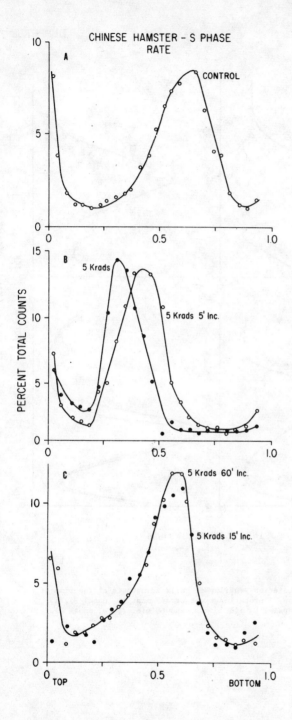

Fig. 2. The sedimentation profiles of cells in S phase at the time of irradiation. Incubation times were 5 min. (●, panel B), 15 min. and 60 min. (●, o; panel C).

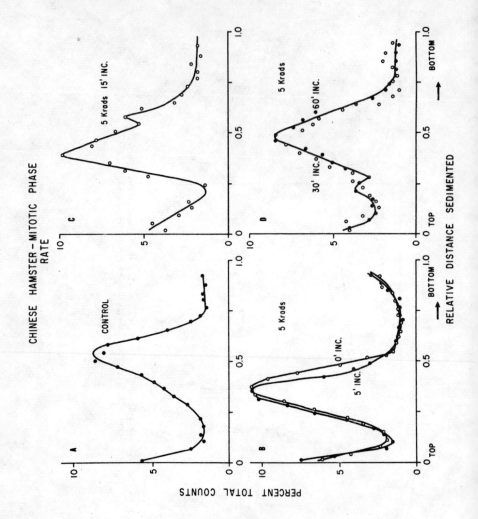

Fig. 3. The sedimentation profiles of cells in mitosis at the time of
         irradiation. Incubation times were 5 min. (o, panel B), 15
         min. (o, panel C) and 30 min. and 60 min. (o, •; panel D).

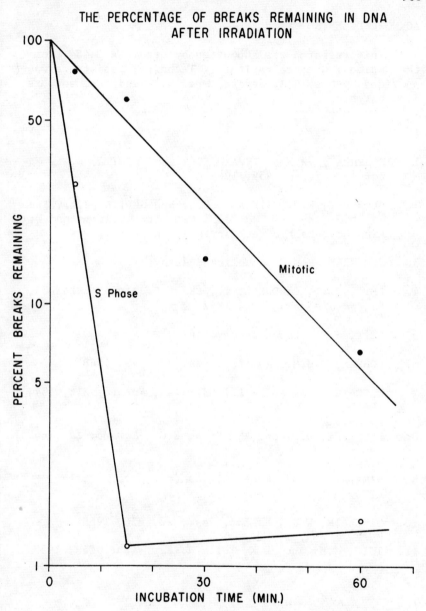

Fig. 4. The percentage of breaks remaining in the DNA versus the time of incubation in normal medium at 37° F. The mitotic population was 98.5% cells in metaphse and the S phase population was 100% cells in DNA synthesis at the time of irradiation (5,000 rads).

ACKNOWLEDGEMNTS

    This research was supported by grant CA 04484 from
the National Cancer Institute. Technical assistance was
provided by Mrs. B.A. Sedita, Mrs. V. Willingham and Mrs.
J. Winston.

REFERENCES

1.   HUMPHREY, R.M., STEWARD, D.L. and SEDITA, B.A., *Mutation Res.*, *6*, 459, 1968.

2.   HUMPHREY, R.M., STEWARD, D.L. and SEDITA, B.A., In: *Genetic Concepts and Neoplasia*, The Williams and Wilkins Co., Baltimore, Maryland, in press.

3.   HUMPHREY, R.M., unpublished data.

4.   LETT, J.T., CALDWELL, I., DEAN, C.J. and ALEXANDER, P., *Nature*, *214*, 790, 1967.

5.   LETT, J.T., these proceedings.

6.   LOHMAN, P.H.M., *Mutation Res.*, *6*, 449, 1968.

7.   McGRATH, R.A. and WILLIAMS, R.W., *Nature*, *212*, 534, 1966.

8.   PETERSEN, D.F. and ANDERSON, E.C., *Nature*, *203*, 642, 1964.

9.   SAWADA, S. and OKADA, S., *Radiat. Res.*, *51*, 145, 1970.

10.   SINCLAIR, W.K., *Radiat. Res.*, *33*, 620, 1968.

11.   TJIO, J.H. and PUCK, T.T., *J. Exp. Med.*, *259*, 1958.

CELL CYCLE DEPENDENT ULTRAVIOLET LIGHT SURVIVAL AND ITS RELATION TO X-RAY RESPONSE

ANTUN HAN

Laboratory of Cellular Radiobiology, Institute "Rudjer Bošković", Zagreb, Yugoslavia

INTRODUCTION

It is well established to-day that radiation responses of cultured mammalian cells depend on the age of cell
at the time of irradiation. This is true for both, X-
rays and ultraviolet light (UVL). Using various methods
of synchronization, as well as the labeling in asynchronous populations, at least four responses to UVL were
shown to depend in magnitude on the position of the cell
in its generation cycle at the time of exposure. These
include: cell survival [5, 7, 8, 12, 13], division delay
and progression [2, 4, 5, 17], inhibition of DNA synthesis and induction of thymine dimers [4, 16], and chromosomal aberrations [10].

The effects of UV-irradiation have been studied in
different types of cultured mammalian cells, and the differences in the properties and in the synchronization
methods used, caused difficulties in comparing the responses of different cell lines. Further complication
comes from the fact, that the physical state (shape and
size) of cells at the time of exposure may contribute
significantly to the amount of UVL absorbed in the cells.
Therefore, specifying the incident UVL dose does not
necessarily correspond to the actual UV flux at different parts within the cell, e.g. cells in suspension vs.
attached cells. Despite the fact that the results in

905

different cell lines are not easy to compare an attempt is
made first to compare the age dependent UVL-lethality of
Chinese hamster cells with those available for some other
cell lines and second, to consider the evidence for similarities and differences in the nature of UVL and X-ray
lesions.

AGE RESPONSE FOR LETHALITY AFTER UVL

The UVL sensitivity of synchronized Chinese hamster
cells was first described by Sinclair and Morton [13] who
found that cells were more sensitive in S than in G_1 and
G_2 and that survival increases some time after DNA synthesis begins.   The timing of survival changes and the
sensitivity of different phases of the cycle in Chinese
hamster cells were established more precisely by Han and
Sinclair [8].   Chinese hamster cells are resistant in G_1,
sensitive throughout S, and become resistant again in G_2.
They further show that cells are the most sensitive 5.5
hr after synchronization, which corresponds to the middle
of the DNA synthetic phase.   The survival curves, made at
selected stages of the generation cycle, revealed that
mitotic cells are most resistant, much more resistant
than S and more resistant than either G_1 or G_2 cells.
Survival curves for G_1 and G_2 cells indicate that their
sensitivity to UVL is about the same.   The survival curve
parameters are summarized in Table 1.

The age response data for Chinese hamster cells are
in good agreement with those reported for HeLa S3 cells
by Djordjevic and Tolmach [5].   The data reported earlier
for D98/AG cells [7] and for L cells [12] differ in some
respects from those reported for Chinese hamster cells
(and HeLa cells as well).   These differences, however,
may reflect either the differences in experimental conditions (e.g. cells in suspension vs. attached cells,
FUdR synchronization and H^3-TdR "suicide" vs. mitotic
selection), or fundamental differences in age dependent
UVL-sensitivity between these strains.   Our recent results indicate that the UVL-sensitivity of mouse L cells
is not different from those described for Chinese hamster
and HeLa cells.   Figure 1 shows the age response for

TABLE 1. PARAMETERS OF SURVIVAL CURVES AFTER UVL IRRADIA-
TION

Time and synchronization	Phase	Single cell extra-polation number	D_0
hr			ergs/mm^2
0	M	2	105
1.25	G_1	6	45
5.5	S	20	35
8.5	G_2	5	55

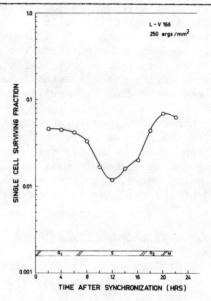

Fig. 1. UVL age response for colonly formation of mouse L cells, clonal isolation L-V166, after exposure to 250 ergs/mm^2.

lethality of L-V166 cells. Synchronous populations at or near division were obtained by harvesting mitotic cells from a log-phase cultures under controlled condition (the method has been described in detail elsewhere [11]). The general pattern of this response is in good agreement

with those reported for Chinese hamster cells [8, 13] and
for HeLa S3 cells [5]. Therefore, it would seem that
differences in the methods of synchronization and experimental condition can account for the differences in response reported thus far. Consequently, it appears that
mouse L-cells do not differ fundamentally, with regard
to their UVL-sensitivity from both Chinese hamster and
HeLa S3 cells.

Mitotic cells were found most resistant in Chinese
hamster cells [8], but before a definite conclusion can
be reached it should be determined whether the mitotic
cells of the other cell lines display the same low UVL
sensitivity. The available age response data also
indicate that the survival of G_2 cells increases with
age, but more specific measurements are required before
a general conclusion can be made, since the presence of
a small fraction of resistant mitotic cells (assuming
their low UVL-sensitivity for all established cell lines)
can affect the measurement of G_2 sensitivity.

Following summarizes, therefore, broadly the principal features of the UVL age response for lethality in
cultured mammalian cells; cells are resistant in G_1,
sensitive throughout S and most sensitive in the middle
of the DNA synthetic phase, sensitivity then decreases
towards the end of the cell generation cycle.

ULTRAVIOLET LIGHT SURVIVAL AND *DNA* SYNTHESIS

Age response studies have established that maximum
sensitivity of Chinese hamster cells to UVL is in the
middle of the DNA synthetic phase [8]. This suggests a
role of DNA synthesis in controlling the sensitivity of
the cell to UVL. Djordjević and Tolmach have shown [5],
that in HeLa S3 cells DNA synthesized during the first
half of S is not followed by a decrease in sensitivity,
and that survival does not drop significantly faster in
cultures prevented from entering S by FUdR. In Chinese
hamster cells, the acquisition of S-period sensitivity
by G_1 cells is not prevented by Hydroxy-urea [8], but
is prevented, at least partially, by TdR (Fig. 2A, open

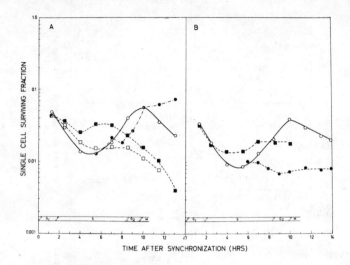

Fig. 2.   A - The effect of hydroxyurea and excess TdR on the age response
           for colony formation of synchronous V79-S171 cells. Open circles,
           cells exposed to 270 ergs/mm^2. Open squares, age response of cells
           treated with 1.0 mM HU at 1.25 hr and exposed to 270 ergs/mm^2,
           closed squares, age response of cells treated with 7.5 mM TdR at
           1.25 h, and exposed to 270 ergs/mm^2 at different times. Closed
           circles, 7.5 mM TdR added at 5.5 and 270 ergs/mm^2 at different
           times.

           B - The effect of cyclohexymide (CH) on the age response. Open
           circles, the same as in 2A, closed squares, 5.0 µg/ml of CH
           added to G_1 cells and 270 ergs/mm^2 at different times, closed
           circles, the same treatment as before, except that CH was added
           to mid-S cells.

           In all experiments, inhibitors were removed immediately after
           exposure.

and closed squares, respectively) or cyclohexymide (Fig.
2B). These findings indicate that not DNA synthesis but
some process concomitant with it is responsible for the
sensitivity of S cells. The development of G_2 resistance after S, however is prevented by hydroxyurea or TdR
and partially by cyclohexymide.

     The addition of excess TdR to the cells in the
middle of S did not prevent the development of the resistance normally observed in G_2, although it was somewhat slower (Fig. 2A, closed circles). This increase in
survival was prevented when cyclohecymide is added to

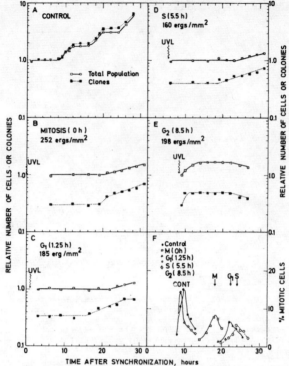

Fig. 3. UVL - induced division delay in V79-S171 cells with exposures adjusted to reduce survival to about 0.3 level, at all stages of teh cycle. Exposures applied, and symbols are explained on each panel.

mid-S cells. Therefore the maximum survival, exhibited by uninhibited cells, can be achieved if DNA synthesis proceeds for at least part of S, but this resistance can be prevented by a protein inhibitor added at the middle of S. Further discussion of these changes is reported elsewhere [8]. The dependence of UVL survival upon macromolecular synthesis is evidently complex, and is related only partially to DNA synthesis. Since both the development of S sensitivity and G_2 resistance can be prevented by a protein inhibitor, it is tempting to think of the process involved being the formation of specific protein.

The results of postirradiation application of inhibitors to asynchronous Chinese hamster cells [1] or to synchronized cells in G_1 or S [8], indicate that post-irradiation inhibition of either DNA or DNA and protein syntheses, does not affect cell survival, but maintains it at a level characteristic of the uninhibited cells. Hanawalt and coworkers [9] have shown that the polymerases involved in semiconservative replication and the repair replication may not be identical, and Cleaver [3] has demonstrated that only inhibitors that bind to DNA are capable of inhibiting DNA repair replication. Therefore, it seems that the inhibitors tested do not prevent unscheduled DNA synthesis from providing the necessary repair. If actinomycin D is applied to G_1 or S cells after exposure, and removed as a function of time thereafter, cell survival decreases sharply (Sinclair and Han, unpublished results).

DIVISION DELAY

The measurement of division or mitotic delay of Chinese hamster cells as a function of age of the cells with exposures were adjusted to yield approximately 0.3 survival at different stages of the cycle is shown in Fig. 3. The results of cell number and surviving cells show that cells irradiated in the middle of S suffered the longest division delay, cells irradiated in G_1 or mitosis have about the same delay in division, and cells in G_2 were not delayed. Interesting features of this study are the absence of division delay for cells exposed in G_2 and shorter delay for surviving cells than that for total population (nonsurvivors). The results for mitotic index (panel F of Fig. 3) versus time agree best with those for the total population, whereas the delay for viable cells is somewhat shorter than these. This suggests, that all cells reach mitosis. The increase in the total number of cells, however, can be accounted for by the increase in size of the viable cell population. Thus, the nonsurviving cells presumably are present during most of the experiment and apparently are stopped at mitosis and do not divide.

The division delay data for Chinese hamster V79 cells are in good agreement with those reported for HeLa [5], T and DON cells [3], and for L cells [4]. No specific measurements of the induced division delay for surviving and nonsurviving cells have been made so far. Most of the data on the other cell lines were obtained after exposures which rendered most of the cells as survivors.

Summarizing the age response for UVL-induced lethality and division delay in Chinese hamster cells it can be concluded, that largest effects occur when cells are irradiated in S.

THE RELATION OF ULTRAVIOLET LIGHT AND X-RAY RESPONSES

Studies of Chinese hamster cells by Sinclair and Morton [13] indicated a markedly different age response for survival after UVL from that of X-rays. The responses to the two types of radiation differ in that the maximum and minimum sensitivity to UVL occur later in the cycle than the corresponding change in X-ray response. The most significant difference between the responses is the sensitivity of mitotic cells, which were found most sensitive fraction toward X-rays [13, 14] and least sensitive toward UVL [8]. Closer analysis of the X-ray and UVL sensitivity of interphase cells shows that peak sensitivity and resistance to UVL occur 2.5-3 hours later than the corresponding changes after X-rays. Although it may appear that X-ray and UVL age responses for lethality are almost "mirror" picture of each other, closer examinations reveal that maximum and minimum sensitivity for UVL do not occur appreciably later than that for X-rays. In HeLa S3 cells, in which G_1 is of a considerable length, cells are relatively resistant to both types of radiation during the early part of G_1 [5].

The dependence of either X-ray or UVL survival upon macromolecular synthesis, as shown so far, is evidently complex [15, 8]. The changes in X-ray survival during the cycle occur in the absence of DNA synthesis [15]. The acquisition of resistance in late S is partially prevented when DNA synthesis is arrested in synchronous cells in G_1 by hydroxyurea or excess TdR [15]. The greatest survival, however, can only be achieved when

DNA has progressed to a certain stage. The development
of G_2 resistance after UV-irradiation is completely prevented when DNA synthesis is arrested in G_1 cells by the
same inhibitors [8]. Arresting DNA synthesis, after it
has progressed to a certain stage, has a negligible effect upon survival after either type of radiation.
Therefore it appears that the development of resistance
after X-rays depends partially on DNA synthesis, but
after UVL-irradiation it depends completely on DNA synthesis. The inhibition of protein synthesis by adding
cycloheximide to G_1 cells suppressed completely the peak
normally seen in late S after X-irradiation, and partially affects the UVL resistance. The resistance in G_2
normally seen after UVL, can be prevented by protein inhibitor added in the middle of S. Therefore, this resistance also depends on protein synthesis, i.e. it develops only if DNA synthesis has proceeded for at least
part of S, and in the presence of protein synthesis. All
these data indicate that after both types of irradiation,
maximum survival depends on whether the DNA and protein
syntheses have progressed to a certain stage. The association between DNA synthesis and X-ray survival does not
seem to be direct, while it could be the case for UVL
irradiation, at least as far as the development of resistance is concerned. Since protein inhibitor added prior
to UVL exposure can prevent both the development of S
sensitivity and G_2 resistance, and when added prior to
X-rays can prevent the development of resistance in late
S, it is tempting to think of the process involved being
the formation of specific proteins. It is likely that
fundamentally different kinds of damage can be expressed
in the same way, and if DNA is important target molecule
for both types of radiations, a common expression of
damage would be facilitated. This in turn suggests that
there could be a partial overlap in the damage, and overlap of expressed damage after UVL and X-irradiation has
been shown in systems other than mammalian cells [6].

The results on the age response for lethality and
the effect of various inhibitors upon it, were obtained
in collaboration with Dr. Warren K. Sinclair, and those
on UVL-induced division delay in collaboration with
Dr. W.K. Sinclair and Dr. C.K. Yu. The work was carried

out at the Division of Biological and Medical Research, Argonne National Laboratory, Argonne, Illinois, and was supported by U.S. Atomic Energy Commission. The experiments with L-cells were performed at Laboratory of Cellular Radiobiology, Institute "Ruder Bošković", Zagreb, Yugoslavia, in collaboration with V. Habazin, M. Sci. The work was supported from the Federal Research Fund.

REFERENCES

1.   ARLETT, C.F., *Int. J. Radiat. Biol.*, *13*, 369, 1967.

2.   BOOTSMA, D. and HUMPREY, R.M., *Mutation Res.*, *5*, 289, 1968.

3.   CLEAVER, J.E., *Radiat. Res.*, *37*, 334, 1969.

4.   DOMON, M. and RAUTH, A.M., *Radiat. Res.*, *40*, 414, 1969.

5.   DJORDJEVIĆ, B. and TOLMACH, L.J., *Radiat. Res.*, *32*, 327, 1967.

6.   ELKIND, M.M. and SUTTON, H.A., *Radiat. Res.*, *10*, 296, 1959.

7.   ERIKSON, R.L. and SZYBALSKI, W., *Radiat. Res.*, *18*, 200, 1963.

8.   HAN, A. and SINCLAIR, W.K., *Biophys. J.*, *9*, 1171, 1969.

9.   HANAWALT, P.O., PETTIJOHN, D.E., PAULING, E.C., BRUNK, C.F., SMITH, D.E., KANNER, L.C. and COUCH, J.L., *Cold Spring Harbor Symp. Qant. Biol.*, *33*, 187, 1968.

10.   HUMPHREY, R.M., DEWEY, W.C. and CORK, A., *Radiat. Res.*, *19*, 247, 1963.

11. PETROVIĆ, D., FERLE-VIDOVIĆ, A., HABAZIN, V. and
     VUKOVIĆ, B., *Int. J. Radiat. Biol.*, 1970, (in press).

12. RAUTH, A.M. and WHITMORE, G.F., *Radiat. Res.*, *28*,
     84, 1966.

13. SINCLAIR, W.K. and MORTON, R.A., *Biophys. J.*, *5*,
     1, 1965.

14. SINCLAIR, W.K. and MORTON, R.A., *Radiat. Res.*, *29*,
     450, 1966.

15. SINCLAIR, W.K., *Proc. Nat. Acad. Sci. USA*, *58*,
     115, 1967.

16. STEWARD, D.L. and HUMPHREY, R.M., *Nature*, *212*, 299,
     1966.

17. THOMPSON, L.H. and HUMPHREY, R.M., *Radiat. Res.*, *41*,
     183, 1970.

PLATEAU PERIOD CELLS AND CELL CYCLE EVENTS

G.M. HAHN and S-J. YANG

Department of Radiology,
Stanford University School of Medicine,
Stanford, California 94305, U.S.A.

I. INTRODUCTION

At first glance the title of this paper contains a self-contradiction. Cyclic cellular events are associated with exponential growth. It is the progression from mitosis to G1 to S to G2 and then again to mitosis which is a characteristic of unlimited growth. However, if one follows the increase in cell number of a culture *in vitro*, the cell number tends to level off reaching a plateau after the cell density has reached a specified value. *In vitro* this is readily observable and many growth curves have been presented in the literature. For example, in a line originating from Chinese hamster ovary cells (HA1) the growth curve levels off (plateau period) at a cell density of about 2×10^5 cells/cm^2 if the cells are not presented with changes of nutrients (Fig. 1). On the other hand, if the nutrient supply is changed frequently then the cell density increases by about a factor of 10 [1]. Thus it is clear that the behavior of the cell number is determined to a large extent by the metabolic milieu. This milieu is influenced by the type of medium used and the amount and type of serum added to the medium; furthermore, different cell lines seem to respond differently to their surroundings. In the present paper, we will discuss the behavior of a line of Chinese hamster cells (HA2) either under plateau conditions owing to nutrient exhaustion ("unfed" cultures) or under con-

ditions where nutrients do not limit growth ("fed" cultures). The reasons why cells stop multiplying in the
presence of adequate nutrients are not well understood.
Our experimental procedures and origins of the cell line
have been described in detail [1,2,3]. Briefly, cells
are grown as monolayers in 60 mm plastic Petri dishes
(Falcon). The medium is Eagle's MEM (Difco, powdered)
supplemented with 15% fetal bovine serum. Unfed cultures are given 5 cc of such medium at the time of
plating. The medium is not changed during the course
of the experiment. Fed cultures have their medium
changed daily once the cell number exceeds about 10^6
cell/dish. Control experiments have shown that more
frequent exchanges of medium do not change the growth
rate not the final cell density [1]. In neither the
fed nor the unfed cultures do the cells form multiple
layers. The fed cultures represent a cell renewal system. Approximately 10% of the cells die and lyse per
day; these are replaced by newly born cells. The cell
cycle of the cycling cells (i.e., those proliferating
to replace the dying cells) in plateau period shows
an extended duration of S and a slightly extended G2.
The duration of the G1 phase is essentially not measurable. Unfed cells have only a very small fraction
of their cells in cycle (at least as determined by pulse
labeling experiments) and the S phase of cells so determined may not be too different from that of exponentially growing cells [4]. Cell death among the unfed cultures is rare. The plateau period cultures
have many properties in common with populations of
solid tumor cells *in vivo*. For this reason we have
been studying various properties of plateau period
cells. In this paper we examine the question: to
what extent are concepts and designations developed
for cycling cells applicable to plateau period cultures?

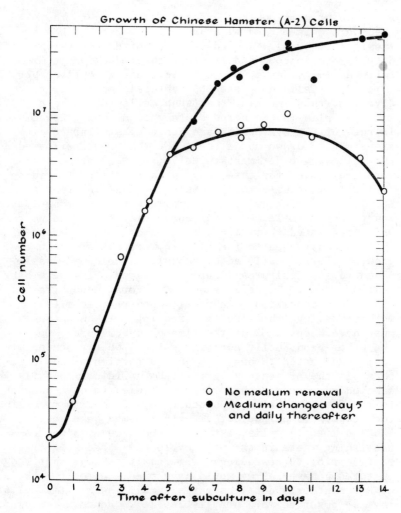

Fig. 1. Growth of Chinese hamster cells (HA2). Cells were plated on replicate dishes. Each day cells from two (or four) dishes were trypsinized and counted on a Coulter electronic cell counter. Points represent averages of eight (or sixteen) counter readings. The maximum cell number and the growth rate of "fed" cultures is not exceeded if feeding rate is doubled. (From reference[1]).

II.   WHERE DO THE CELLS LEAVE THE CYCLE WHEN THEY ENTER
      THE PLATEAU PERIOD?

     The transition from exponential growth to the pla-
teau period is marked by a drop in the rate of DNA synthesis (per cell). In fed cultures of HA2 cells this
drop is precipitous and precedes the reduction in mitotic activity (as measured by increase in cell number)
(Fig. 2). Cells complete DNA synthesis and go on to
division, thus implying that such cells leave the cycle
in G1. Cells in the unfed state show a more gradual drop
in rate of DNA synthesis, and hence no similar conclusions can be drawn about them. We therefore performed
the following experiments. Cells in the plateau period
were prelabeled for three days with tritiated thymidine
(0.1 μCi/ml, 6 Ci/m mole). This was done in order to
label any cycling cells. The cells were then subcultured
and plated into large dishes containing fresh medium to
which tritiated thymidine was added as before. Most of
the cells attached to the plastic were able to resume
growth. Periodically after subculture colcemide was
added to some cultures; four hours later cells were harvested and mitotic cells examined autoradiographically.
Under such conditions, any cell which reached mitosis
without having label incorporated into its chromosomes
must have been in G2 at the time of subculture. On
the other hand, cells containing label when reaching mitosis had passed through at least a portion of the S
phase in the presence of tritiated thymidine. Heavily
labeled mitoses may therefore be assumed to have been
in the G1 phase prior to subculture. From data recording
the numbers of unlabeled, lightly labeled, and heavily
labeled mitotic cells, estimates could be obtained es-
tablishing where in the cell cycle cells had been arrested prior to reseeding. Our results showed that fed
cultures behaved as we would have predicted on the basis
of DNA synthesis data: essentially all the mitotic cells
that we observed were heavily labeled. Hence we concluded
that in fed cultures essentially all the cells not cycling
had left the cycle in G1. On the other hand, the picture
in the unfed cultures was more complicated. First of all,
analysis of the autoradiographs of the early plateau period cultures and late plateau cultures differed. Early

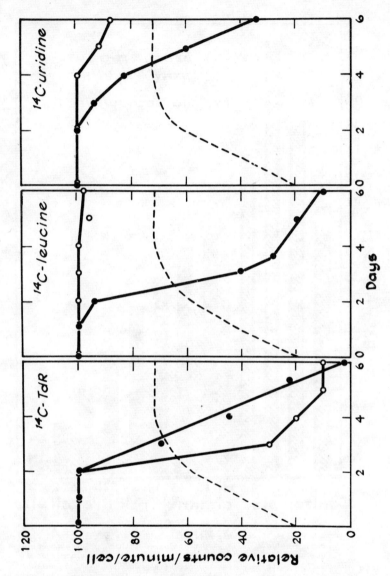

Fig. 2. Incorporation of labeled precursors by cultures growing into
         plateau period. Cells were plated into plastic petri dishes
         and exposed (30 min periods) to indicated ^{14}C labeled pre-
         cursors of DNA (TdR), protein (leucine) and RNA (uridine).
         The incorporated radioactivity was assayed by punching out
         the bottoms of the dishes and counting on a planchet gas flow
         Geiger-Müller counter (for details see reference [1]). Cell
         number was obtained from replicate cultures and the data are
         presented as counts/min/cell. The dotted lines show the be-
         havior of the cell number (on logarithmic scale, not shown).
         0——0 fed cultures; ●——● unfed cultures.

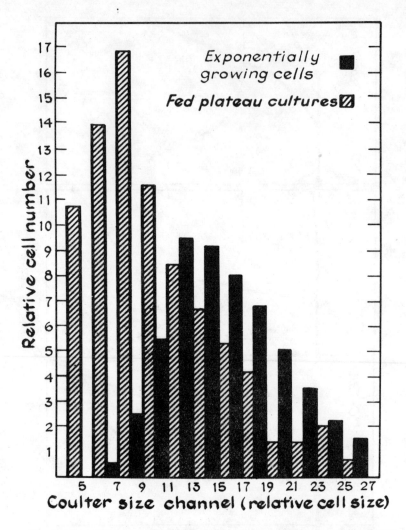

Fig. 3. Comparison of cell sizes of exponentially growing and fed plateau
period cells. Cells were trypsinized either during exponential
growth (solid bars) or during the late plateau period (shaded
bars). Cell size measurements were made on a model B Coulter
size analyzer. Total cell number: ~10^6 during exponential growth;
~2×10^7 during the plateau period. Histograms of unfed cultures
(not shown) closely resemble histograms of fed cultures.

plateau period cultures had between 10-20% and some-
times even more unlabeled mitotic cells indicating
arrest of some cells in G2. On the other hand, similar autoradiographs from late plateau period cultures
showed no unlabeled mitosis; however, many mitotic cells
harvested shortly after subculture were lightly labeled.
This is illustrated in Fig. 3, which shows histograms
of grain counts from such mitotic cells harvested within the first 12 h after subculture. For comparison,
Fig. 3 also shows data obtained from the first harvest
of fed cells. The lightly labeled cells from the unfed
cultures presumably traversed only a portion of the S
phase in the presence of tritiated thymidine. Therefore
during the plateau period these cells were arrested in
S. The near-absence of lightly labeled cells in the
12 h group indicates that essentially all the cells
which had been arrested in S reached mitosis within 8 h
after resuming growth. This result, plus the early appearance in mitosis of lightly labeled cells, shows that
cells arrested in S resume progression around the cell
cycle almost immediately after being subcultured. The
fate of the G2 cells found in early plateau (but not
in late plateau) is not clear. Either they slowly
moved through G2, divided, and were finally arrested in
G1, or else they lost their ability to initiate mitosis
and were therefore not scored in our experiments.

III. COMPARISON OF EXPONENTIALLY GROWING AND PLATEAU
      PERIOD CELLS

    In the last section we showed that plateau period
cells are largely in the G1-like part of the cell cycle.
The question arises: if cells remain in plateau period
for some time, to what extent do the non-cycling cells
then still resemble G1 cell? To answer this question
we compared exponentially growing and late plateau period cells in a variety of ways to determine whether
or not parameters characterizing various aspects of
plateau period cells were consistent with those of exponentially growing cells in the G1 phase.

924

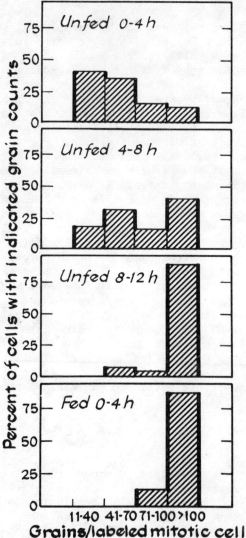

Fig. 4. Histograms of grain counts of mitotic cells obtained from subcultured late plateau period cells. Cells were labeled with
tritiated thymidine in plateau period for three days, then subcultured into fresh medium also containing ^{3}HTdR. Colcemide
was added for the periods indicated, the cells harvested and
autoradiographs scored for grain counts/labeled mitotic cell.
Lightly labeled mitotic cells in the early harvests of unfed
cultures arise from cells arrested in S. By 12 h few if any
lightly labeled cells are seen; heavily labeled cells traversed
entire S and hence were arrested in G1. Note difference between 0-4 h results from unfed cells *vs* those from fed cells.

a) *Cell size*

Fig. 4 shows histograms of cell sizes from exponentially growing cells and from fed plateau period cells. Histograms from unfed late plateau period cells did not differ significantly from those of fed cells. The histogram of exponentially growing cells is consistent with theoretical expectations if one assumes that the smaller cells are G1 cells. The vast majority of the plateau period cells are considerably smaller than even the smallest of the exponentially growing cells. Hence, it is clear that far as size is concerned, the plateau period cells cannot be characterized as G1 cells.

b) *RNA and protein metabolism*

We examined uptake of precursors of RNA (^{14}C-uridine) and protein (^{14}C-leucine) by the cells in experimential growth and in plateau period (Fig. 2). The results indicate that fed cultures have rates of uptake of these two precursors not too different from exponentially growing cultures. Particularly because of the reduced cell size, this implies a very high turnover rate of both RNA and protein, probably much higher than in normal Gi cells; however, the synthesis rates may be quite similar to those of G1 cells. The very low incorporation of labeled precursors into unfed cells shows that these are truly in what might be called a "stationary" state.

c) *Protein-free sulfhydryls*

Several authors have really recently shown that the contents of protein-free sulfhydryls varies with the position of the cell in the cell cycle [5]. We therefore examined the sulfhydryl contents of plateau period cultures to see if the values obtained were consistent with those of exponentially growing cultures. Fed cultures had, on the average, one third as much protein-free sulfhydryl per cell as did the exponentially growing cultures, and if this was corrected for differences in amount of protein per cell, the sulfhydryl content per cell per unit of protein was still lower by at least a factor of 2 than that of the exponentially growing cultures [6]. However, variations

of better than 2:1 during the cell cycle have been shown
to occur in mammalian cells [5], and furthermore at the G1/S
interphase cells are particularly low in protein-free sulfhydryl content. Therefore, if we assume that in late plateau period the fed cultures are in a state similar to
that of exponentially growing cultures in the G1/S interphase, then the protein-free sulfhydryl values are consistent with those of exponentially growing cultures. On the
other hand, unfed cultures show sulfhydryl contents not
significantly different from the mean value of that observed
from exponentially growing cultures (Hahn, unpublished data).

d) *Radiation response*

Survival of cells X-irradiated in the plateau period
was examined in detail [2]. In early plateau period, the
D_O of survival curves was somewhat higher than that of exponentially growing cultures and in late fed plateau period again approached that of exponentially growing cultures,
and at times was even below that. Concomitantly, the extrapolation number remained constant during early plateau
period but then asymptotically approached a value of 1 [2].
Cells in early fed plateau period were still able to repair
sublethal damage, while those in the late plateau period
(presumably because they were no longer able to sustain
sublethal damage) were also not able to repair it. This
latter fact was assayed by performing split dose survival
experiments [3]. Elkind has presented data which indicates
that Chinese hamster cells at the G1/S interphase may also be incapable of repairing sublethal damage [7] and this
again may indicate that during late plateau, fed cells resemble cells at the G1/S interphase. Radiation response
of unfed cultures did not differ significantly from that
of exponentially growing cultures. Such unfed cells were
also capable of sustaining and repairing sublethal damage.
There is, however, one way in which the radiation response
of plateau period cells is significantly different from
that of exponentially growing cultures. Plateau period
cells are able to repair potentially lethal damage, provided they remain in plateau period after irradiation [8].
By this we mean that cells irradiated in platieau in dense
cultures and subcultured at increasing times post-irradiation, will show increasing survival levels. With unfed

cultures, this is true even at low doses (300-500 R) while
with fed cultures repair of potenially lethal damage only
becomes obvious at appreciably higher doses (1000 R or
higher) (Hahn, Bagshaw, and Gordon, in preparation). Repair of potenially lethal damage is an important feature
of dense cell cultures and may have considerable bearing
on the radiosensitivity of some tumor systems.

III. CONCLUSION

The data we have presented show that cells, in the
presence of adequate nutrients, leave the cell cycle in
the G1 phase. Most of such cells (unless subcultured)
never enter S; it is therefore reasonable to assume that
the growth-limiting control is along the pathway of DNA
synthesis. Our data throw no light on how this control
operates; it appears that no contact related phenomenon
is directly involved.

In the absence of adequate nutrients, some cells
leave the cycle during phases other than G1. Those cells
that exit from the cycle during G2 either progress slowly
through mitosis and are arrested again in G1 or else die.
Cells leaving during S may be arrested in that phase for
considerable time (alternatively cells arrested in S during late plateau period may be G1 cells attempting to
cycle but not quite making it through S).

To the major question we posed, do non-cycling cells
remain the same as G1 cells, our data supply an equivocal
answer. In some ways (e.g., radio-response of unfed cells,
synthesis of RNA and protein of fed cells) they do; in o-
ther ways (e.g., cell size) they do not. This is perhaps
not surprising. Many cellular processes are not coupled
to the DNA-synthetic pathway; there is no reason to sup-
pose that because DNA synthesis in inhibited that other
important cellular events may not continue.

_____

Work performed under USPHS research grants CA-10372
and CA-04542 from the National Cancer Institute, National
Institutes of Health. George M. Hahn is holder of a Dern-
ham Senior Fellowship in Oncology from the American Cancer
Society, California Division.

REFERENCES

1. HAHN, G.M., STEWART, J.R., YANG, S-J., and PARKER,
    V., *Exper. Cell Res.*, *49*, 285, 1968.

2. STEWART, J.R., HAHN, G.M., PARKER, V., and BAGSHAW,
    M.A., *Exper. Cell Res.*, *49*, 293, 1968.

3. HAHN, G.M., *Nature*, *217*, 741, 1968.

4. HAHN, G.M., in: (Conference) Proc. on Time and
    Dose Relationships in Radiation Biology as Ap-
    plied to Radiotherapy, *Carmel*, Calif., U.S.A.
    Sept. 1969.

5. MAURO, F., GRASSO, A., and TOLMACH, L.J., *Biophys.
    J.*, *9*, 1377, 1969.

6. HARRIS, J., PAINTER, R.B., and HAHN, G.M., *Int.
    J. Radiat. Biol.*, *15*, 289, 1969.

7. ELKIND, M.M., in: (Conference) Proc. on Time and
    Dose Relationships in Radiation Biology as Applied
    to Radiotherapy; *Carmel*, Calif., U.S.A. Sept. 1969

8. LITTLE, J.B., *Nature*, *224*, 804, 1969.

9. HAHN, G.M., and KALLMAN, R.F., *Radiat. Res.*, *30*,
    707, 1967.

THE EFFECT OF RADIATION ON CELLS IN THE STATIONARY PHASE OF THEIR GROWTH

NICOLAS J. McNALLY

Medical Research Council, Experimental Radiopathology Unit, Hammersmith Hospital, DuCane Road, London, W.12, England

Many tumours have a growth rate which is only in-directly related to the rate at which their cells di-vide. This may be due to a number of factors. There may be death of the tumour cells, or cells may be in a non-proliferative state resulting in a growth fraction of less than one, with only a fraction of the tumour cell population in exponential growth. Cells in tissue culture in the stationary phase of their growth may be considered as a model system of these tumour cells by virtue of the fact that they are non-proliferating but potentially colony forming cells.

Cells can become stationary either because of nutrient depletion (unfed) or because of a lack of space but not nutrients (fed). I have studied both types of population using a cell line derived from a benzopyrene-induced sarcoma in rats, tumour RIB$_5$. The cells are grown in Eagle's minimum essential medium with 10 per cent foetal calf serum added. For both radiation and growth studies replicate 5 cm polystyrene petri dishes were inoculated with cells from a suspension in log-arithmic growth. The cells had a population doubling time of 17 hours and were treated either 30 hours after inoculation of 4×10^5 cells, when they were in log-arithmic growth, or after about 50 hours in the sta-tionary phase, corresponding to a period of growth of

929

either 120 hours (unfed) or 160 hours (fed). Following
irradiation in the dishes in which they had grown, the
cells were trypsinised and appropriate dilutions were
plated into new petri dishes. Except for fractionation
studies, the medium was removed at the time of irradiation. Irradiations were by a Phillips X-ray machine
operating at 250 Kv., 15 ma., H.v.1. 0.3 mm Cu. In all
experiments the plating efficiency was in the range 60
to 80 per cent.

Uptake of ^{3}H-thymidine was used to study DNA synthesis. Cells were grown on glass cover-slips and
after exposure to the label and subsequent cell growth,
were fixed and stained, and autoradiographs were prepared by standard techniques. The cell cycle parameters were measured by scoring labeled mitoses at times
after pulse labelling, while the growth fraction was determined by counting labeled cells after continuous exposure to the label.

The only survival curve parameter to change significantly with the state of growth of the cell culture
was the extrapolation number (n) which was reduced from
four to one as cells moved from the logarithmic to the
stationary phase regardless of whether they had been fed
or not (Fig. 1). There was no change in the oxygen
enhancement ratio (o.e.r.) or the value of D_0. When the
radiation was delivered in two equal doses separated in
time, the logarithmic cells were able to recover from
their sub-lethal damage (Fig. 2). Fed stationary phase
cells showed no sparing effect of fractionation (Fig. 2).
However unfed stationary cells showed an apparent sparing effect. This was only apparent because if they were
exposed to a single dose of radiation and then held for
a period in the medium in which they had grown, prior
to replating into fresh medium, then the same increase
in survival was seen as when the dose was fractionated
(Fig. 2). The cells were recovering from potentially
lethal rather than sub-lethal damage.

Cells in the logarithmic phase of growth had a
mean cell cycle time of 17 hours and a DNA synthetic
period of 9 hours (Fig. 3). The growth fraction was

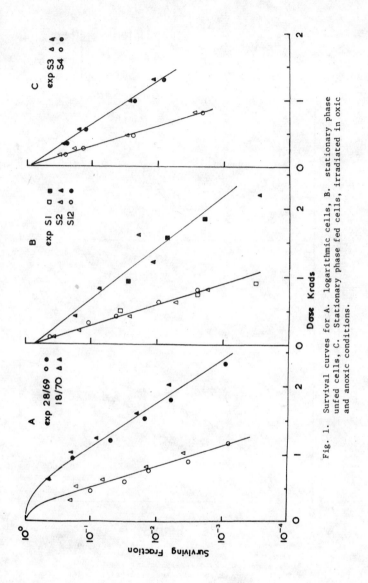

Fig. 1. Survival curves for A. logarithmic cells, B. stationary phase unfed cells, C. Stationary phase fed cells, irradiated in oxic and anoxic conditions.

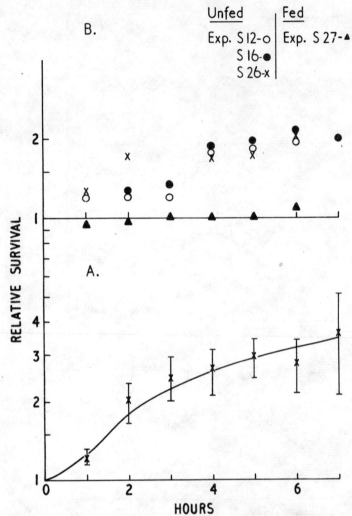

Fig. 2. Recovery from sub-lethal and lethal damage. A. logarithmic cells,
mean of three experiments, with standard errors (500 r + 500 r).
B. fed and unfed stationary cells. Expts. S 12, S 16, S 27-500 r
+ 500 r. Expt. S 26-500 r and held prior to replating.

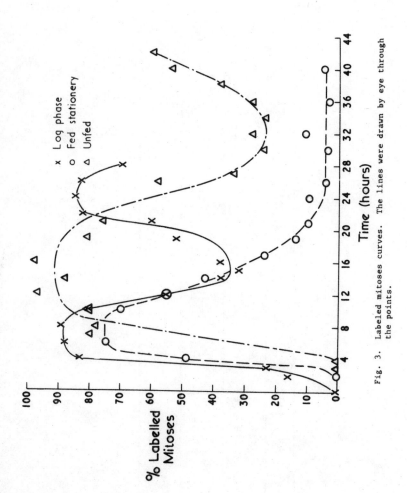

Fig. 3. Labeled mitoses curves. The lines were drawn by eye through the points.

TABLE 1.

Population	Do (air)	n	o.e.r	T_C	T_S	T_{G1}	T_{G2}	G.F.
Logarithmic	134 (119-154)	4.50 (2.17-9.28)	2.12 (1.97-2.28)	17	9	3½	3½	100%
Stationary unfed	136 r (120-157)	0.74 (0.42-1.32)	2.42 (2.12-2.77)	33	18	8	7	56%
Stationary fed	136 r (128-146)	0.88 (0.72-1.12)	2.07 (1.95-2.21)	—	9	>25	3	8%

near one as measured by continuous labelling. In the
stationary phase of the fed population this fraction was
8 per cent (Table 1). Those cells which underwent mitosis appeared to synthesise DNA and then enter a prolonged
G_1 period (Fig. 3). Unfed stationary cells showed a different pattern of movement through the cell cycle to
that of the fed cells. The cell cycle increased due to
a doubling in all stages of the cell cycle (Fig. 3), while
the fraction of cells labeled following continuous exposure to the label increased slowly to a value of 56 per
cent at 30 hours (Table 1). The lack of an increase in
cell number was due to a combination of decrease in the
growth fraction together with an increase in the occurance
of pyknosis and cell degeneration.

DISCUSSION

Exponential survival in the stationary phase was
first demonstrated by Hahn [2] using Chinese Hamster
cells, and these results with RIB_5 cells are in agreement with his. They are in contrast to those of Madoc-
Jones [5] using cells derived from a benzpyrene induced
sarcoma in rats, and of Little [4] using Chang liver
cells, both of whom found changes in the value of Do and
an increase in the value of n as cells entered the stationary phase. Berry [1] has reported a change in the
o.e.r. for unfed HeLa cells grown in medium 199 and
irradiated in the stationary phase. The same cells
showed no change in the o.e.r. when irradiated in medium
F10 which, unlike 199, contained thymidine, asparagine
and a high concentration of folic acid. The medium used
in the present study, in which there was no change in
the o.e.r., contained folic acid but no thymidine or
asparagine.

It is well established that the shape of the radiation survival curve depends on the stage of the cells
in the cell cycle, and that exponential survival may be
observed at certain stages, for instance in mitosis with
Chinese Hamster cells. This phenomenon might account for
the exponential survival of fed stationary phase cells
encountering a block in G_1 (Fig. 3), but seems unlikely

to apply to the unfed cells which did not encounter such
a block. The stationary phase of these cells was char-
acterised by an overall doubling in the stages of the
cell cycle together with a fall in the growth fraction
to 56 per cent, an effect similar to that reported by
Lala [3] using Ehrlich Ascites Tumour cells in mice. It
may be that the non-cycling cells in the unfed population are in a prolonged G_1 phase as in the Ascites
tumour [3] and that they do exhibit exponential survival
to radiation, but they represent less than 50 per cent
of the population and cannot alone account for the exponential survival curves seen when unfed stationary phase
RIB_5 cells are irradiated.

   The absence of a sparing effect of fractionation for
cells in the stationary phase was to be expected in view
of the exponential nature of the survival curves. However the recovery from lethal damage in the unfed cells
was not. There is a paucity of evidence for the recovery of lethal X-ray damage in mammalian cells. Recently Little [4] has demonstrated the occurrence of
such recovery in fed stationary phase Chang liver cells,
though I have found it only with unfed RIB_5 cells. The
removal of cells from the stationary phase (fed or unfed)
quickly restored their ability to absorb some radiation-
induced lesions as sub-lethal, since within one hour
of replating the extrapolation number had returned to
its logarithmic phase value.

   If cultured cells in stationary phase are a reasonable model for non-proliferative cells in solid tumours,
the absence of a sparing effect of fractionation would
be beneficial from a radiotherapeutic point of view,
though any recovery from lethal damage might counteract
such a benefit. However, results of labeled mitoses experiments on a number of solid tumours have not revealed
cell populations with extended cell cycle times. Furthermore, a number of workers have found an increase in cell
cycle with cell number in ascites tumours qualitatively
similar to that which occurs in unfed stationary RIB_5
cells (see Lala [3] for instance). These observations
would suggest that cells in vitro which have become
stationary because of nutrient depletion are a better
model for ascites than for solid tumours.

SUMMARY

    Cells in culture were irradiated in the lograithmic
and stationary phases of growth. The only survival
curve parameter to change was the extrapolation number
which was reduced from four to one. Fed stationary cells
encountered a block in G_1, while unfed ones experienced
a doubling in the cell cycle time. Unfed stationary
cells, unlike fed ones, were able to repair potentially
lethal radiation damage. Though synchrony might be the
explanation for the reduced extrapolation number of fed
cells, this is not so for the unfed ones.

REFERENCES

1. BERRY, R.J., *Brit. J. Radiol.*, *43*, 81, 1970.

2. HAHN, G.M., *Nature, 217*, 741, 1968.

3. LALA, P.K., In: *Effects of Radiation on Cellular
    Proliferation and Differentiation,* p. 463, I.A.E.A.,
    Vienna, 1968.

4. LITTLE, J.R., *Nature, 224*, 804, 1969.

5. MADOC-JONES, H., *Nature, 203,* 983, 1964.

INFLUENCE OF GROWTH PHASE AND CULTURAL CONDITIONS ON SURVIVAL OF IRRADIATED MAMMALIAN CELLS *IN VITRO**

JOHN. B. LITTLE

*Department of Physiology, Harvard University School of
Public Health, Boston, Massachusetts, U.S.A.*

When cultured mammalian cells growing in monolayer
are detached and explanted into new flasks at low concentration they are characterized by lag, exponential and
stationary or plateau phases of growth. In the stationary phase, the mitotic index and all-over DNA synthesis
are considerably decreased, while cell division is balanced by cell loss into the culture medium [4]. In the
present investigation, we have studied some of the factors which determine ultimate cell survival following irradiation in the various phases of growth. A most interesting finding is that stationary phase cultures release
a diffusible substance into the culture medium which promotes the repair of potentially lethal radiation damage
in exponentially growing cells.

MATERIALS AND METHODS

Chang liver cells were grown and plated for colony
forming ability in 25 CM^2 plastic "Falcon" flasks with
Eagle's minimal essential medium supplemented with Earle's
salts and 10% 56°C inactivated calf serum. Details concerning the preparation and maintenance of cultures and
the experimental methodology have been described [5].

*Supported by grant CA-11751 from the National Can-
cer Institute, U.S. Public Health Service.

Culture medium was changed daily, and experiments with stationary cultures performed after 8-10 days of growth when the cell numbers had reached a plateau of about 10^7 cells per flask. All conditioned media were centrifuged at ambient temperature and the supernatant used on the day of collection; plating efficiencies were obtained with the supernatant medium to make sure it contained no colony forming cells. The cells were irradiated with 250 KvP X-rays at 100 R/min at room temperature; otherwise, all incubations were carried out at 37°C.

RESULTS

Experiments in which the effects of the time of trypsinization and plating in relation to irradiation were studied are shown in Table 1. Survival parameters showed little change when the cells were irradiated immediately (about 30 min) before rather than immediately after trypsinization; the D_0 was consistently about 5R higher and $\tilde{n}$ slightly lower with irradiation before plating. When

Table 1. Effect of Time Between Platings and Irradiation on Survival Parameters

Time of irradiation in relation to plating	Exponential Cultures			Stationary Cultures		
	D_0	$N\tilde{n}$	N	D_0	$N\tilde{n}$	N
30 min before	156	1.8	---	127	3.1	---
30 min after	151	2.3	1.01	123	5.4	1.03
6 hrs after	160	2.0	1.10	133	5.0	1.08
24 hrs after	158	3.4	1.83	158	3.5	1.63

cultures were irradiated in the lag phase (30 min after plating), the D_0 was 5-10 R lower and $\tilde{n}$ slightly higher as compared with irradiation during exponential growth (24 hours). The most marked difference, however, was between cultures irradiated in stationary as compared with exponential growth.

It has been shown that if trypsinization and plating are delayed for 6 hours after irradiation of stationary phase cultures, these cultures will repair potentially lethal radiation damage [6]; this phenomenon is described in detail by Mauro in this symposium [8]. In Table 2, the results of an experiment are presented in which complete survival curves were obtained by exposing replicate groups of stationary and exponentially growing cultures to various doses of radiation following which trypsinization and plating were carried out either immediately or delayed for 6 hours after exposure. In both growth phases, survival was consistently enhanced when trypsinization was delayed, but the relative effect was considerably greater

Table 2. Effect of Time of Trypsinzation and Plating (Explant) After Irradiation and of Post-irradiation Medium Change on Survival Parameters.

Growth Phase	Time of Explant After Ir- radiation	Medium Change	Survival Parameters	
			D_0	$\tilde{n}$
Station- ary	Immediate	None	125	4.7
"	6 hrs	None	152	4.2
"	6 hrs	Fresh Medium	132	4.9
Exponen- tial	Immediate	None	145	4.5
"	6 hrs	None	160	4.2
"	6 hrs	Fresh Medium	158	4.3
"	6 hrs	Plateau Medium	185	3.3

in stationary as compared with exponential cultures. In the initial experiments, the culture medium was not changed on the day of the experiment (before the final trypsinization and plating). When the medium was changed immediately after irradiation, and the cells incubated in fresh medium for the 6 hour post-irradiation interval, the enhanced survival found with stationary cultures was markedly diminished whereas no change in ultimate survival occurred in exponential cultures.

These results suggested that the enhanced survival seen in irradiated cultures allowed to remain in the stationary phase of growth for 6 hours before trypsinization and plating was actually related to some factor either present or lacking in the culture medium in which the cells had been growing. This hypothesis is supported by the final results tabulated in Table 2; when exponentially growing cultures were incubated for 6 hours after irradiation and before trypsinization with conditioned medium from stationary cultures (Plateau Medium), the D_0 of the survival culture was increased by about 20%.

In order to elimate possible effects of trypsinization on these results, experiments were performed in which cells were irradiated 24 hours after plating while in optimal exponential growth. Immediately after irradiation, the cultures were incubated with conditioned medium from stationary cultures (Plateau Medium). Six hours later, they were changed to fresh medium and returned to the incubator for 12-14 days to assay for colony forming ability. The results of a typical experiment are shown in Fig. 1. The exposure of exponentially growing cells to plateau medium for a 6 hour interval after irradiation consistently enhanced net survival, primarily by increasing the slope of the dose-response curve.

It is known that cells incubated in balanced salt solution after irradiation will repair potentially lethal damage [2]. The restorative effect of plateau medium may likewise be due to the lack of some nutrient factor. In order to test this hypothesis, exponential cultures (plated 24 hours before) were incubated for 6 hours after irradiation in a 50-50 mixture of fresh and plateau medium and ultimate survival compared to that in cultures incubated with either medium alone. It was reasoned that

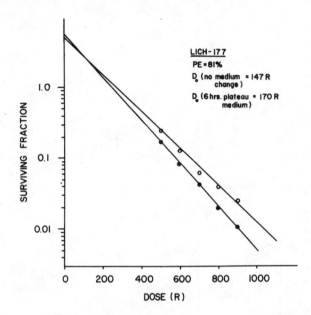

Fig. 1. Effect of conditioned medium from plateau phase cultures on
survival of exponentially growing cells. Cells were irradiated
24 hours after plating and either returned directly to the incubator to assay for colony forming ability (lower curve, closed
circles), or incubated for 6 hours after irradiation in medium
from stationary cultures (upper curve, open circles).

if some factor was lacking from the plateau medium, the
fresh medium in the 50-50 mixture should supply this substance in sufficient quantity to largely inhibit repair.
On the other hand, if repair was due to the presence of a
substance in plateau medium, the enhanced survival should
not be greatly affected by dilution of the plateau medium
with fresh medium.

The results of 2 such experiments are tabulated in
Table 3. In 4 out of 5 experiments in which cultures
were exposed to single doses of 800 or 1000 R, survival
of cells incubated with the 50-50 mixture approached that
of cells incubated with plateau medium alone, suggesting
that cells in stationary phase cultures release a difus-
sible substance into the culture medium which promotes

Table 3. Effect of Incubation for 6 Hours After Irradiation With Various Media on Surviving Fraction (%)*.

Experime (Dose)	No Medium (change)	Fresh Medium	Plateau Medium	1/2 Fresh 1/2 Plateau	56° inactivated Fresh Medium	56° inactivated Fresh Medium
LICH-177 (800 R)	2.01 ± 0.04	1.95 ± 0.04	4.04 ± 0.12	3.58 ± 0.10	---	---
LICH-187 (1000 R)	0.35 ± 0.04	0.44 ± 0.03	1.06 ± 0.16	0.83 ± 0.02	0.41 ± 0.05	0.51 ± 0.03

*Percent survival ± 1 S.D.

the repair of potentially lethal radiation damage. As is
also shown in Table 3, its activity appeared to be largely
inactivated if the plateau medium was incubated for one
hour at 56° C prior to use. Preliminary studies suggest,
furthermore, that relative survival become disproportion-
ately greater with higher radiation doses, and in one experiment several colonies grew out in cultures initially
containing 2×10^5 cells which were irradiated with 2000
R and incubated with plateau medium for 6 hours. If these
results can be confirmed, they may at least partially explain why surviving cells are occasionally found when
crowded cultures are irradiated with doses as high as
20,000 rads [7].

DISCUSSION

     It is obvious that cultural conditions play an import-
ant role in the apparent radiosensitivity of cultivated
mammalian cells and may explain in part the variations in
the results reported by different laboratories for similar
cell lines. As for the effect of plateau medium, it is
well known that conditioned media from mammalian cells
possess certain growth enhancing effects and recently it
has been shown that crowded or stationary phase cultures
may release into the medium substances which inhibit protein synthesis [1], and can depress both cell multipli-
cation and DNA synthesis in exponentially growing cells
[3]. The relationship between these observations and the
evidence presented here that stationary phase cultures may
also release a diffusible substance which promotes the repair of potentially lethal radiation damage is not clear
at the present time.

     If net survival of cells in a tissue can be influ-
enced by the presence of stationary cells which release a
substance which promotes repair, this phenomenon could be
of significance in the radiotherapy of malignant tumors.
Experimental evidence suggests that as tumors grow, hypoxic areas appear, the cells become crowded and many of them
stop proliferating and are arrested in some stage of the
life cycle. Tumors therefore have certain features in com-

mon with stationary phase cultures; as tumor growth proceeds and many of its cells become stationary, the tumor might likewise become more "resistant" to a single dose of radiation owing to the repair phenomenon. With a fractionated course of exposure, however, gradual cell depletion could lead to reoxygenation of hypoxic areas and less cell crowding; as a consequence stationary cells would begin cycling and the repair potential would be reduced. By such a mechanism, fractionated exposure might have a preferential killing effect as compared with single dose irradiation in tissues containing a substantial fraction of stationary but potentially clonigenic cells.

SUMMARY

The radiosensitivity of cultured mammalian cells varies with the growth phase of the culture, as well as with the time of trypsinization and plating in relation to irradiation. If plating is delayed for 6 hours after irradiation of stationary phase cultures, net survival is considerably enhanced. This effect appears to be due to the release by the cells of a diffusible substance which promotes the repair of potentially lethal damage in both stationary and exponentially growing cells.

ACKNOWLEDGMENT

I express my appreciation to Mrs. Helen Vetrovs for her expert technical assistance in these experiments.

REFERENCES

1.   BELANGER, F. and HAREL, L., *C.R. Acad. Sc., Paris, 269*, 113, 1969.

2.   BELLI, J.A. and SHELTON, M., *Science, 165*, 490, 1969.

3.   GARCIA-GIRALT, E. and MACIEIRA-COELHO, A., *C.R. Acad. Sci. Paris, 268*, 2316, 1969.

4.   HAHN, G.M., STEWART, J.R., YANG, S.J. and PARKER, V., *Exp. Cell Res.*, *49*, 285, 1968.

5.   LITTLE, J.B., *Radiology*, *93*, 307, 1969.

6.   LITTLE, J.B., *Nature*, *224*, 804, 1969.

7.   LUND, E. and ROSENGREN, B., *Internat. J. Radiat. Biol.*, *11*, 99, 1966.

8.   MAURO, F. and LITTLE, J.B. (This Book).

REPAIR OF POTENTIALLY LETHAL RADIATION DAMAGE IN PLATEAU PHASE CULTURES OF MAMMALIAN CELLS*

F. MAURO** and JOHN B. LITTLE

*Division of Radiation Biology, Institute of Radiology,
Washington University School of Medicine,
St. Louis, Mo. 63110, U.S.A.*

and

*Department of Physiology, Harvard University School of
Public Health, Boston, Mass. 02115, U.S.A.*

Repair of potentially lethal radiation damage, reported originally in bacteria and yeasts, has been observed in several lines of cultured mammalian cells in
which ultimate survival after a single radiation exposure
can be modified by a variety of pre- or post-irradiation conditions [1, 2, 11, 13]. This phenomenon
must be distinguished from the repair of sublethal damage between fractionated radiation doses, although this
distinction is experimental and does not imply differing mechanisms [3]. Studies of repair kinetics have
generally been performed with exponentially growing populations of mammalian cells. Recently, one of us [8]
has reported on the repair of potentially lethal damage

---

*This investigation was supported by Public Health
Service Research Grants CA-04483, CA-10435 and CA-11751
from the National Institutes of Health.

**Present address: Laboratorio di Radiobiologia
Animale Centro Studi Nucleari della Casaccia Comitato
Nazionale Enerbia Nucleare, C.P. 2400, 00100 Rome, A.D.
Italy.

949

in plateau phase cultures of a line of cells derived from
normal human liver (Chang). Plateau phase populations
differ in radiosensitivity from exponentially growing
cells and display different shapes of their survival
curves [5, 8, 10, 12]. As plateau phase cultures of mammalian cells have some interesting features in common with
in vivo systems such as tumors and normal renewal tissues
[6], it seemed of interest to explore in detail the kinetics of the repair of potentially lethal damage in several different cell lines.

MATERIALS AND METHODS

        Three lines of cultured cells were used: A line
derived from normal human liver (Chang), HeLa S3, and
Chinese hamster V79 (sub-line V79-735B-SL1). All lines
were grown as monolayer cultures (at 37°C, in an atmosphere of 5% CO_2 in air) in different media: Eagle's
Minimal Essential Medium with Earle's balanced salt solution, supplemented with non-essential amino acids and
10% heat-inactivated calf serum for Chang cells [8];
N16 medium supplemented with 20% human and 10% horse
serum for HeLa cells [7]; and HUT medium supplemented
with 15% fetal calf serum for Chinese hamster cells [4].
The cells had a mean generation time of approximately
24 h, 22 h, and 11 h respectively. The mitotic indices
and fraction of labelled cells following pulse-labelling
with tritiated thymidine are tabulated in Table 1.

        For the experiments, cells were grown in plastic
vessels (Falcon). "Fed" cultures of Chang cells were
initially implanted with 5.0×10^5 cells in 5 ml of
medium, the nutrient medium was then changed daily and
the experiments performed 8 to 10 days later when the
cells were in the plateau phase, at a concentration of
$1.0-1.2 \times 10^7$ per bottle. "Unfed" cultures of Chang
cells were implanted with 5.0×10^4 cells, with no subsequent medium changes. By the 8th day, when the experiments were performed, the cell concentration had
reached a plateau of approximately 1.5×10^6 cells.

        In the case of HeLa and Chinese hamster cells, the

TABLE 1. Survival and Proliferation Parameters of Log and Plateau Phase Cultures

Cell line	Phase	t between irradiation & plating	Fraction labelled cells*	Fraction mitotic cells**	Survival parameters D_0 (rads)	D_q (rads)
Chang ("fed")	log	0 h	0.34	0.034	155	91
	plateau	0 h	0.14***	0.012†	123	190
		6 h			152	225
		12 h			156††	228
HeLa S3	log	0 h	0.42†††	0.033	89	203
	plateau	0 h	0.086††††	0.0086	74	10
		6 h			82	6
		12 h			102	4
Chin. hamster V79	log	0 h	0.51†††	0.050	134	383
	plateau	0 h	0.0096†††	0.0031	121	58
		5 h			140	78
		10 h			155	95

*1 h tritiated thymidine pulse.
**Scored as rounded-up cells.
***The value for "unfed" cultures is 0.012.
†The value for "unfed" cultures is 0.010.
††In one of three experiments, the D_0 was 173 rads.
†††In collaboration with H. Madoc-Jones.

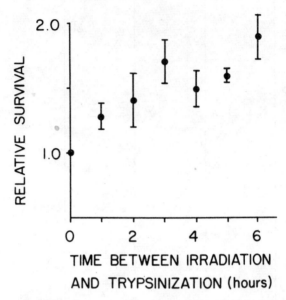

Fig. 1.   The effect of various intervals of incubation after irradiation
and before plating on the survival (500 rads) of plateau phase
cultures of Chang cells. Mean results from 6 different experiments ± 1 S.E.   Although the degree to which survival was enhanced by allowing the cells to remain in the stationary phase
after irradiation varied among experiments, the surviving fraction after 4 hours was always less than that found after either
3 or 6 hours.

initial inoculum was either 1.5×10^4 or 1.5×10^5 cells
per dish in 13 ml of medium and the medium was left unchanged.   For HeLa cells the experiments, according to
the initial inoculum, were performed 8 to 9 or 4 to 5
days later when the cells were in the plateau phase, at
a concentration of $1.5-2.0 \times 10^6$ cells per dish.   For
Chinese hamster cells the experiments were performed,
according to the initial inoculum, 6 to 7 or 4 to 5 days
later when the cells were in the plateau phase, at a
concentration of $1.2-1.5 \times 10^6$ cells per dish.

In a typical experiment, plateau phase populations
were irradiated at room temperature in flasks or dishes
containing the growth media indicated.   Immediately or

at the desired interval of time after the irradiation,
the cells were trypsinized, diluted with fresh medium to
the desired concentration and replated. Cell survival
was then determined from counts of macroscopic colonies.

RESULTS

Repair of Potentially Lethal Damage in Chang Cells

Figure 1 shows the mean data from 6 different experiments in which replicate plateau phase cultures ("fed")
of Chang cells were irradiated with 500 rads, returned to
the incubator for 0-6 h, then trypsinized and plated for
colony-forming ability. Survival was enhanced by a factor of approximately two when 6 h elapsed between irradiation and plating. Enhanced survival was observed in
"unfed" as well as in "fed" cultures and the major component of repair occurred within the first 6 hours.

Repair of Potentially Lethal Damage in HeLa S3 Cells

The lower curve in Fig. 2 represents the results of
an experiment in which plateau phase HeLa cells were irradiated with a single dose of 200 rads, returned to the
incubator for different intervals of time (0 to 120 h),
then trypsinized and plated for colony-forming ability.
Survival as a function of the time interval starts to
rise immediately and by 24 h is enhanced by approximately
a factor of 6. The curve has two components with the
change in slope taking place at around 24 h. The second
component indicates a further continuous increase in
survival up to an enhancement factor of about 14 by
120 h.

The upper curves in Fig. 2 show the results of the
same type of experiments when the cells were monitored
under the microscope. Previous observations had shown
that unirradiated HeLa cells maintain the same cell concentration for 5 days after entering the plateau phase.
During this period of time, however, some of the cells
detach from the surface (presumably loosing viability)
and are replaced in the population by proliferating cells
(H. Madoc-Jones, personal communication). It was

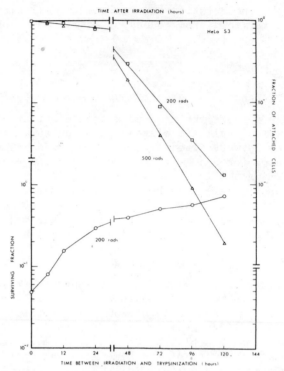

Fig. 2.   Lower curve (circles): The effect of various intervals of in-
          cubation after irradiation and before plating on the survival
          (200 rads) of plateau phase cultures of HeLa S3 cells. Upper
          curves: Fraction of cells still attached to the dish as a
          function of time after irradiation with 200 rads (squares) or
          500 rads (triangles).

necessary, therefore, to exclude the possibility that the
increase in survival could be due to selective cell detachment of "doomed" cells. Such a possibility can be
excluded in the case of Chang cells because of the shorter intervals of time before plating; in the case of
Chinese hamster cells, it can be discarded on other
grounds (see below). The results in Fig. 2 indicate
that after irradiation the number of cells attached to
the surface is maintained nearly constant up to 24 h.

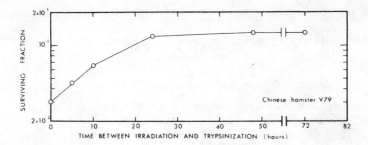

Fig. 3. The effect of various intervals of incubation after irradiation
         and before plating on the survival (500 rads) of plateau phase
         cultures of Chinese hamster V79 cells.

After that, the number of attached cells begins to decrease exponentially with time and in a dose-dependent
fashion. It can be concluded that the initial increase
in survival (0 to 24 h) represents the true repair of
potentially lethal damage, whereas the secondary increase
may be due to the preferential presence of surviving
cells in the fraction of the populating which is still
attached and therefore is ultimately plated for colony
forming ability. This possibility is supported by the
fact that survival as a function of time does not seem
to reach a final plateau, in contrast to the case of
Chinese hamster cells described below.

*Repair of Potentially Lethal Damage in Chinese Hamster
V79 Cells*

Figure 3 shows the results of an experiment in
which plateau phase Chinese hamster cells were irradiated with a single dose of 500 rads, returned to the
incubator for 0 to 72 h, then trypsinized and plated
for colony-forming ability. Once again, survival as a
function of time starts to rise immediately and reaches
a final plateau by approximately 24 h with an enhancement factor of 4-5. In the case of Chinese hamster
cells, there are no complications due to cell detachment or cell turnover. The fraction of proliferating
cells in unirradiated cultures is very small and after
irradiation with 500 rads no cell detachment is observed

by 48 h; 20% or less are detached, but not replaced, by
72 h. Enhanced survival can therefore be considered to
result entirely from the repair of potentially lethal
damage.

Lack of Effect of Trypsinization on Repair

In several control experiments utilizing all 3
lines, asynchronous logarithmically growing cells were
irradiated and then trypsinized and replated at different times after irradiation. With the exception of a
small increase in survival with the Chang cells [9], no
significant changes in survival were observed when cells
were replated immediately or at various times after if-
radiation. The possibility still existed that the repair could be due to an effect of trypsinization on
plateau phase cells only. Experiments were therefore
performed in which cells were removed at different times
after irradiation by mechanical detachment. The enhanced survival still took place regularly, and its
kinetics were indistinguishable from those described
above, indicating that trypsinization itself was not a
significant factor in the repair phenomenon.

DISCUSSION

The phenomenon of repair of plateau phase cells has
been also analyzed in terms of survival curves obtained
with graded doses of radiation. The findings are summarized in Table 1 where the parameters describing proliferative characteristics as well as the survival curves
are given for the three lines in both exponentially growing and plateau phase cultures. The characteristics of
the survival curves for plateau phase cells seem to be
dependent on the cell line tested: HeLa cells exhibit no
initial shoulder; Chinese hamster cells also have a very
small or absent shoulder as originally reported by Hahn
[5], whereas Chang cells show a considerable shoulder
(the D_q is more than twice the value for log populations)
as well as the ability to recover from sublethal damage
[8]. In all three lines, however, the slope of the survival curve (D_0) is smaller in the plateau phase than in

the log phase and probably similar to that of logarithmically growing populations synchronized at the G_1/S
transition.

The survival parameters for different intervals of
time between irradiation and replating (Table 1) clearly
indicate that the variations in survival are characterized
by an increase in slope rather than by changes in shoulder
width of the survival curve. It is interesting to note
that by 10-12 h the slope of the curve for plateau phase
cells of all three lines is already the same or higher
than that for logarithmically growing cells. The repair of potentially lethal damage appears to be a similar phenomenon in all three lines, despite the differences in the nutritional status and the degree of proliferative activity taking place in the respective
plateau phase populations (Table 1). The presence of a
shoulder on the survival curve also seems to be independent of the proliferation characteristics of the cell
line. The major difference among the 3 cell lines as to
potentially lethal damage repair seems to be in the maximum repair they can achieve: Chang cells reach a maximum survival by 6 to 12 h after irradiation (and before
replating) whereas HeLa and Chinese hamster cells continue
to show a survival increase up to about 24 h. Preliminary observations related to serum concentration and HeLa
cell growth (M. Logie and H. Madoc-Jones, personal com-
munications), however, suggest that this factor may also
influence the time course for this repair.

If these observations obtained with plateau phase
cultures can be applied to the *in vivo* situation, then
repair of potentially lethal damage must be added to
the other factors (proliferation characteristics, clo-
nogenicity, degree of oxygenation, presence of the
shoulder) affecting the overall response of malignant
tumors to fractionated radiotherapy.

SUMMARY

The repair of potentially lethal radiation damage
has been shown to occur in 3 lines of cultures mammalian

cells if they are allowed to remain in the plateau phase
of growth for 2 to 24 hours after irradiation. Enhanced
survival was characterized by an increase in slope of
the survival surve, and the amount of repair was similar
in all 3 cell lines, despite significant differences in
their proliferative activities.

REFERENCES

1.   BEER, J.Z., LETT, J.T. and ALEXANDER, P., *Nature*,
     199, 193, 1963.

2.   BELLI, J.A. and BONTE, F.J., *Radiation Res.*, *18*,
     272, 1963.

3.   ELKIND, M.M., KAMPER, C., MOSES, W.B. and SUTTON-
     GILBERT,H., *Brookhaven Symp. Biol.*, *20*, 134, 1968.

4.   ELKIND, M.M. and SUTTON, H., *Radiation Res.*, *13*,
     556, 1960.

5.   HAHN, G.M., *Nature*, *217*, 741, 1968.

6.   HAHN, G.M., (This symposium).

7.   HAM, R.G. and PUCK, T.T., *Methods Enzymol.*, *5*, 77,
     1962.

8.   LITTLE, J.B., *Nature*, *224*, 804, 1969.

9.   LITTLE, J.B., (This symposium).

10. MADOC - JONES, H., *Nature*, *203*, 983, 1964.

11. MAURO, F. and ELKIND, M.M., *Science*, *155*, 1561.

12. PHILLIPS, R.A. and TOLMACH, L.J., *Radiation Res.*,
     29, 413, 1966.

13. RÉVÉSZ, L. and LITTBRAND, B., *Exptl. Cell Res.*,
     55, 283, 1969.

14. WHITMORE, G.F. and GULYAS, S., Abstract 253, Intern.
     Congress, *Radiation Res.*, Cortina d'Ampezzo
     (Italy) 1966.

CELL SYNCHRONIZATION BY RELEASING CONTACT INHIBITION AND ITS APPLICATION TO THE STUDY OF RADIATION EFFECTS ON DIFFERENT STAGES OF THE CELL CYCLE

H. YOSHIKURA

Institut du Radium, Biologie, Faculté des Sciences, Bâtiment 110, 91 Orsay, France

C3H2K cell line originating from the kidney tissues of a newborn C3H/He mouse is sensitive to contact inhibition: the cell replication stopped in the G_1 phase when confluent monolayer was formed, and resumed in a synchronized fashion when cell-cell contact was removed by scraping the monolayer or when culture medium (Eagle's MEM + 10% calf serum + 10% tryptose phosphate broth) was renewed [7]. Serum factor(s) are responsible for the induction of cell replication in the latter case. After medium change, DNA synthesis began at 10 hr and reached its maximum at 20 hr; mitosis occurred 10 hr later than DNA synthesis. There were two peaks of RNA synthesis, immediately after medium change and just before the DNA synthesis (Fig. 1, bottom). These properties are quite similar to those of 3T3 cells [5]. Synchronization index calculated by Blumenthal and Zahler's method [1] was 39%. The characteristics of this synchronization method are its physiologicalness and availability of a large amount of farily synchronized cells.

EFFECT OF X-RAYS AND ULTRAVIOLET LIGHT (UV) ON THE GROWTH OF THE CELLS AT DIFFERENT STAGES OF THE CELL CYCLE

Estimation of cell survival by colonial growth was unsuccessful because of low plating efficiency (lower

959

960

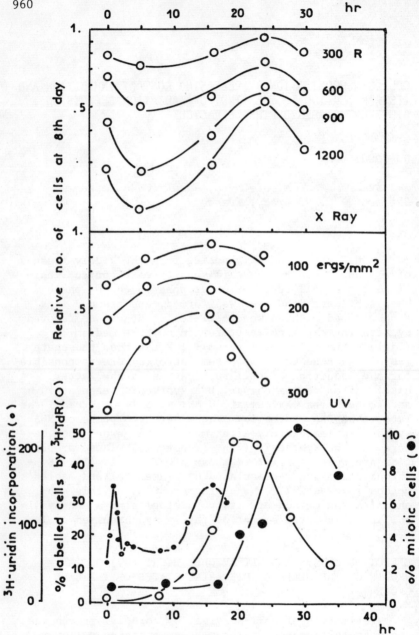

Fig. 1. Sequence of DNA and RNA synthesis and also of mitosis during the synchronized cell division (bottom) and effects of radiations on the growth of the cells irradiated at different stages of the cell cycle (upper 2 figures).

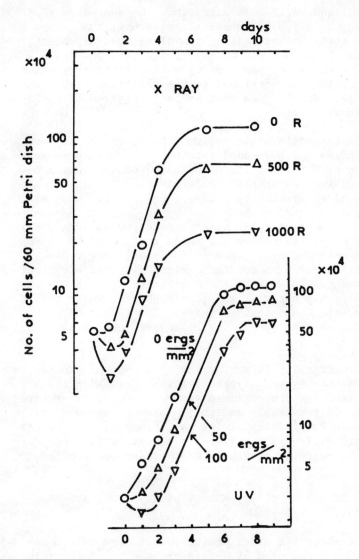

Fig. 2. Growth curve of the irradiated cells.

than 5%) and rapid cell migration. So another method
was sought. Figure 2 shows the growth of the irradiated cells. There was an immediate dose-dependent
cellular loss followed by the growth at normal rate.
Then the cells stopped growing at a cell density which
was inversely proportional to the radiation dose. This
final cell density was used as an indication of radiation sensitivity.

At intervals after medium change, the cells were
trypsinized and suspended into the medium to a concentration of 5×10^4 cells/ml. The suspension was distributed into 60-mm plastic Petri dishes in an amount of
1 ml, and irradiated by X-rays (Vega 250 kV X-ray machine; dose rate, 60 R/min) or by UV (a low pressure
mercury lamp, λ = 2,537 Å; dose rate, 10 ergs/mm^2/sec).
Then 2 ml of the medium was added to each dish. After
8 days when the cells were in the stationary phase,
the cell number was counted. Figure 1 shows a typical
experiment. To X-rays, the maximum resistance was observed in the early G_1 and late S phases, while to UV
in the late G_1 to early S phase. The result is similar to the one reported by Djordjevic and Tolmach in
HeLa cells [2].

A difficulty in performing this type of experiment in this system is the fact that detaching the
cells from the dishes immediately before or after irradiation is inevitable and this procedure may modify the
intrinsic sensitivity of the cells in a given stage of
the cell cycle. The difficulty of estimating cell survival by colonial growth is another serious problem.

EFFECT OF γ-RAYS (^{60}Co) AND UV LIGHT ON DNA AND RNA
SYNTHESIS

At intervals after medium change, the cell monolayer was irradiated by γ-rays or by UV. ^{3}H-thymidine
incorporation (for 1 hr) of all the samples was measured
23 hr after medium change. For RNA synthesis, ^{3}H-uridine
incorporation (for 1 hr) was measured just after medium
change. The results shown in Fig. 3 show:

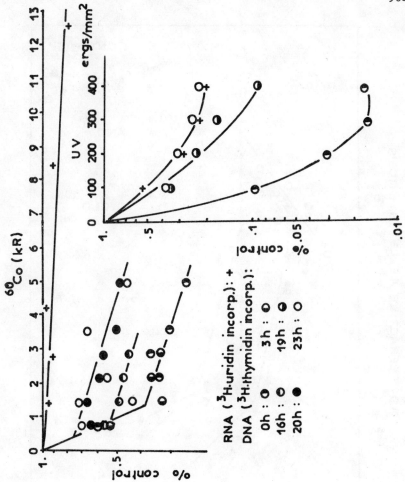

Fig. 3. Radiation effects on DNA and RNA (first peak) synthesis.

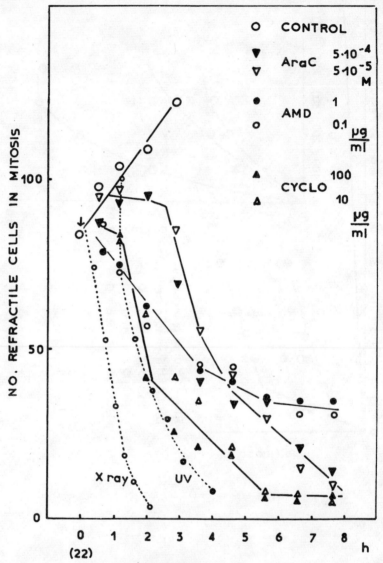

Fig. 4. Mitotic inhibition by radiations or by antimetabolites. The
cells were irradiated or contacted with an antimetabolite at
the time indicated by an arrow.

CYCLO: cycloheximide; AMD: actinomycin D; AraC: cytosine
arabinoside.

1) All γ-ray dose-response curves for DNA synthesis
were biphasic in accordance with the classical data [3,
4]. The resistant portion of the curves was gradually
elevated as the interval between medium change and irradiation increased, suggesting the fact that population of the cells whose DNA synthesis is radioresistant
increased as the cell cycle proceeded from the G_1 to S
phase. The radiosensitive portion probably represents
the sensitivity of initiation of DNA synthesis, while the
radioresistant portion, that of DNA synthesis already in
progress.

With UV, an essentially similar phenomenon was
observed.

2) The radiosensitivity of RNA synthesis is low,
but is not so widely different from that of DNA synthesis already in progress. This may suggest that
common radiation damages are responsible for arresting
continuation of DNA duplication and transcription of
DNA.

3) Within physiological doses, UV inhibits DNA or
RNA synthesis more strongly than γ-rays.

4) It is difficult to correlate the cell-cycle-
dependent radiation sensitivity of cell growth and
that of DNA synthesis.

EFFECT OF X-RAYS AND UV LIGHT ON MITOSIS

Figure 4 shows the time course of mitotic inhibition by radiation or by antimetabolites at 23 hr. The
slope of the curves was independent of the radiation
dose, if the dose was higher than 100 R in the case of
X-rays and 100 ergs/mm^2 in the case of UV. When the
cells were incubated in the medium containing any one
of the antimetabolites after irradiation, the curve was
nearly identical to the one produced by radiation alone.
The onset of radiation-induced mitotic block was abrupt,
while the one induced by antimetabolites insidious. The
time delay between X-ray irradiation and the onset of

mitotic inhibition was actually zero (shorter than 20 min, if any), while there was 1 hr of time delay between cycloheximide (protein inhibitor) addition and the onset of mitotic inhibition. This is in contradiction to Walters and Petersen's data [6] and may suggest that the radiation-induced mitotic inhibition is not simply due to a translation defect. On the other hand, mitotic recovery from γ-ray radiation damage seems to require the protein synthesis: partial mitotic recovery occurred in the presence of cytosine arabinoside (10^{-5} M), DNA inhibitor, or actinomycin D (0.1 μg/ml), RNA inhibitor, but not in the presence of cycloheximide (10 μg/ml).

After UV irradiation, mitosis proceeded completely normally for 80 min, and then mitotic cells sharply decreased in number. This UV-induced mitotic block is probably not the one brought about by over-all inhibition of DNA synthesis, because mitotic inhibition by cytosine arabinoside was about 2 hr later than UV-induced mitotic block.

The work reported in this paper was undertaken during the tenure of a Research Training Fellowship awarded by the International Agency for Research on Cancer. I thank Dr. Ethel Moustacchi and Dr. R. Latarjet for their advice.

SUMMARY

I presented a cell synchronization method by releasing the cells from contact inhibition. Cell cycle-dependent variations in radiation sensitivity of macro-molecular synthesis and cell growth were described.

REFERENCES

1.   BLUMENTHAL, L.K. and ZAHLER, S.A., *Science*, *135*, 724, 1962.

2.   DJORDJEVIC, B. and TOLMACH, L.J., *Radiation Res.*, *32*, 327, 1967.

3. LAJTHA, L.G., OLIVER, R., BERRY, R. and NOYES, W.D., *Nature, 182*, 1788, 1958.

4. ORD, M.G. and STOCKEN, L.A., *Nature, 182*, 1787, 1958.

5. TODARO, G.J., LAZAR, G.K. and GREEN, H., *J. Cell Comp. Physiol., 66*, 325, 1966.

6. WALTERS, R.A. and PETERSEN, D.F., *Biophys. J., 8*, 1487, 1968.

7. YOSHIKURA, H. and HIROKAWA, Y., *Exp. Cell Res., 52*, 439, 1968.

RADIOSENSITIVITY OF NON-DIVIDING CELLS *IN VIVO*

N.F. KEMBER

Dept. of Medical Physics, Royal Free Hospital, School of Medicine, London, W.C. 1, England

INTRODUCTION

The survival system based on the recovery of irradiated growth cartilage offers the possibility of examining the relative radiosensitivities of the phases of the cell cycle *in vivo*. Three methods suggest themselves for the production of synchrony or partial synchrony in this system:

1.   The use of radiation: if a conditioning dose produces partial synchrony by preferential killing of cells in one phase, then the sensitivity round the cell cycle may be tested by giving second doses at a range of time intervals. A split dose experiment was tried (Kember 1967) and some variation in sensitivity with time following the conditioning dose was found. It was not clear, however, if this was a result of synchronisation since examination of the mitotic index following the conditioning dose used (1600 rads), showed no significant degree of synchrony. It is possible that this experiment should be repeated using a lower conditioning dose.

2.   The use of physiological controls: the cells in growth cartilage might be induced to some degree of synchrony by reducing the rate of division by hypophysectomy and subsequently giving growth hormone to 'trigger off' cell division. This approach has been tried and is described in this paper.

3.   The use of drugs such as hydroxyurea: this system
does not appear to be suitable for the use of drugs which
kill or block cells selectively at one stage in the cycle
since the generation time of the cartilage cells is of the
order of 40 - 50 hours and therefore any drug treatment
would have to be extended over a large fraction of this
period in order to produce a reasonable degree of cell
synchrony when the drug is discontinued. It is then likely that a lethal dose would have been administered to the
more rapidly dividing cells in the gut and bone marrow.
Pilot experiments are now in progress using hydroxyurea
and the results will be reported elsewhere.

RADIATION EXPERIMENTS ON GROWTH CARTILAGE IN HYPOPHYSEC-
TOMISED RATS

Young male Wistar rats were hypophysectomised by the
transaural route and the success of hypophysectomy was
judged from inspection of the excised pituatries and from
daily weighings of the animals. Rats were taken at intervals of one day to twelve weeks after hypophysectomy and
the labelling index, that is the percentage of cartilage
plate nuclei labelled at one hour after injection of tritiated thymidine, was measured. It was found that the
percentage of labelled cells dropped rapidly from the
normal level of 10% over the first four days after operation, and then continued at a steady reduced level of
2% thereafter. This continued proliferation of the cells
of the growth cartilage in hypophysectomised rats implies
either a large fraction of the cells out of cycle (G_0) or
an increase in the average length of G1.

By giving the hypophysectomised rats a week's course
of 5 mg per day Thiouracil, an anti-thyroid drug, the percentage labelling index was reduced to less than 0.5 percent. The first series of radiation experiments was carried out on animals under this condition, although it
should be remembered that the labelling index by itself
does not describe the state of proliferation of a population. It is also necessary to know the length of the
synthesis period and there was some evidence from work
with labelled mitoses that the synthesis time in hypophy-
sectomized animals was longer by 50 - 100% than in normal
young rats.

It was found possible to carry out radiation experiments on these hypophysectomised animals if a course of daily injection of growth hormone (100 µgm/day) was given after the irradiation. By twenty-five days, recovery clones could be counted as usual in histological sections.

Doses of 1700 and 1800 rads of 250 kV X-rays were localised to the hind legs. These doses produced a survival level in the growth cartilage of 10^{-3} to 10^{-4}. In Table 1 the survival level in hypophysectomised rats is compared with that in normal rats of the same age but one would hesitate to say that the doubling in survival is significant since the experiments are not directly comparable. The number of recovery clones seen in the growth cartilage of the hypophysectomised rats was similar to that observed in the normal rats, but there is a reduction in the number of cells at risk due to the decrease in the densities of columns in the cartilage plates of hypophysectomised animals. This reduction in the cells at risk is about 50%. In one experiment normal rats were given growth hormone during the twenty-five day period following irradiation but no increase in the number of recovery clones was detected following this treatment.

Split dose experiments were also carried out on the hypophysectomised rats, single doses of 1800 rads being given to one leg of an animal and split doses of 900 + 900 rads to the other leg with a six hour interval between. If the recovery ratio is defined as the number of clones in the leg receiving a split dose divided by the number following a single dose, then the recovery ratio in hypophysectomised rats was not significantly different from that found in normal animals (See Table). Thus in hypophysectomised animals treated with Thiouracil the rate of cell division in the growth cartilage is reduced by a factor of at least 20 but there is no significant change in either radiosensitivity or in the ability of the cells to recover between split doses. This does not agree with published results of similar, if not strictly comparable, experiments in other systems. Hahn (1968) found no recovery in cells during the stationary

phase of culture growth and Coggle (1968) who investigated chromosome damage in liver, found no recovery until
the tissue was induced to regenerate following hepatec-
tomy.

ATTEMPTS TO PRODUCE SYNCHRONY OF CELL DIVISION IN HYPOPHY-
SECTOMISED ANIMALS

Following the injection of bovine growth hormone to
hypophysectomised rats it was found that the labelling index increased after a delay of about 8 - 12 hours (Kember
1971). However the maximum labelling, which occurs at
about twenty-four hours following a single dose of growth
hormone, was not increased above 18%, that is about twice
the normal labelling index in animals of this age.
Thiouracil was given as a pre-treatment for a week and
Thyroxine was adminstered with the growth hormone, the
maximum labelling index was increased to 25%. The effect
was dependent on the dose of growth hormone given, up to
400 µg, but beyond this no further increase in labelling
occurred.

Some radiation experiments were carried out under
these conditions of partial synchrony. Rats were irradiated with 1700 rads to one leg and then the growth
hormone was given, the other leg being irradiated with a
similar dose at intervals of twelve or twenty-four hours
after the growth hormone. There was no detectable change
in the sensitivity of cells at these intervals after
growth hormome injection (See Table).

One split dose experiment was also carried out at
twenty to twenty-six hours following growth hormone but
the recovery ratio was not different from that found in
normal animals (see Table).

These radiation experiments have little value since
no useful degree of synchrony occurred in these experiments. Not only was the number of cells in the synthesis
phase increased little above the normal levels, but the
rate of increase was slow so that at the time of irradiation cells would be found in both early and late S

Table of Results

	Normal	Hypophy-sectomy + Thiour-acil	12 hrs after Growth Hormone	24 hrs after Growth Hormone
Labelling Index 10%		0.5%	2%	25%
Compara-tive sur-vival Single Dose	1.0	2.6 ± 2.3 (5) 1.0	0.5 ± 0.2 (4)	0.9 ± 0.4 (9)
Split dose ratio: 6 hour interval	4.4 ± 1.5 (5)	3.8 ± 1.3 (10)	-	5.1 ± 1.6 (6)

Results with standard deviations. Number of rats per experiment in brackets.

phase. Higher labelling indices have been reported following injections of repeated doses of growth hormone, but here again the overlap of cells in early and late S is likely to be large. It is difficult to imagine any method of producing a good degree of synchrony in this system.

SUMMARY

    In hypophysectomised rats the rate of cell division can be reduced by a factor of 20. Under these conditions there may be some decrease in cell radiosensitivity but there is no detectable change in the ability of cells to recover between split doses.

ACKNOWLEDGEMENT

    This work was supported by a grant from the British Empire Cancer Campaign for Research.

REFERENCES

1.   COGGLE, J., *Nature, 217*, 180, 1968.

2.   HAHN, G., *Nature, 217*, 741, 1968.

3.   KEMBER, N., *Brit. J. Radiol., 40*, 496, 1967.

4.   KEMBER, N., In: *Clinical Orthopaedics, 76*, 213, 1971.

ALTERED RECOVERY IN NON-CYCLING BONE MARROW STEM CELLS*,**

GERALD E. HANKS

*Department of Radiology,Division of
Radiation Therapy, The University of
North Carolina, School of Medicine,
Chapel Hill, North Carolina 27514, U.S.A.*

High specific activity tritiated thymidine suicide
and Vinblastine experiments have demonstrated that the
colony-forming unit (CFU) compartment of mouse bone marrow contains a group of cells that do not undergo mitosis or DNA synthesis in a 24 hour period [1,7]. These
non-cycling CFU may play a particularly important role
in re-populating bone marrow after depletion with cycle-
active chemotherapeutic agents, and the existence of this
compartment has partially provided the basis for logical
programs of cyclic chemotherapeutic administration.

The radiation single-dose response curve of this
non-cycling CFU compartment was shown to have a D_0 similar to CFU as a whole, but no shoulder on the dose response curve [3,6]. When Chinese hamster cells were irradiated in the stationary phase of growth and compared
with exponentially growing cells, they had a reduced
shoulder, similar D_0, and a reduction in early recovery

---

*This work was supported in part by the American
Cancer Society #T-472 and the National Cancer Institute,
2 RO1 CA 11284-02.

**A portion of this work was performed in the Ra-
diobiology Laboratories of Stanford University, Palo
Alto, California.

975

as measured by split-dose radiation studies [2]. More recent observations have indicated the complexity of this *in vitro* system and indicate nutritional factors or post-irradiation conditions may influence this response [5].

The current experiments extend the previous radiation dose response observations on non-cycling bone marrow cells and demonstrate the split-dose radiation response of these cells.

MATERIALS & METHODS

C57 Black Male Mice between 100 and 110 days of age weighing 25 plus or minus·2 grams were used for bone marrow donors in these experiments. Non-cycling cells were quantitatively removed from the tibia of donor mice 24 hours after 0.75 mgs. of Vinblastine was given intraperitoneally. Previous studies indicate a further increase in Vinblastine resulted in no further depression of CFU content (16% of control). Control cells were obtained from the tibia of carefully matched untreated mice and quantitatively transplanted by previously published techniques [8]. Recipient mice received 700 R total body exposure for hours prior to bone marrow transplantation, and recipient and donor mouse irradiation was delivered with 250 KVP; 15 ma., H.V.L. 1.1 mm. Cu., dose rate 32R/Min.

In both the single and split-dose studies of non-cycling and control marrow, the irradiation dose was given to the donor animal prior to quantitative trans plantation. Spleens were harvested 8 days after bone marrow transplantation, counted by a double blind technique, and surviving fractions calculated.

EXPERIMENTAL RESULTS

Suvival Curve for Control and Non-Cycling CFU:

1. Figure 1 shows the single dose response curve for control and non-cycling bone marrow colony-form-

ing units. There is no difference in D_0 between control
and non-cycling bone marrow CFU, and non-cycling CFU
have no shoulder on the single dose response curve.

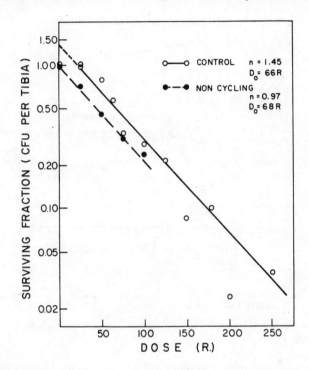

Fig. 1. Single dose-response curves for control and non-cycling CFU.

Early Repair in Control and Non-Cycling CFU:

   Figure 2 shows the surviving fraction observed in
control and non-cycling CFU after selected single radiation doses, and the result of dividing these doses into two equal fractions separated by 1,2, or 4 hours.
There was no significant difference in surviving fraction in the non-cycling cells when the dose was split,
while there is a significant increase in survival when
the dose is delivered in two equal fractions to control
CFU. The asterisks indicate split-dose surviving frac-

tions that differ from their respective single dose surviving fractions at the 95% confidence levels.

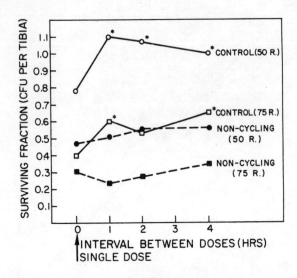

Fig. 2.   Selected single and split-dose responses of control and non-
          cycling bone marrow CFU.

DISCUSSION

     The radiation responses of non-cycling compartments
are of great interest in clinical radiation therapy as
experimental and human tumor systems have been shown to
contain large variable fractions of cells that may be
called non-cycling. The present studies indicate that
non-cycling bone marrow colony-forming units do have a
differential response as compared to control cells.
This differential lies in a reduction in their ability
to repair sub-lethal injury, although it remains to be
proven whether this phenomenon is common to other mammalian cells *in vivo* , particularly tumor cell populations.

     If non-cycling tumor cell populations exhibit a
similar response, the reduced ability to repair sub-

lethal injury would result in a major advantage in the response of the tumor to fractionated radiation therapy.

REFERENCES

1.   BRUCE, W.R. and MEEKER, B.E., *J. Nat. Cancer Inst.*, *34*, 849, 1965.

2.   HAHN, G.M., *Nature*, *217*, 741, 1968.

3.   HANKS, G.E., *Radiation Research*, *35*, 570, 1968.

4.   HANKS, G.E. and AINSWORTHE, E.J., *Nature*, *215*, 20, 1967.

5.   LITTLE, J.B., *Nature*, *224*, 804, 1969.

6.   SILINI, G., ELLI, R., SIRACUSA,G., and POZZI, L.Z., *Cell and Tissue Kinetics*, *1*, 111, 1968.

7.   VALERIOTTE, F.A., BRUCE, W.R., and MEEKER, B.E., *J. Nat. Cancer Inst.*, *36*, 21, 1966.

RECOVERY AND REPAIR OF RADIATION DAMAGE IN YEAST CELLS

W. POHLIT

Gesellschaft für Strahlenforschung mbH. Abteilung Biophysikalische Strahlenforschung, Frankfurt/Main, W. Germany

TARGET THEORY

In the classical target theory it is assumed that an irradiated object is transformed from a state "A" into another state "B". For obtaining dose effect curves with a shoulder, multiple hits or multiple targets are assumed. A comparison of experimental curves for surviving diploid yeast cells with calculated curves as in Fig. 1a results in a target number of about n = 3. There is, however, no other indication for the presence of three targets in a yeast cell. Therefore a less formalistic model should be derived for the explanation of dose effect curves for living cells.

RADIATION SENSITIVITY

During irradiation with sparsely ionizing radiation radicals are produced from water molecules in the cell. These radicals can diffuse through the cell and can inactivate organic molecules. As a working hypothesis it should be assumed that the DNA is the essential molecule, responsible for the cell to be in state "A" or in "B". The probability of a radical reaction with this essential molecule depends on the concentration of other organic molecules in its surrounding medium, which can compete with the DNA in radical reactions. If this concentration is high, the "radiation sensitivity" of the essential molecule is low,

and vice versa. Due to irradiation this radiation sensitivity may increase due to reduction of the surrounding
molecules. This transforms the cell from the original
state "A" into a more sensitive state "A' ".

Using this model a simple formula can be derived for
the decrease of cells in state "A" (see Fig. 1b). From

with
$$\frac{dC_A}{C_A} = -\eta_{AB}^*(D) \cdot dD$$

$$\eta_{AB}^*(D) = \eta_{AB} \left[1 - \exp\left[-\eta_{AA'} \cdot D \right] \right]$$

it follows
$$\frac{C_A}{A_0} = \exp \left\{ -\eta_{AB} \cdot D + \frac{\eta_{AB}}{\eta_{AA'}} \left[1 - \exp\left[-\eta_{AA'} \cdot D \right] \right] \right\}$$

where η_{AB} is the maximum value of the reaction constant
for the transformation from state "A" to "B" and $\eta_{AA'}$ is
the reaction constant for the surrounding molecules. A
comparison with experimental values for diploid yeast results in values for $\eta_{AB} / \eta_{AA'}$ of about one. This means
that the reaction rate of radicals with the essential molecule is of the same order as with the surrounding organic
molecules. Since both are organic macromolecules, this result seems reasonable.

Changes in the structure of the essential molecule
due to irradiation would lead also to an increase in radiation sensitivity. The same mathematical formalism can be
used in this case, but the meaning of $\eta_{AA'}$ is then different.

RECOVERY

The radiation sensitivity of the essential molecule
is assumed to increase during irradiation. A reversed reaction, called "recovery", can be seen in cells which were
irradiated with two fractions of absorbed dose. As shown
in Fig. 2a, after a first irradiation with $D_1 = 60$ krad an
interval of t_{rec} without irradiation is introduced. If
the cells were supplied with an energy source they repro-

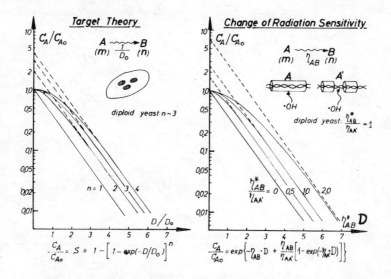

Fig. 1. a) Dose effect curves calculated by using the multitarget theory.

b) Dose effect curves calculated by using a changing radiation sensitivity.

produce the destroyed molecules and recover their initial low radiation sensitivity of state "A". The subsequent dose effect curve with various D_2 starts again with a shoulder. By varying the interval t_{rec}, the time constant $\varepsilon_{A'A}$ of this reversed reaction can be determined quantitatively as shown in Fig. 2b. If no energy is supplied to the cells the recovery is negligible during this time.

REPAIR

The radiation damage at the essential molecule is produced with a reaction constant η_{AB}. This damage can be repaired by the cell if the repair enzymes are present and the cell is not forced to perform cell division immediately after irradiation. To fulfill these conditions the cells are kept in a buffer solution after irradiation for time intervals t_{rep}. By varying this interval t_{rep} the time constant of this reversed reaction, called "repair", can be determined quantitatively (see Fig. 3b).

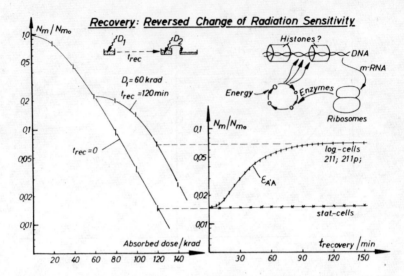

Fig. 2. a) Relative concentration of m-cells, N_m/N_{mo} as a function of
             absorbed dose, D, for diploid yeast, strain 211 in nutrition
             medium.

         b) Change of N_m/N_{mo} as a function of time t_{rec}, present between
             the two absorbed dose fractions for yeast cells in nutrition
             medium (log cells) and in buffer solution (stat cells).

Cells which are respiratory deficient cannot perform
repair of this type. However, they also show an initial
shoulder in the dose effect curve. This is an indirect
confirmation of the fundamental assumption of this model
that the shoulder is not due to repair but due to changes
in radiation sensitivity.

Experiments with different absorbed dose rates from
30 rad/min up to 100 krad/min have shown that only this repair process with a reciprocal time constant of $1/\varepsilon_{BA}$ = 25
hours could be observed in yeast cells. Other repair processes with $1/\varepsilon_{BA}$ from 10 seconds up to 100 hours are not
present in these cells [1].

The difference in the dose effect curves between the
wild type strain 211 and its respiratory deficient mutant

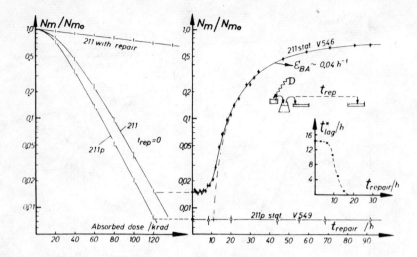

Fig. 3.   a)   Relative concentration of m-cells, N_m/N_{mo}, as a function of
                 absorbed dose for wild type yeast cells, strain 211, and its
                 respiratory deficient mutant, 211p, in buffer solution.

          b)   Increase of N_m/N_{n}, due to repair during storage of the cells
                 in buffer for time t_{rep}. Insert: Change of lag time, t_{lag},
                 due to storage in buffer for time t_{rep}.

211p in Fig. 3a can be explained by the repair effect
which is performed by the wild type on the nutrition agar
during the radiation induced lag time. As can be seen
from the insert in Fig.4b this lag time is constant during
the first 10 hours in the buffer and seems to be longer
than the time until the repair process is initiated at
this absorbed dose.

A MODEL FOR RADIATION REACTIONS IN YEAST

        All the facts described in the previous sections can
be combined in one model shown in the insert of Fig. 4.
Cells in the normal state "A" and in the sensitive state
"A' " belong to the population of m-cells, which can grow
to a macrocolony (concentration N_m). The cells in state B
are not able to grow to a macrocolony, but their damage is
repairable. Added to this model is the possibility of an
irrepairable damage. Cells with such a damage are in state

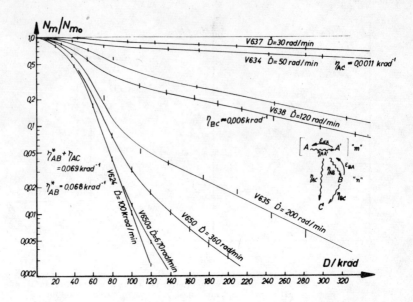

Fig. 4. Dose effect curves for diploid yeast cells, strain 211, in buffer
solution for different absorbed dose rates. Insert: Model for
radiation reactions in living cells.

"C". This state can be reached from state "B" by a second
radical reaction (η_{BC}) or from state "A" by a direct radiation reaction (η_{AC}).

The experimental determination of $\varepsilon_{A'A}$ and ε_{BA} can
be performed as demonstrated in Fig. 2 and 3. The quanti-
tative determination of η_{AB}, η_{BC} and η_{AC} must be done using extremely small and extremely high absorbed dose rates.
If the absorbed dose rate is extremely small, then due to
repair the concentration of cells in state "B" tends to
zero and from the dose effect curve (see Fig. 4) η_{AC} can
be read. For very high absorbed dose rates the repair
(ε_{BA}) can be neglected and the reduction of N_m is due to
$\eta_{AC} + \eta_{AB}$. The value of this sum can be read at the exponential part of this dose effect curve. The value of η_{BC}
can be determined from the slope of the curves at intermediate absorbed dose rates for high absorbed doses. A
more precise determination can be done from the dose ef-

fect curve with repair after irradiation with high absorbed dose rates in Fig. 3a. The slope of this curve gives
η_{BC} directly as can be seen from a more extensive analysis
of the model used here [1]. *

The model developed here has been checked up to now
only with sparsely ionizing radiation and with diploid
yeast cells. It can be assumed, however, that it is valid also for other types of radiation and other types of
living cells.

REFERENCES

1.   KAPPOS, A., and POHLIT, W., A cybernetic model for
      radiation reactions in living cells. I. Sparsely
      ionizing radiations; stationary cells. (In prepar-
      ation).

CORRELATION BETWEEN SENSITIVITY TO IONIZING RADIATION AND DNA REPLICATION IN PHYSARUM POLYCEPHALUM

ODDVAR F. NYGAARD, EUGENE N. BREWER, THOMAS E. EVANS, and JONATHAN R. WOLPAW

Division of Radiation Biology,
Department of Radiology,
Case Western Reserve University,
Cleveland, Ohio 44106, U.S.A.

In the synchronously dividing plasmodial slime mold, *Physarum polycephalum*, the period of greatest sensitivity to ionizing radiation, as measured by mitotic delay, occurs at the preceding mitosis. The division delay curve falls sharply to a minimum over the next 2 - 2 1/2 hours which coincides with the period of nuclear DNA replication in this organism. Nuclear reconstruction, a readily identifiable cytologic phase, also takes place during this time. During the remaining 2/3 of the division cycle there is a steady increase in the division delay curve until shortly before mitosis, at which time radiation produces no delay of the ensuing mitosis. Fig. 1 shows the effects of 10,000 and 20,000 rad of Co^{60} γ-radiation, given at different times during the division cycle of *Physarum*. Results similar to these have also been obtained by W. Sachenmaier and co-workers with 10,000r of 25 kv x-radiation (personal communication).

This organism, because of its natural synchrony of nuclear division, offers an excellent opportunity for interpreting the variability of radiation sensitivity in terms of damage inflicted upon specific cellular processes (or "events") occurring at different stages of the division cycle. For the current report we have chosen to concentrate on the effect of radiation delivered early

in the division cycle, with specific emphasis on the relationship between observed mitotic delays and the effect on DNA structure and function. (Elsewhere at
these meetings, W. Sachsenmaier and E. Bohnert will report on the effect of ionizing radiation on the induction of thymidine kinase in *Physarum polycephalum*).

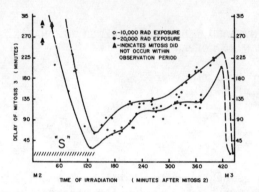

Fig. 1.

Since nuclear reconstruction and nuclear DNA replication both begin immediately after mitosis (there is
no G_1 period in the division cycle of *Physarum*), we first
wanted to determine if either of these "events" correlated with the early high sensitivity to radiation. Our
approach to this problem was to create an artifical G_1-
period through selective inhibition of DNA synthesis
with 5-fluorodeoxyuridine (FUdR, $2 \times 10^{-5}M$) in the presence of uridine (UR, $4 \times 10^{-4}M$). Exposing the mold to
FUdR for limited periods starting prior to Mitosis 2 and
extending into the next division cycle, we found that the
effect of the inhibitor was easily reversible leading to
reproducible delays of the subsequent division (Mitosis
3) only slightly longer than the time that the mold was
exposed to FUdR beyond Mitosis 2.

As seen in Fig. 1, the mold was least sensitive to
radiation at 120 - 140 min. after mitosis. To achieve
the most clear-cut effect, we decided to delay DNA synthesis for approximately this length of time, and to
irradiate control as well as FUdR treated plasmodia with
10,000 rad at 140 min. after Mitosis 2, i.e., just prior

to removal of FUdR from the treated plasmodia. (Since
the plasmodia can easily be subdivided, and the various
pieces serve as mutual internal controls, quarter-sec-
tions were left untreated, treated with FUdR, exposed
to γ-radiation, or exposed to both FUdR and radiation,
respectively; the time of Mitosis 3 was determined for
each section). A second set of plasmodia was irradiated
280 min. after Mitosis 2, i.e. 140 min. after removal
of FUdR from the treated molds.

Fig. 2 shows that for the FUdR treated molds, irradiation at 140 min. after Mitosis 3, indicated that
the sensitivity curve had been shifted corresponding
to the delay of DNA synthesis. This is also
borne out by the occurrence of a minimal delay after irradiation of FUdR-treated plasmodia at 280 min.
after Mitosis 2, at a time when the sensitivity of the
control plasmodia was increased. The effect of a 140
min. shift in the sensitivity curve is indicated by the
dotted curve in Fig. 2; the solid curve represents the
10,000 rad curve transposed from Fig. 1. (From studies
with incorporation of labeled deoxyadenosine into DNA
in the presence of FUdR and UR at the given concentrations, it has been established that inhibition of DNA
synthesis is only 85% complete. Allowing for 15% synthesis of DNA the projected shift in the sensitivity
curve would be somewhat less, as indicated by the short
dotted line in Fig. 2, which corresponds very closely
to the observed points).

Having established that the early portion of the
sensitivity curve is somehow linked to the synthesis
of nuclear DNA, we were intrigued by the apparent in-
verse relationship between sensitivity in terms of mitotic delay and the degree of completion of nuclear DNA
replication; i.e., the delay seemed to be related to the
amount of unreplicated DNA present at the time of irradiation. Several interpretations of this relationship
were considered.

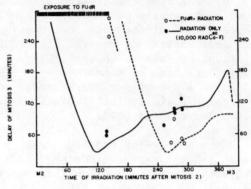

Fig. 2.

1) *The irradiated DNA may undergo repair which must be completed before the damaged site is replicated* -- Imperative for this interpretation would be the demonstration of DNA repair in *Physarum* within the same division cycle in which it was exposed to ionizing radiation. Two slightly different approaches were employed in an attempt to demonstrate "repair synthesis" of DNA in plasmodia exposed to 10,000 rad of γ-radiation. In the first and simpler approach plasmodia were irradiated during the G_2 period of the division cycle, at which time there is no interference by replication of the major nuclear DNA fraction. The molds were subsequently exposed to medium containing H^3-thymidine (H^3-TdR) for one hour, either immediately or 2 1/2 hours after irradiation, and then harvested prior to the next Mitosis (and hence before the next S period). DNA was isolated and subjected to density gradient centrifugation in CsCl, to allow separation of the major nuclear DNA from the mitochondrial and heavy nuclear satellite DNAs. Unlabeled bulk *Physarum* DNA was added to allow identification of the major peak by optical density measurements. If "repair synthesis" had occurred there should be "unscheduled" incorporation of radioactive thymidine into the major nuclear DNA of the irradiated molds. No such incorporation was detected in the several experiments of this type that were performed.

A second protocol was used to test for the possi-

bility that repair synthesis of DNA might occur during
the regular S period. Plasmodia were allowed to undergo replication in the presence of 5-bromodeoxyuridine
(BUdR) and tracer levels of H^3-deoxyadenosine (H^3-AdR),and
were also exposed to radiation during the early part of
the same S period. FUdR and UR were included in the medium to improve the efficiency of the BUdR incorporation.
In the course of normal DNA replication each newly synthesized DNA strand would be density labeled (with BUdR)
as well as radioactivity labeled (with H^3AdR), whereas
the old (parental) strand would remain unlabeled. If
the parental DNA was damaged by irradiation and repair
synthesis occurred, small amounts of H^3AdR would be incorporated into the parental strand, (together with a-
mounts of BUdR insufficient to significantly alter the
buoyant density of the parental DNA). At the end of
the S-period DNA was isolated and subjected to density
gradient sedimentation in alkaline CsCl to allow separation of the heavy and light strands of DNA. Bulk,
unlabeled *Physarum* DNA was added to provide a reference
standard by optical density measurements. In the samples that were analyzed by this technique, essentially
all incorporated radioactivity was recovered in the
heavy (BUdR-labeled) strand Fig. 3, suggesting that no
"repair synthesis" of DNA had occurred in the parental
strand as a result of the irradiation.

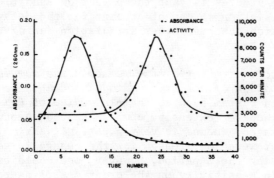

Fig. 3.

Our results indicate that repair synthesis does
not occur after irradiation of *Physarum*. It may be
pertinent to mention that McCormick and Nardone sim-

ilarly were unable to demonstrate "repair synthesis" of
DNA in *Physarum* after exposure to nitrogen mustard [1].
We realize that the absence of unscheduled incorporation
of measurable amounts of radioactive DNA precursors does
not preclude the repair of damaged DNA by other mechanisms.
For this reason we have looked for repair of single-strand
breaks in DNA after irradiation. Our preliminary results
indicate that strand breaks do occur, but we have no
data as yet relating to the subsequent repair of these
breaks.

   2) *The completion of nuclear DNA replication may be
delayed by irradiation* --Earlier data [2] suggested that
DNA synthesis was not substantially inhibited following
irradiation during the S period, as evidenced by incorporation of C^{14}-orotic acid into DNA-thymine. In other,
more recent experiments, replication was monitored by
the decrease, during the S period, in the specific activity of pre-labeled DNA. After irradiation with 10,000
rad immediately after mitosis, the completion of DNA synthesis, by this criterion, was delayed by approximately
one hour. We have also tested the effect of radiation
in vivo on the *in vitro* template activity of *Physarum*
nuclear DNA using *E. coli* DNA polymerase. The results
indicated no significant effect of DNA in this test system with a dose of 10,000 rad. Our tentative conclusion
from these studies is that the effect of radiation on
DNA synthesis *per se* cannot account for the delay of nuclear division observed after irradiation during the S
period.

   3) *The intermitotic time reflects the degree of
complementation of active, undamaged genes*--In a mul-
tinucleated system such as the plasmodium of *Physarum*,
the likelihood of extensive complementation among partially damaged genomes is very great. If a simple gene-
dose effect were the reason for the change in sensitivity during the S period, however, one could expect
a change in sensitivity on the order of 2:1 as replication is completed, rather than the fairly extreme
ratio observed. One possible explanation is that after mitosis in *Physarum* part of the parental genome may
be inactive prior to its replication; this interpreta-

tion receives support from the observations of Rao and Gontcharoff [3] which suggest that in *Physarum* a significant portion of RNA required early in the cell cycle is not transcribed until replication of DNA has occurred. If radiation damages the activation process as well as the structural genes, one might readily visualize a greater differential than 2:1 for the complementation of active, undamaged genes in plasmodia of *Physarum* irradiated early and late during the period of nuclear DNA replication.

Our present results do not allow us to rule out any of the above hypotheses for the rapid decrease in radiation sensitivity of *Physarum* as the plasmodia progresses through the S period. With continued investigations, however, we hope eventually to identify some of the critical events responsible for the pattern of radiation sensitivity in this organism.

SUMMARY

During the period of DNA replication the radiation sensitivity of the synchronously dividing plasmodial slime mold, *Physarum polycephalum*, in terms of delay of nuclear division, appears to be proportional to the amount of unreplicated DNA present at the time of irradiation. We have discussed this result in terms of 1) repair of damage to the DNA, 2) inhibition of DNA synthesis, and 3) complementation among active, undamaged genes.

(This work was supported by Contract W-31-109-ENG-78 with the U.S. Atomic Energy Commission, Report No. COO-78-228.)

REFERENCES

1.   McCORMICK, J., and NARDONE, R., *Exptl. Cell Res.*, *60*, 247, 1970.

2.   NYGAARD, O., and GUTTES, S., *Internat. J. Radiation Biol.*, *5*, 33, 1962.

3.   RAO, B., and GONTCHAROFF, M., *Exptl. Cell Res.*, *56*, 269, 1969.